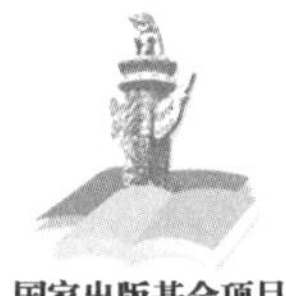

An Intensively Compiled Practical English-Chinese Library of Traditional Chinese Medicine

(英汉对照)精编实用中医文库

Chief General Compilers CHEN Kaixian LI Qizhong(Executive) HE Xinghai

总主编 陈凯先 李其忠(执行) 何星海

Chief General Translators SHI Jianrong HU Hongyi XU Yao(Executive)

总主译 施建蓉 胡鸿毅 徐 瑶(执行)

Pediatrics of Traditional Chinese Medicine

中医儿科学

Chief Editor YU Jian'er

Chief Translator DONG Jing

主 编 虞坚尔

主 译 董 晶

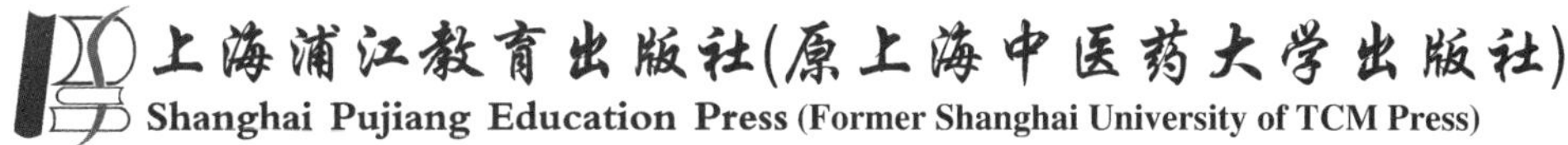

An Intensively Compiled Practical English-Chinese Library of Traditional Chinese Medicine

Compilation Board of the Library

Compilation and Translation Committee of the Library

Pediatrics of Traditional Chinese Medicine

Chief Editor YU Jian'er

Deputy Chief Editor XUE Zheng

Chief Translator DONG Jing

《(英汉对照)精编实用中医文库》

编纂委员会

总　主　编　陈凯先　李其忠(执行)　何星海

编　　　委(按姓氏笔画为序)

马烈光　何建成　余小萍　沈雪勇

张婷婷　陈红风　陈德兴　赵　毅

郭　忻　黄　平　虞坚尔　詹红生

缪晚虹

编译委员会

总　主　译　施建蓉　胡鸿毅　徐　瑶(执行)

编　译　者(按姓氏笔画为序)

朱爱秀　杨　渝　肖元春　张亿萍

诸建民　黄国琪　董　晶　韩丑萍

《中医儿科学》

主　　　编　虞坚尔

副　主　编　薛　征

主　　　译　董　晶

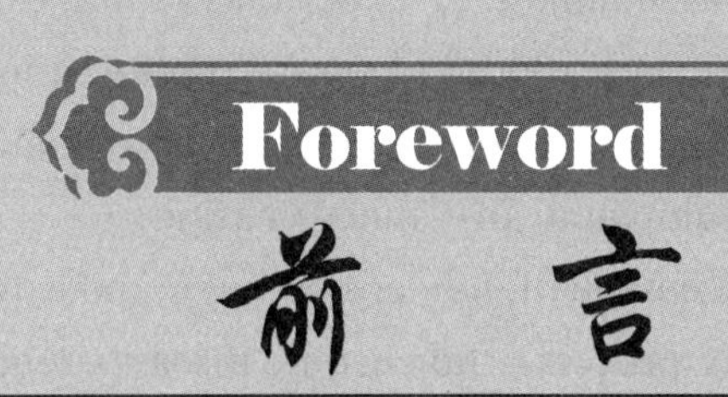
Foreword
前　言

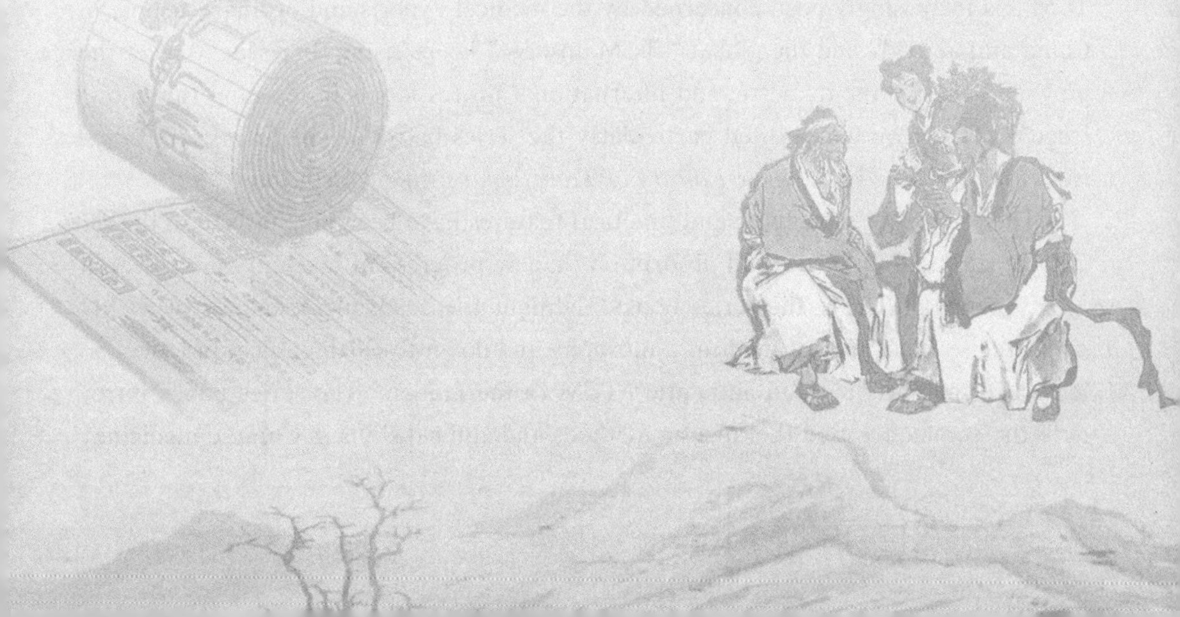

With the traditional medical philosophy and clinical experience as the principal body, the science of Traditional Chinese Medicine (TCM) is a comprehensive subject to study the rules of life activities and the disease prevention, diagnosis, treatment, rehabilitation as well as healthcare. The science of TCM has a long history of development and belongs to a summary of experiences that Chinese nation has fought against diseases for over several thousand years, is also an important component part of Chinese outstanding traditional culture and has contributed greatly to the health-care undertaking and development of Chinese nation.

By increasing enhancement of modern living standard, change of living modes and acceleration of ageing process, the chronic diseases represented by tumors, cardiovascular diseases and diabetes become gradually the important factors in impacting the health of mankind, but TCM presents the better therapeutic effects. Nowadays, the modern medical mode of "society-psychology-biology" has been advocated in medical science, changing from the medical idea of "disease treatment" to "health promotion". The more and more patients in China and abroad have chosen natural and low side-effect Chinese herbal medicine for their problems. With the changes in medicine modes and in spectrum of diseases in the recent several dozens of years, TCM has increasingly been concerned by the medical experts and ordinary people in China and abroad, and the global " TCM upsurge" keeps rising. In order to meet the growing needs of the domestic and international professionals in learning the knowledge of TCM, we have edited particularly the series books of *An Intensively Compiled Practical English-Chinese Library of Traditional Chinese Medicine*.

The scientific, systematic and practical features have been emphasized in the series books. Based upon the full absorption of new progress in teaching and research achievements of TCM, the series books highlight the academic essentials of TCM, with precise exposition of medical philosophy and down-to-earth clinical practice, to introduce the "original and authentic" TCM to the readers. The series books introduce the commonly used therapeutic methods and clinical skills in Chinese medicine, by the clinically encountered and frequently seen diseases and the relevant ailments predominantly effective by Chinese medical therapies.By studying the series books, the readers can learn the knowledge and techniques of TCM on gradual progress and become proficient gradually in TCM.

The series books highlight "the precise features in three aspects" —capable in authors, refined in contents and accurate in translation. The majority of the authors of the series books are senior experts from the related faculties of Shanghai University of Traditional Chinese Medicine. The translator team is composed of the senior teachers with plentiful expertise in translation of TCM from international education college and foreign language center of Shanghai University of Traditional Chinese Medicine. In order to meet the needs of the readers in China and abroad, the basic and clinical core contents are selected and the latest research achievements are consulted based upon the principle "to seek its essentials but its completion" in the series books.

The series books can satisfy the beginners with certain knowledge of English language in studying TCM systematically and can also be used as the textbooks for education of TCM and pharmacy for foreign students. We sincerely hope the publication of the series books plays its promoting role for TCM going to the world.

Editors

June, 2017

中医学是以传统医学理论与实践经验为主体，研究人体生命活动规律和疾病预防、诊断、治疗、康复以及保健的一门综合性学科。中医学历史悠久，源远流长，是中华民族几千年来同疾病作斗争的经验总结，也是中国传统文化的重要组成部分，长期以来为中国人民的健康保健事业和民族繁衍作出了巨大的贡献。

随着现代生活水平的不断提高、生活方式的改变以及老龄化进程的加快，以肿瘤、心血管疾病和糖尿病等为代表的慢性病日渐成为影响人类健康的重要因素，而中医药显示了良好的治疗效果。当今的医学倡导“社会—心理—生物”的现代医学模式，医学理念从“疾病治疗”向“健康促进”转变，国内外越来越多的患者选择天然、毒副作用低的中医药治疗疾病。近几十年来，随着医学模式的转变和疾病谱的改变，中医学日益引起越来越多的海内外医学专家和普通民众的关注，全球性的“中医热”正在持续升温。为了满足海内外人士日益高涨的学习中医学知识的需求，我们特地编撰了《(英汉对照)精编实用中医文库》丛书。

本丛书注重“三性”——科学性、系统性、实用性。丛书在充分吸取近年中医教学、科研进展的基础上，突出中医学术精华，理论阐述准确、临床切合实际，向读者介绍“原汁原味”的中医学；丛书介绍中医学常用的治疗方法和临床技能，所涉及的病证均为临床常见病、多发病和中医优势病种。丛书的 13 个分册涵盖了中医基础与临床的主干课程，通过阅读本丛书，读者可以由浅入深、循序渐进地学习中医药知识和技能。

本丛书突出“三精”——作者精干、内容精炼、翻译精准。丛书的中文作者绝大部分为上海中医药大学各相关教研室的资深专家，翻译团队由上海中医药大学国际教育学院和外语中心具有丰富的中医药学翻译经验的骨干教师组成。为了适合海内外读者的需求，丛书本着“求其精而不求其全”的原则，选取了基础和临床的核心内容，翻译上参考了最新的研究成果。

本丛书既可满足具有一定英语水平的初学中医者系统学习中医所用，也可供中医药留学生教育作为教材使用，衷心希望本丛书的出版在中医药走向海外进程中发挥应有的推动作用。

编者

2017 年 6 月

Note for Compilation

编写说明

As a clinical discipline under the guidance of traditional Chinese medicine theories, pediatrics in traditional Chinese medicine studies infantile growth and development, preventive measures and health care of infants, and diagnosis and treatment of infant diseases. With its long history, very rich clinical practice and systematic theories, it is popular with child patients and their parents. In recent years, pediatrics in traditional Chinese medicine develops quite quickly, and gets attention from more and more overseas specialists. On account of this, the book is compiled.

The whole book includes General Introduction and Specific Introduction. There are three chapters in General Introduction which respectively deal with the physiological and pathological characteristics of infants, key to diagnosis and treatment of pediatrics in traditional Chinese medicine. For Specific Introductions, there are 13 chapters based on the nature of diseases, which include over 30 diseases like acute upper respiratory infection and 6 disease patterns in traditional Chinese medicine like sweat pattern. For each disease or pattern, firstly there is a general description of its basic concept, its characteristics and key to prevention and treatment, then the focus is on the etiology and pathogenesis, key points to diagnosis, and key points to the treatment based on pattern differentiation. For certain diseases or patterns, alternative treatment methods are also introduced. To help readers understand, in "Key to diagnosis", both the key points of four inspections in traditional Chinese medicine and the main lab exam index in Western medicine are introduced; in "Treatment based on Pattern Differentiation", key to diagnosis and treatment principles comes first, then concrete methods for treatments of specific patterns are discussed; in alternative treatment methods, the focus is on acupuncture and moxibustion, external application of traditional Chinese medicine, Chinese patent medicine and diet therapy, etc.

中医儿科学是在中医理论指导下，研究小儿生长发育、预防保健和疾病诊治的临床学科，具有悠久的历史、系统的理论和丰富的临床实践，深受患儿及其家长的欢迎。近年来，中医儿科学得到了较快的发展，并受到了越来越多的海外医学专家的关注。有鉴于此，编写了本书。

全书分总论和各论两大部分。总论共有 3 章，分论小儿生理病理特点、中医儿科诊断要点、中医儿科治疗要点。各论按疾病的性质分为 13 章，共收载急性上呼吸道感染等 30 种疾病和汗证等 6 个中医病证。每一病或证均在概述其基本概念、特点、防治要点等的基础上，重点介绍其病因病机、诊断要点、辨证论治，有的病、证还介绍了其他疗法。为了便于读者的理解，在"诊断要点"中同时介绍中医的四诊要点和西医的主要实验室检查指标；在"辨证论治"中先介绍辨证要点和治疗原则，再介绍其分型论治的具体方法；在"其他疗法"中着重介绍针灸、推拿、中药外敷、中成药及饮食疗法等。

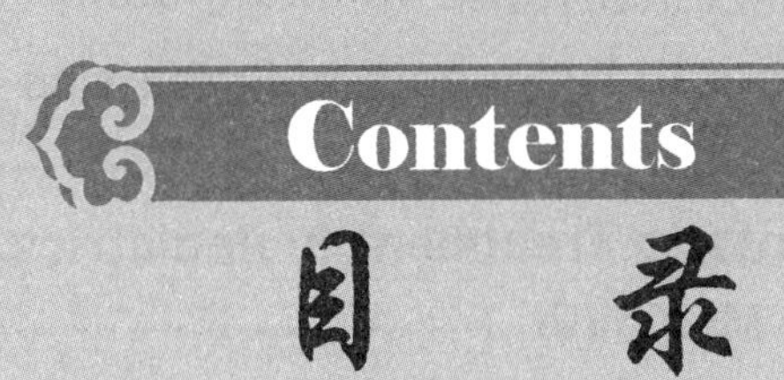
Contents
目 录

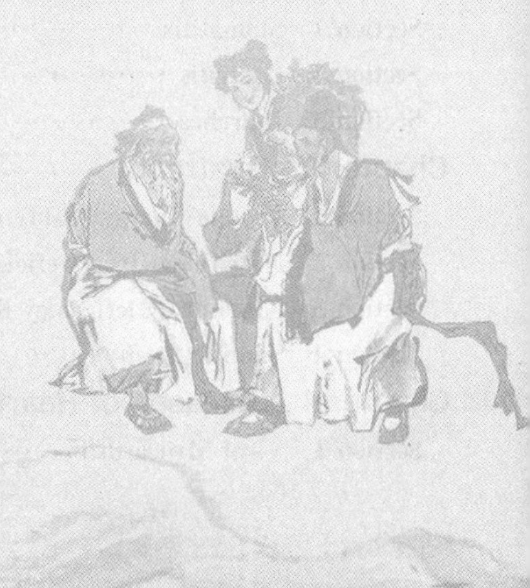

General Introduction

Specific Introduction

总 论

各 论

General Introduction

总 论

Chapter 1 Physiological and Pathological Characteristics of Infants

第1章 小儿生理病理特点

Section 1 Physiological Characteristics

第1节 生理特点

As infants keep growing from the time they are born till they are adults, infants have their own physiological characteristics, different from those of the adults. The younger the age, the more obvious the differences are.

小儿自出生至成人，处于不断的生长发育过程中，因此有不同于成人的生理特点，年龄越小，差异越显著。

1 Delicate bowels and viscera and unfilled physique and qi

1 脏腑娇嫩，形气未充

The bowels and viscera are the five viscera and six bowels; "delicate" means weak, soft and less resistant to attack. Physique refers to the tangible matters like physical structure, four limbs and hundred bones, essence, blood and body fluids. Qi means physiological functions and activities. "Filled" suggests full and strong. "Delicate bowels and viscera and unfilled physique and qi" means that infants are at a growing stage, when the physical body, the form and bearing of organs have not matured and physiological functions have not come into full play.

脏腑，指五脏六腑；娇嫩，指娇弱柔嫩，不耐攻伐；形，指形体结构、四肢百骸、精血津液等有形物质；气，指各种生理功能活动；充，指充实旺盛。脏腑娇嫩，形气未充，是指小儿处于生长发育时期，机体脏腑的形态尚未成熟、各种生理功能尚未健全。

The bowels and viscera of infants are both defi-

小儿五脏六腑的形与气

cient in physique and qi, and the lung, spleen, and kidney are especially weak, manifested by a tender lung, a frequently insufficient spleen and a frequently deficient kidney.

皆属不足,其中又以肺、脾、肾三脏不足更为突出,常表现出肺脏娇嫩、脾常不足、肾常虚的特点。

The lung of the infants is delicate with thin and weak fleshy exterior and loose interstices. It is insufficient in governing qi, and there is a quicker and shallower breath than adults. When exterior defense is insecure, external evils will easily enter from the exterior, attack the lung and cause diseases.

小儿肺脏娇嫩,肌表薄弱,腠理不实,主气功能不足,呼吸较成人浅快,卫外功能未固,外邪每易由表而入,侵袭肺脏,发生疾病。

The spleen of the infants is often insufficient, not yet vigorous in transforming ability; but infants, due to their rapid growth and great demand in nutrition of essence, blood and body fluids, are likely to be damaged by diet, which results in diseases in the spleen and stomach.

小儿脾常不足,运化功能尚未健旺,但生长发育迅速,对精血津液等营养物质的需求比成人多,因此易为饮食所伤,出现脾胃疾病。

The kidney of the infants is often insufficient, manifested by kidney essence not being fully filled and insufficient kidney qi. Girls before adolescence have no "monthly matters coming on due time", and boys have no "spilling and discharging of essential qi". Infants are unable to self-control or weak in self-controlling urination and stool, etc.

小儿肾常虚,表现为肾精未充,肾气不盛,青春期前的女孩无"月事以时下"、男孩无"精气溢泻",婴幼儿二便不能自控或自控能力较弱等。

Moreover, the heart and liver of the infants have not fully grown and are not strong. They are still insufficient in their function. Heart governs the blood and blood vessels, and governs the spirit and mind. The heart qi of the infants is not filled and heart spirit is timid and weak, shown by rapid pulse, susceptibility to fright, poor control of mind and conduct. Liver governs free coursing and sinews. The liver qi of the infants is not filled. When yin blood is lack of nourishment, and the meridians and tendons are not mutually supported, there will

此外,小儿心、肝两脏同样未臻充盛,功能尚不健全。心主血脉、主神明,小儿心气未充、心神怯弱,表现为脉数,易受惊吓,思维及行为的约束能力较差;肝主疏泄、主筋,小儿肝气尚未充实,阴血失养,经筋刚柔未济,表现为好动、易搐。

be signs of restlessness and susceptibility to convulsion in infants.

Medical practitioner, Wu Jutong, in Qing Dynasty generalized the physiological characteristics of infants as "tender yang not filled and tender yin not grown". "Yin" here refers to tangible physical matters like essence, blood, body fluids, bowels and viscera, sinews and bones, brain marrow, blood vessels, skin and flesh, etc. "Yang" refers to various physiological functions of internal organs. "Tender" means young and immature. Tender yin and tender yang include features like tender physique, weak qi and blood, weak spleen and stomach, insufficient kidney qi, loose interstices, timid spirit qi, and weak sinews and bones, etc.

清代医家吴鞠通将小儿这种生理特点概括为"稚阳未充，稚阴未长"。这里的"阴"，指机体的精、血、津液及脏腑、筋骨、脑髓、血脉、肌肤等有形之质；"阳"指脏腑的各种生理功能；"稚"指幼嫩尚未成熟。稚阴稚阳包括了机体柔嫩、气血未盛、脾胃薄弱、肾气未充、腠理疏松、神气怯弱、筋骨未坚等特点。

2　Vigorous life and rapid growth

In the course of growth and development, infants rapidly and continuously grow towards maturity and improvement, both in physical form and structure and physiological functions. The younger, the faster the speed is. Infants under one year old change obviously in weight, height, head and chest circumference, teething, etc. For instance, the height of a one-year-old infant is 1.5 times higher than that of the newborn while the weight is 3 times more. There is also a rapid growth in the abilities of thinking, language and motion, etc.

The medical practitioners in the ancient times used "pure yang", a word in *Book of Changes* (Yi Jing), to describe the physiological features of vigorous life and rapid growth of infants.

2　生机蓬勃，发育迅速

小儿在生长发育过程中，无论是机体的形态结构，还是各种生理功能活动，都在迅速地、不断地向着成熟、完善方面发展。年龄越小，这种发育的速度愈快。周岁内的小儿在体重、身长、头围、胸围、出牙等方面，每个月都会有明显的变化，如周岁时的身长是初生时 1.5 倍，体重则达初生时 3 倍，小儿的思维、语言、运动能力等也随年龄增加而迅速发育。

古代医家借用《易经》中"纯阳"一词来表述小儿生机蓬勃、发育迅速的生理特点。

2 Pure visceral qi and easy recovery

The body constitution of the infants is of pure yang, and the infant is full of life. The bowels and viscera are clear and vigorous. The infants are quick in response to various treatments. They have relatively few deep-rooted diseases. The causes of diseases are relatively simple and there are relatively few emotional and mental influences and disturbances. Therefore, although there are such disadvantages as easy attack and rapid transmission, generally speaking, as long as the diagnosis and pattern identification are correct, the treatment is in time and proper, and the medication and attending are proper, the infants will recover quickly.

2 脏气清灵，易趋康复

小儿体禀纯阳，生机蓬勃，脏腑清灵，活力充沛，对各种治疗反应灵敏；小儿宿疾较少，病因相对单纯，疾病过程中情志因素的干扰和影响相对较少。因此，小儿虽有发病容易、传变迅速不利的一面，但一般说来，只要诊断无误，辨证准确，治疗及时，处理得当，用药合理，护理适宜，疾病康复也较快。

Chapter 2 Key Points to Diagnosis in Pediatrics of Traditional Chinese Medicine

第2章 中医儿科诊断要点

Diagnosis is a general term for a variety of clinical examinations. The diagnostic methods for infantile diseases are the same as those used for diagnosis and pattern identification by other clinical departments, which include inspection, listening and smelling, inquiry and pulse examination. However, because the infants are different from adults in constitution, physique, physiology and pathology, the four examinations used are different from those used for adults.

诊法是临床诊察疾病的各种方法的总称。小儿疾病的诊断方法,与临床其他各科一样,均用望、闻、问、切四种不同的诊查手段进行诊断和辨证。由于小儿与成人在体质、形态、生理及病理等方面均有差异,所以在四诊的运用上也与其他学科有别。

1 Inspection

1 望诊

Inspection mainly includes that of spirit and complexion, of form and bearing, of physiological indicators, of macules and papules, of urine and stool, and of fingerprints.

主要包括望神色、望形态、审苗窍、辨斑疹、察二便、看指纹。

1.1 Inspection of spirit and complexion

1.1 望神色

Spirit manifests externally whether there is enough yin, yang, qi, blood, essence and body fluids in the bowels and viscere and whether these are in accord. It is especially important for the infants. To judge whether a child patient is full of spirit or low spirit, the inspection of spirit may fall on the following aspects: the change of look in eyes, the consciousness of mind, the quickness in response,

神是脏腑阴阳气血精津是否充足、和调的外在表现之一,在小儿尤为重要。望神应主要从目光的变化、意识是否清楚、反应是否敏捷、躯体动作是否灵活协调等方面去判断患儿有神、失神等不同情况。凡小儿有神则表

the quickness and coordination of body movements, etc. When a child has bright eyes, a clear mind, quick response, quick and coordinated movements, then there is spirit, otherwise, there is a loss of spirit.

现为目光炯炯，意识清楚，反应敏捷，躯体动作灵活协调，反之则为失神。

Complexion refers to the color and luster of skin. The inspection of complexion mainly refers to that of face.

色，是指皮肤的颜色和光泽，主要以望面部的颜色为主。

Normal complexion for Chinese infants usually is a slight yellowish ruddy complexion with luster. The newborn are tender-red all over, which is a manifestation of harmony in qi and blood. The pattern identification of the five colors of facial complexion usually has the following laws.

正常面色：中国小儿的常色为微黄红润而有光泽，新生儿则全身皮肤嫩红，是气血调和的表现。面部五色诊病辨证，一般符合以下规律。

A green-blue facial complexion is often seen in patterns of cold, pain, blood stasis, and convulsive epilepsy. A somber grayish green-blue facial complexion indicates yang qi deficiency. Alternate blue and pale complexion indicates severe internal cold. Green-blue in pain pattern is often seen in internal pain of abdominal pain. Seizure of infantile convulsion and epilepsy often manifests a somber green-blue facial complexion. Green-blue facial complexion and purple lips with rapid breathing are often a sign of lung qi blockage and obstruction of qi and blood. In most cases, green-blue facial complexion of the infants indicates severe illness and needs more observation.

面色青，多见于寒证、痛证、瘀证、惊痫。面色青灰晦暗为阳气虚，乍青乍白为里寒甚；痛证色青多见于里寒腹痛；惊风和癫痫发作常见面青而晦暗；面青唇紫，呼吸急促为肺气闭塞，气血瘀阻。大凡小儿面呈青色，病情一般较重，应多加观察。

A red facial complexion often indicates heat pattern. Red face and eyes, fever, aversion to cold and floating pulse indicate infection of exogenous wind and heat. Interior heat is often indicated by red face, rough breathing, high fever, vexation and thirst. Deficiency heat often involves flushed

面色赤，多为热证。若面红目赤、恶寒发热、脉浮为外感风热；里热常见面赤气粗、高热烦渴；虚热常见颧红潮热、低热起伏；若两颧艳红如妆、面白肢厥、冷汗淋漓为

cheeks, tidal feverish sensation and fluctuating low-grade fever. When there are flushed cheeks, bright like make-up, pale facial complexion, cold sensation in the limbs and dripping cold sweat, it is a upward floating of deficient yang, a critical condition due to collapse of yang qi deficiency. Normal complexion should be tender red in the newborn or rosy and ruddy in the infants.

虚阳上越，是阳气虚脱的危重证候。新生儿面色嫩红，或小儿面色白里透红，为正常肤色。

A yellow facial complexion often indicates spleen deficiency pattern or the existence of damp turbidity. A sallow yellow facial complexion indicates qi deficiency in the spleen and stomach. A puffy swelling yellow face is spleen deficiency with dampness stagnation. A dry yellow one indicates exhaustion in qi and blood. A pronounced yellow eyes and facial complexion often indicate yang jaundice due to internal accumulation of dampness and heat. A somber yellow face and eyes indicate yin jaundice due to obstruction of dampness and heat. The jaundice that appears shortly after birth is fetal jaundice, which can be physiological or pathological.

面色黄，多为脾虚证或有湿浊。面色萎黄，是脾胃气虚；面黄浮肿，是脾虚湿滞；面色枯黄，是气血枯竭。面目色黄而鲜明，是湿热内蕴之阳黄；面目黄而晦暗，是湿热阻滞之阴黄；小儿生后不久出现的黄疸为胎黄，有生理性与病理性之分。

A pale facial complexion often indicates patterns of deficiency and cold. A pale and lusterless face with pale lips indicates blood deficiency. An intermittent pale face and incessant crying often suggest abdominal pain due to central cold. A facial complexion as pale as sheet, and cold limbs with sweating, often suggest fulminant collapse of yang qi.

面色白，多为虚证、寒证。面白少华、唇色淡白为血虚；阵阵发白，啼哭不宁，常为中寒腹痛；面色惨白、肢冷汗出，多为阳气暴脱。

A black facial complexion often indicates patterns of cold, pain, blood stasis and retained fluid. Green-blue black face and cold sensation in the limbs are signs of internal preponderance of yin cold. A dull and grey-black face often indicates de-

面色黑，多为寒证、痛证、瘀证、水饮证。小儿面色青黑，四肢厥冷，为阴寒内盛；面色灰黑暗滞，多为肾气虚衰；面唇黧黑，多为心阳虚

bilitation of kidney qi. Soot-black face and lips are a sign of prolonged debilitation of heart yang. Purple-black lips and fingers suggest debilitation of heart yang and obstruction of stagnant blood. A puffy, light and floating pale face often indicates kidney yang depletion and internal retention of water and fluid.

衰；唇指紫黑，多为心阳虚衰，瘀血阻滞；面色浅淡虚浮，常是肾阳亏虚，水饮内停。

1.2 Inspection of form and bearing

Form refers to the physical body and bearing refers to the dynamic posture. Inspection of form and bearing means to observe whether an infant is strong or weak, fat or thin, and to observe the movement and posture of the infants.

The infants who grow normally, with strong bones and sinews, bountiful muscles, moist skin, lustrous black hair, and active movement are well-nourished and healthy. The infants whose development is retarded and slow, with weak bones and sinews, emaciation, poor form, dry skin, withered yellow hair, delayed closure of the fontanel and dull movement are undernourished and mostly are unhealthy.

For instance, square head with sparse hair, wide fontanel with delayed closure can be found in five types of retardness. The sunken anterior fontanel and orbital socket, dry skin can be found in the infants sick with diarrhoea due to yin damage and humor desertion. Rising chicken chest is often found in rickets and asthma. Loose flesh, withered yellow skin is often found in anorexia, predilection for certain food and recurrent cold. Distending sensation in the abdomen, emaciation, sparse hair, and prominent blue veins on the forehead often belong to infantile malnutrition. Withered yellow hair, or standing sparse hair, or easy hair loss are manifesta-

1.2 望形态

形指形体，态指动态。望形态就是观察患儿形体的强弱胖瘦和动静姿态。

凡发育正常、筋骨强健、肌丰肤润、毛发黑泽、姿态活泼者，为营养良好，属健康表现；若生长迟缓、筋骨软弱、肌瘦形瘠、皮肤干枯、毛发萎黄、囟门逾期不合、姿态呆滞者，为营养不良，多属病态。

如头方发稀，囟门宽大，当闭不闭，可见于五迟证；前囟及眼窝凹陷，皮肤干燥，可见于婴幼儿泄泻阴伤液脱；胸廓高耸形如鸡胸，可见于佝偻病、哮喘病；肌肉松弛，皮色萎黄，多见于厌食、偏食、反复感冒；腹部膨大，肢体瘦弱，发稀，额上有青筋显现，多属疳积；毛发枯黄，或发竖稀疏，或容易脱落，均为气血亏虚表现。

tions of qi and blood depletion.

When an infant prefers to lie on his face, it may indicate interior retention of milk feeding. When an infant prefers to lie with his legs curled, it mostly indicates abdominal pains. Rigidity of the neck and nape, spasm and contracture in the limbs, and opisthotonos often indicate infantile convulsion. Restless rolling, screaming and crying, hands holding the abdomen often result from abdominal pain. Sitting with hasty breathing, phlegm rale and wheezing often indicate asthma.

如小儿喜俯卧者，为乳食内积；喜蜷卧者，多为腹痛；颈项强直，四肢拘急抽搐，角弓反张，是为惊风；若翻滚不安，呼叫哭吵，两手捧腹，多为腹痛所致；端坐喘促，痰鸣哮吼，多为哮喘。

1.3 Inspection of tongue

1.3 望舌

Tongue is a mirror of the heart. To examine the tongue is a major part of diagnosis by inspection. It includes observing the tongue body and tongue coating. A normal tongue in the infants manifests free and natural movement of tongue body, light red tongue, and a moist thin white coating.

因舌为心之苗，察舌是望诊的主要内容。包括观察舌质与舌苔。正常小儿舌象表现为舌体灵活，活动自如，舌质淡红，舌苔薄白质润。

Inspecting the tongue body mainly includes observing the color, the form and the body of the tongue. A light red and moist tongue reflects a normal state of bowels and viscera, qi and blood. A pale tongue indicates insufficiency of qi and blood, mainly deficiency and cold. A bright red tongue indicates heat pattern. A dark red tongue indicates excessive heat pattern, often found in acute heat diseases. A red and dry tongue is caused by heat damaging yin fluid. A red tongue tip often indicates febrile disease in the Upper Energizer or upward flaming of heart fire. A red tongue margin indicates heat in the liver and bladder. A tender-soft red but dry tongue indicates heat due to yin deficiency. A crimson tongue indicates heat entering Ying-nourishing system and blood, and mixture of blood stasis

察舌质，主要观察舌色、舌形和舌体。舌色淡红质润，多为脏腑气血功能正常。舌色淡白不荣，多为气血不足，主虚主寒；舌色鲜红主热证；舌质老红为实热证，多见于急性热病；舌红干为热伤阴津；舌尖红多为上焦温病或心火上炎；舌边红为肝胆有热；舌嫩红，伴质干不润者，为阴虚有热；舌色红绛主热入营血、瘀热互结，质干者为热灼阴津；深绛为血瘀夹热；舌质紫暗为气滞血瘀。舌形胖嫩为脾气不足；舌起芒刺为热入营血；舌生裂纹

and heat. If combined with dryness, then it is heat scorching yin fluid. A dark crimson indicates blood stasis with heat. A dark purple tongue indicates qi stagnation and blood stasis. An enlarged tender tongue indicates insufficient spleen qi. A prickly tongue indicates heat entering Ying-nourishing system and blood. A tongue with cracks means consumption and damage of yin fluid. A deviated tongue indicates an involvement of the collaterals by the pathogenic wind. A flaccid tongue indicates a debilitated spleen qi. To lick the lips repatedly with the tongue, followed by rolling back the tongue immediately is termed a waggling tongue. To protrude the tongue outside of the mouth without rolling it back is termed spitting of the tongue, which often indicates heat in the heart and spleen. A waggling tongue can be a sign of infantile convulsion. Both can be found in those with prenatal insufficiency of natural endowment and mental subnormality.

多为阴液耗伤;舌体歪斜为风邪中络;舌体萎软为脾气衰弱。舌反复伸出舐唇,旋即回缩为弄舌;舌常伸出口外,久不回缩,为吐舌。吐舌常为心脾有热,弄舌可为惊风先兆,二者均可见于先天禀赋不足及智能低下者。

Inspecting the tongue coating: A thin tongue coating is normal or indicates mild or shallow diseases, like initial onset of infection of exogenous pathogens. A thick tongue coating indicates interior disease or severe and deep diseases like food retention or accumulation of phlegm and dampness. Moist coating means the existence of body fluid. Slippery and moist coating indicates dampness stagnation. Dry coating suggests damage of body fluid. Sticky coating is phlegm and dampness. Putrid and grimy coating indicates turbidity in the stomach. A white coating is normal or indicates cold and dampness. White and thin coating is an infection of exogenous wind and cold or initial onset of wind and heat. Sticky and white coating indicates an internal

察舌苔:舌苔薄主正常或病轻浅,如外感初起;舌苔厚主病在里或深重,如食积痰湿。苔质滋润为有津;苔质滑润为湿滞;苔质干燥为津伤;苔质黏腻为痰湿;苔质腐垢为胃浊。舌苔白为正常或寒湿;薄白为外感风寒或风热初起;白腻为痰湿内蕴。舌苔黄主热证、里证,薄黄为风热在表、风寒化热或热邪入里;黄腻为脾胃湿热或痰热;老黄干燥主热甚耗伤气阴。舌苔花剥如地图主脾胃病,舌淡胖有津主脾胃气虚,

accumulation of phlegm and dampness. Yellow coating indicates heat pattern and interior pattern. Thin and yellow coating indicates wind heat in the exterior, wind cold transforming into heat or heat evil entering the interior. Sticky and yellow coating indicates dampness and heat or phlegm and heat in the stomach and spleen. Old, yellow and dry coating indicates consumption and damage of qi and by preponderant heat. Patchy and peeled map-like coating indicates diseases in the spleen and stomach. Pale and enlarged tongue with body fluid indicates qi deficiency of the spleen and stomach. Red tongue with little body fluid and scant coating is yin deficiency of the spleen and stomach. Tongue without coating indicates yin damage and body fluid exhaustion or nearly exhaustion of stomach qi. Note that children tend to have stained coating easily, which should not be considered pathological. Usually the stained coating is shallow and uneven.

舌质红少津、少苔为脾胃阴虚。舌光无苔，主阴伤液竭或胃气将竭。儿童容易出现染苔，须注意不可误认为病态，一般染苔比较浮浅而不均匀。

1.4 Inspection of throat

Throat is the opening of the lung and stomach and the passage for breath and food. Red throat, aversion to cold and fever indicate infection of exogenous pathogens. Red throat and tonsillitis indicate infectin of exogenous wind and heat or upward flaming of fire in the lung and stomach. Pyorrhea in tonsillitis is termed rotten flesh due to accumulation of heat. Enlarged tonsil without redness means hypertrophic, mostly indicating incomplete elimination of blood stasis and heat or failed healing due to qi deficiency.

1.4 望咽喉

咽喉为肺胃之门户，是呼吸与饮食通道。咽红、恶寒、发热是外感之象；咽红、乳蛾肿痛为外感风热或肺胃之火上炎；乳蛾溢脓，是热壅肉腐；乳蛾大而不红，多为瘀热未尽，或气虚不敛。

1.5 Inspection of fingerprint

Fingerprint refers to the superficial veins at the radial side of the index finger. Infants' skin is thin and tender. The veins can show up easily. There-

1.5 望指纹

指纹是指食指桡侧的浅表静脉，婴幼儿皮肤薄嫩，络脉易于显露，故 3 岁以下小

fore, for children under 3, to observe the finger veins is one of the inspecting methods.

儿看指纹为望诊内容之一。

Location of fingerprint refers to the apparent veins from tiger's mouth (the region between the thumb and the index finger) along the index finger to its tip. The three knuckles of index finger are respectively termed Pass of Wind, Pass of Qi and Pass of Life. The first knuckle at the base of index finger is Pass of Wind. The second knuckle is Pass of Qi, and the third is Pass of Life. The fingerprint should be inspected at a bright place and the doctor uses the radial side of his thumb to push slightly the index finger of the infants several times from Pass of Life to Pass of Wind, to make the finger veins appear. Normal fingerprint of the infants should be faintly purple and invisible over Pass of Wind. The inspection can be generalized as this: "Floating or sinking is used to differentiate between the exterior and interior; red or purple color is used to differentiate between cold and heat; light color or stagnation is used to differentiate between deficiency and excess; three Passes are used to differentiate the severity of disease."

指纹的部位,是从虎口沿食指桡侧所显现的脉络,以食指三指节分风、气、命三关,食指根的第一指节为风关,第二指节为气关,第三指节为命关。看指纹时要将患儿抱于光线充足处,医生用拇指桡侧,从命关到风关,轻轻推几次,使指纹显露。正常小儿的指纹应当是淡紫隐隐,不显露于风关之上。其内容可以概括为:"浮沉分表里,红紫辨寒热,淡滞定虚实,三关测轻重。"

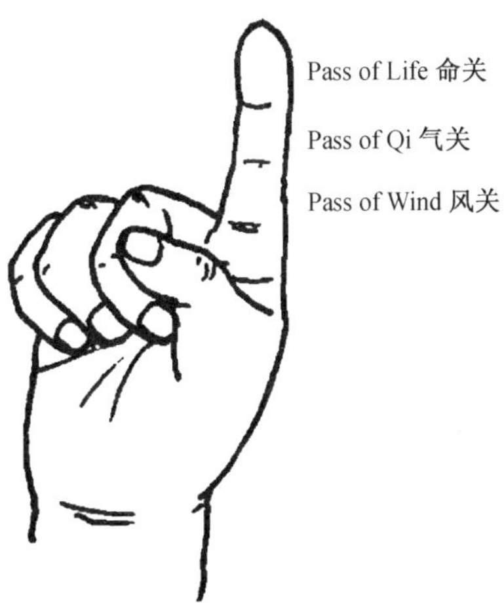

Finger prints of children
小儿指纹部位图

Floating or sinking is used to differentiate between the exterior and interior: floating means visible fingerprint, which indicates that the pathogenic evils are in the exterior; sinking means fingerprint is deep and hidden, and the pathogenic evils are in the interior.

浮沉分表里:浮为指纹显露,主病邪在表;沉为指纹深隐,主病邪在里。

Red or purple color is used to differentiate between cold and heat: red means red fingerprint, indicating cold patterns; purple fingerprint indicates heat pattern.

红紫辨寒热:红为红色,即指纹显红色主寒证;紫为紫色,纹显紫色主热证。

Light color or stagnation is used to differentiate between deficiency and excess: light color means smooth by pushing, indicating deficiency; stagnation means unsmooth by pushing and slow in recovery, indicating excess.

淡滞定虚实:淡为推之流畅,主虚证;滞为推之不流畅,复盈缓慢,主实证。

Three Passes are used to differentiate the severity of disease: the severity of disease can be inferred by the places where fingerprint appears. Appearance at Pass of Wind indicates the initial infection of pathogenic evil, and the condition is mild. When it reaches Pass of Qi, it indicates evil is going inward and the condition is relatively severe. When it appears at Pass of Life, it means the pathogenic evil has gone deep and the condition is getting worse. When the fingerprint appears at the tip of the finger, it is called "shooting nail through the Pass" (which means extension of visible veins through the Pass to the nail), which indicates critical condition, if it has never been so before.

三关测轻重:根据指纹所显现的部位判别疾病的轻重。纹在风关,示病邪初入,病情轻浅;纹达气关,示病邪入里,病情较重;纹达命关,示病邪深入,病情加重;纹达指尖,称"透关射甲",如非一向如此,则示病情危笃。

Inspection of fingerprint is of certain diagnostic value in clinic, but when the fingerprint and patterns do not correspond, "it is appropriate to focus on the symptoms by neglecting the observation of finger veins".

指纹诊法在临床有一定的诊断意义。但若纹证不符时,当"舍纹从证"。

2 Listening and smelling examination

Listening and smelling examinations include listening to sounds and smelling odors.

Listening to sounds means listening to the strident or faint sounds of the infant's crying, voice, coughing, and breathing, in a hope to identify the condition of the disease.

Crying is the language of babies. It can be physiological, or indicates certain discomforts or manifests different types of diseases.

Smelling odors includes smelling those of child patient's breath, vomit, urine and stool, etc. Many diseases have special odors, and smelling these odors can assist diagnosis. For example, belching of putrid and sour gas usually indicates milk and food retention. Foul breath often indicates accumulation of heat in the spleen and stomach. Fishy and purulent nasal discharge often indicates rhinorrhea. Sour and malodorous stool mostly indicates food damage.

3 Inquiry

The targets of inquiry in pediatric clinics mainly are the parents, nurses, or the older child patients. Inquiry should cover the following aspects.

3.1 Age

Carefully ask about the exact age of year, age of month or age of day. Newborns should be inquired of the day after birth. Children under two years old should be inquired of the exact age of months. Children over 2 years old should be inquired of the exact years and months. Some infantile diseases are closely related to the age. Age is also of important reference to prescription of medi-

2 闻诊

闻诊包括听声音和嗅气味两个方面。

听声音是听小儿啼哭、语言、咳嗽、呼吸等声音的高亢低微，从而辨别病情。

啼哭是婴儿的语言，有属生理表现的，也有身体不适的表示，还可以是各种病态的表现。

嗅气味包括患儿口中之气味及大小便、呕吐物等的气味。多种疾病可有一定的特殊气味，闻之可协助诊断。如嗳腐酸臭多为乳食积滞，口气臭秽多为脾胃积热，脓涕腥臭多为鼻渊，大便酸臭多为伤食等。

3 问诊

儿科问诊对象多是家长、保育员或年长患儿，应注意询问以下方面情况。

3.1 问年龄

详细询问确切的年龄、月龄或日龄。新生儿应问明出生天数；2 岁以内的小儿应问明实足月龄；2 岁以上的小儿，应问明实足岁数及月数。因儿科某些疾病与年龄有密切关系，年龄大小也是儿童用药的重要参考依据。

cations for the infants.

3.2 Condition of illness

Inquiry of condition includes the symptoms, duration, changes in the course of illness, causes and treatment of the disease. Besides the main symptoms and the accompanied ones, diets, urine, stool, and sleep should also be asked about. Chen Xiu Yuan in the Qing Dynasty made a 10-question song, which concludes inquiry like this: "first question cold and heat, secondly question sweat, thirdly question head and body, fourthly question urine and stool, fifthly question diet, sixthly question chest and abdomen, seventhly question deafness, eighthly question thirst, ninthly question previous illnesses, and tenthly question causes, plus administration of medications for referencecs. Women must be asked particularly about their periods, if delayed, advanced, and stopped or in profuse bleeding. More words should be asked in the pediatric clinics, to confirm smallpox and measles."

3.2 问病情

包括询问疾病的症状及持续时间、病程中的变化、发病的原因及治疗情况等。除主症及伴发症状的询问外，还应注意患儿的饮食、二便、睡眠情况等。清代陈修园将问诊的主要内容归纳为十问歌："一问寒热二问汗，三问头身四问便，五问饮食六胸腹，七聋八渴俱当辨，九问旧病十问因，再兼服药参机变，妇女尤必问经期，迟速闭崩皆可见，再添片语告儿科，天花麻疹全占验。"

3.3 Inquiry of personal history

This includes the following aspects: The first is the history of birth, including the number of pregnancy, the number of delivery, whether the infant is full term infant, whether the delivery is smooth or difficult, whether the mother has a history of abortion, manner of delivery, place of birth, condition at birth, health and nutrition of the mother during pregnancy. The second is the history of feeding, including way of feeding, supplementary food, weaning and conditions after weaning. For older child patients, dietary habits, current food types and appetite should be inquired as well. The third is the history of growth, including both physical and

3.3 问个人史

包括以下几个方面：一是生产史，主要询问胎次、产次，是否足月，顺产或难产，是否有流产史及接生方式、出生地点、出生情况、孕期母亲的营养和健康状况。二是喂养史，包括喂养方式和辅助食品添加情况，是否已经断奶和断奶的情况。对年长患儿还应询问饮食习惯，现在的食物种类和食欲等。三是生长发育史，包括体格生长和智能发育，如坐、立、行、

mental development, for instance, at what time to sit, stand, walk, and speak and to grow teeth, when the fontanel closes, and the condition of body weight and height. For older child patients, psychological, behavioral and learning problems should also be asked about. The fourth is history of vaccination, such as types and time of vaccination, whether there is adverse reaction, etc. In addition, the past history of the infants and family history should also be asked about.

语、齿等出现的时间；囟门闭合的时间；体重、身长增长情况；年长患儿应询问一些心理、行为、学习的情况等。四是预防接种史，询问曾接种过的疫苗种类、接种时间、有无不良反应等。其他方面还应询问患儿既往患病史、家族史等。

4 Palpation

The palpation includes pulse examination and body palpation, which is an important means to diagnose the pediatric diseases.

Pulse examination for child is different from that for adult. ①Method of pulse examination: The pusle would not be checked for children under three usually, but fingerprint would be checked instead. For children over three, one finger is used to determine the three pulse regions. Because the radial part of the infants is too narrow for the medical practitioner to check the pulse by three fingers, the medical practitioners usually use their index finger to press the three pulse regions, respectively Cun region, Guan region and Chi region. Then, based on different forces of the index finger, which are light, moderate or heavy, the medical practitioner may feel the changes of the pulses in the infants, which are light, medium and heavy pressure. ②The morbid pulses in the infants are mainly based upon the following six basic types of pulses, floating, deep, slow, rapid, feeble or forceful. These basic types work as the principle way to identify whether

4 切诊

包括脉诊和按诊两个方面，是诊断儿科疾病的重要手段。

小儿脉诊与成人脉诊不同。①脉诊方法：3 岁以下小儿一般不切脉，而以指纹诊法代替；3 岁以上小儿用一指定三关的方法。因小儿寸口部位较短不能容纳成人三指，故医者用食指同时按压寸、关、尺三部，再根据指力轻、中、重的不同，取浮、中、沉，来体会小儿脉象的变化。②小儿病脉主要以浮、沉、迟、数、无力、有力六种基本脉象为纲，以辨疾病的表里、寒热、虚实。③当“脉证不符”时，可“舍脉从证”。

the disease is in the exterior or in the interior, whether it is cold or heat, and whether it is deficient or excessive. ③If the symptoms and pulses do not match, it is appropriate to ignore the pulses and focus on the symptoms.

Body palpation is also called touching examination. The medical practitioner presses or touches the fontanel, neck and armpits, chest and abdomen, four limbs, and skin, etc, to observe heat, cold, softness, hardness, projection, sinking, or palpable mass or lumps, so as to help diagnose the pathologic situations. The following aspects should be noted: ①For little infants, the vertex and occipital skull should be felt to observe the closure of anterior and posterior fontanel, to observe any convex or concave, and mollification in the skull like a table tennis ball. ②It is advisable to palpate the abdomen at the feeding time or at the time when infants are quiet. ③It is necessary to judge the clinical significance of the information obtained by palpation, in accordance with the infant's age. For instance, the signs can be incorrect, because the infants are too small in age and keep crying when palpating, it is necessary to differentiate the signs carefully.

按诊亦称触诊，是医者用手按压或触摸颅囟、颈腋、胸腹、四肢、皮肤等，以察其冷、热、软、硬、突、陷、有无癥瘕痞块等情况，从而协助诊断病情。须注意以下几方面：①小婴儿须触摸顶部及枕部颅骨，了解前后囟的闭合情况，有无隆起或凹陷，颅骨有无软化呈乒乓球样的感觉等。②小儿腹部的按诊，应尽量在小儿安静时，或在婴儿哺乳时进行。③要根据年龄特点以判断按诊所得资料的临床意义。如小儿年龄小，按诊时若啼哭不止，获取的体征不准确，应加以识别。

Chapter 3 Key Points to Treatment in Pediatrics of Traditional Chinese Medicine

第3章 中医儿科治疗要点

1 Common internal therapies

1.1 Common therapies in pediatrics

(1) Method to expel wind and resolve the exterior This therapy can promote sweating and resolve the flesh, expel wind and promote eruption, and dissipate the pathogenic evils. It is used for patterns of external evils invading the exterior. To resolve the exterior with herbs in warmth and acridity, *Schizonepeta and Saposhnikovia Toxin-Vanquishing Powder* (Jing Fang Bai Du San), and *Scallion and Fermented Soybean Decoction* (Cong Chi Tang) are used often. To resolve the exterior with the herbs in acrid and cool property, *Lonicera and Forsythia Powder* (Yin Qiao San) and *Mulberry Leaf and Chrysanthemum Decoction* (Sang Ju Yin) are often used. To resolve summer-heat and relieve the exterior, *Newly Supplemented Mosla Decoction* (Xin Jia Xiang Ru Yin) is often used. To promote eruption and relieve the exterior, *Toxin-Diffusing Exterior-Effusing Decoction* (Xuan Du Fa Biao Tang) is often used.

(2) Method to diffuse and purify the lung qi This therapy can diffuse the lung qi, depurate and descend the lung qi, and restore the normal respiratory functions of the lung qi. It is used for patterns

1 常用内治法

1.1 儿科常用治法

（1）疏风解表法 具有发汗解肌、疏风透疹、透邪外出作用的治法，用于外邪犯表的证候。辛温解表常用荆防败毒散、葱豉汤；辛凉解表常用银翘散、桑菊饮；解暑透表常用新加香薷饮；透疹解表常用宣毒发表汤等。

（2）宣肃肺气法 具有宣发、肃降肺气，恢复肺正常呼吸功能的治法，用于肺失宣肃的证候。宣肺止咳常用

of impaired diffusion and depuration of the lung qi. To diffuse the lung qi and suppress cough, *Mulberry leaf and Chrysanthemum Decoction* (Sang Ju Yin) and *Apricot Kernel and Perilla Powder* (Xing Su San) are often used. To depurate lung qi and suppress cough, *Melberry Root Bark Decoction* (Sang Bai Pi Tang) and *Three Disobedience Decoction* (San Ao Tang) are commonly used. To reduce the lung qi and calm panting, *Perilla Fruit Qi-Downbearing Decoction* (Su Zi Jiang Qi Tang) and *Ephedra, Apricot Kernel, Gypsum, and Licorice, Decoction* (Ma Xing Shi Gan Tang) are often used. To diffuse the lung qi and disinhibit water, *Ephedra, Forsythia, and Rice Bean Decoction* (Ma Huang Lian Qiao Chi Xiao Dou Tang) is often used.

杏苏散、桑菊饮；肃肺止咳常用桑白皮汤、三拗汤；泻肺平喘常用苏子降气汤、麻杏石甘汤；宣肺利水常用麻黄连翘赤小豆汤等。

(3) Method to dry dampness and dissolve phlegm This therapy is to regulate the spleen and dissolve dampness, to expel phlegm and fluid and to separate the clear from the turbid, used for patterns of damp turbidity and phlegm and fluid. To warm up dryness and dissolve dampness, *Stomach-Calming Powder* (Ping Wei San) is often used. To clear away heat and dispel dampness, *Coptis and Officinal Magnolia Bark Decoction* (Lian Po Yin) is often used. To warm and dissolve phlegm and fluid, *Minor Blue Dragon Decoction* (Xiao Qing Long Tang) is often used. To clear away and dissolve phlegm heat, *Metal-Clearing Phlegm-Transforming Decoction* (Qing Jin Hua Tan Tang) is often used.

(3) 燥湿化痰法　具有调脾化湿、祛除痰饮、分清别浊作用的治法，用于湿浊痰饮的证候。温燥化湿常用平胃散；清热祛湿常用连朴饮；温化痰饮常用小青龙汤；清化痰热常用清金化痰汤等。

(4) Method to clear away heat and resolve toxin This method is to clear heat away and drain fire, cool blood and resolve toxin, clear away and resolve the interior heat, used for pattens of excessive interior heat. *White Tiger Decoction* (Bai Hu

(4) 清热解毒法　具有清热泻火、凉血解毒、清解里热作用的治法，用于里热实证的证候。清气分热常用白虎汤；清营凉血常用清营汤、

Tang) is often used to clear away heat from qi-energy system. *Ying-Nutrient System-Clearing Decoction* (Qing Ying Tang) and *Rhinoceros Horn and Rehmannia Decoction* (Xi Jiao Di Huang Tang) are often used to clear away heat from Ying-Nourient System and cool blood. To drain fire and resolve toxin, *Coptis Toxin-Resolving Decoction* (Huang Lian Jie Du Tang) is often used. To clear away heat from bowels and visceras, *Gentian Liver-Draining Decoction* (Long Dan Xie Gan Tang), *Red-Abducting Powder* (Dao Chi San), *White-Draining Powder* (Xie Bai San), *Yellow-draining Powder* (Xie Huang San), *Pueraria, Scutellaria, and Coptis Decoction* (Ge Gen Huang Qin Huang Lian Tang) are often used.

犀角地黄汤;泻火解毒常用黄连解毒汤;清脏腑热分别采用龙胆泻肝汤、导赤散、泻白散、泻黄散、葛根黄芩黄连汤等。

(5) Method to free the bowels and promote purgation This method is to promote bowel movement, eliminate constipation, expel water and fluid, and clean up excessive heat, used for patterns of interior excess and accumulation. To free the bowels and clear away heat, *Stomach-Regulating Qi-Coordinating Decoction* (Tiao Wei Cheng Qi Tang) is often used. To moisten the intestines and promote bowel movement, *Cannabis Fruit Pill* (Ma Zi Ren Wan) is often used.

(5) 通腑泻下法 具有通便下积、攻逐水饮、荡涤实热作用的治法,用于里实积聚的证候。通腑泻热常用调胃承气汤;润肠通便常用麻子仁丸等。

(6) Method to help digestion and remove stagnancy This method is to digest milk and food, to remove stagnancy and accumulations, and to promote purgation for eliminating obstruction, used for patterns of retention of mild and food. *Milk-Dispersing Pill* (Xiao Ru Wan) is used to digest milk and eliminate food retention. *Harmony-Preserving Pill* (Bao He Wan) is used to digest food and eliminate stagnation. *Unripe Bitter Orange Stagnation-Abducting*

(6) 消食导滞法 具有消乳化食、消痞化积、通导积滞作用的治法,用于乳食积滞的证候。消乳化积常用消乳丸;消食化积常用保和丸;通导积滞常用枳实导滞丸;健脾消食常用健脾丸等。

Pill (Zhi Shi Dao Zhi Wan) is used to relieve and remove stagnation. *Spleen-Fortifying Pill* (Jian Pi Wan) is often used to fortify the spleen and digest food.

(7) Method to quicken the blood, dissolve blood stasis, dredge blood vessles and eliminate stangnancy　This method is to free the blood vessels and eliminate blood stasis and accumulation, used for patterns of stagnancy of blood vessel. *Chinese Angelica Counterflow Cold Decoction* (Dang Gui Si Ni Tang) is used to warm up the channels and quicken the blood. *Rhinoceros Horn and Rehmannia Decoction* (Xi Jiao Di Huang Tang) is used to cool and quicken the blood. *Peach Kernel and Carthamus Four Agents Decoction* (Tao Hong Si Wu Tang) is used to promote the circulation of qi and blood. To break blood stasis and dissolve concretions, *Rhubarb and Ground Beetle Pill* (Da Huang Zhe Chong Wan) is often used.

(7) 活血化瘀法　具有疏通血脉、消除瘀积作用的治法，用于血脉瘀滞的证候。温经活血常用当归四逆汤；凉血活血常用犀角地黄汤；行气活血常用桃红四物汤；破瘀消癥常用大黄蟅虫丸等。

(8) Method to calm down the spirit and open the apertures　This method is to calm down the spirit and stabilize the mind, to settle fright and tranquilize the mind, and to free apertures for opening and closing, used for symptoms and signs of restless mind, and unconsciousness due to closure of apertures. To nourish the heart and quiet the spirit, *Spleen-Returning Decoction* (Gui Pi Tang) is often used. To settle fright and quiet the mind, *Loadstone and Cinnabar Pill* (Ci Zhu Wan) is often used. To clear away heat and open apertures, *Palace-Clearing Decoction* (Qing Gong Tang) and *Peaceful Palace Bovine Bezoar Pill* (An Gong Niu Huang Wan) are often used. *Storax Pill* (Su He Xiang Wan) is often used for warming up and opening the

(8) 安神开窍法　具有安神定志、镇惊宁心、通窍开闭作用的治法，用于神志不宁、窍闭神昏的证候。养心安神常用归脾汤；镇惊安神常用磁朱丸；清热开窍常用清宫汤、安宫牛黄丸；温通开窍常用苏合香丸等。

apertures.

(9) Method to dispel wind and extinguish wind This method is to dispel wind, dredge the collaterals, balance the liver and extinguish wind, used for patterns of wind evil lodging in the collaterals and pattern of liver wind stirring internally. *Impediment-Alleviating Decoction* (Juan Bi Tang) is used to dispel wind and expel dampness. *White Tiger Decoction Plus Cinnamon Twig* (Bai Hu Gui Zhi Tang) is often used to dispel wind and clear away heat, *Antelope Horn and Uncaria Decoction* (Ling Jiao Gou Teng Tang) for cooling the liver and extinguishing wind; *Major Wind-Stabilizing Pill* (Da Ding Feng Zhu) for nourishing yin and extinguishing wind.

(9) 祛风息风法　具有祛风通络、平肝息风作用的治法，用于风邪留络、肝风内动的证候。祛风逐湿常用蠲痹汤；祛风清热常用白虎桂枝汤；凉肝息风常用羚角钩藤汤；养阴息风常用大定风珠等。

(10) Method to secure astringency This therapy is to check sweating and constrain the lung qi, astringe the intestines, reduce urine, secure and contain essence and body fluid, used for patterns of outward discharge of qi, blood, essence and body fluid. To secure the exterior and astrige sweating, *Oyster Shell Powder* (Mu Li San) is often used. To astringe the lung qi and stop cough, *Nine Immortals Powder* (Jiu Xian San) is often used. To astringe the intestines for relieving depletion, *True Man Viscus-Nourishing Decoction* (Zhen Ren Yang Zang Tang) is often used. To secure the bladder and check seminal emission and enuresis, *Mantis Egg-Case Powder* (Sang Piao Shao San) is often used.

(10) 收敛固涩法　具有止汗敛肺、涩肠缩尿、固摄精津作用的治法，用于气血精津外泄的证候。固表敛汗常用牡蛎散；敛肺止咳常用九仙散；涩肠固脱常用真人养脏汤；固脬止遗常用桑螵蛸散等。

(11) Method to supplement and fortify the spleen This method is to supplement spleen qi, warm up and supplement spleen yang and is applied for spleen deficiency patterns. *Special Achievement Powder* (Yi Gong San) is often used to fortify the

(11) 补益健脾法　具有补益脾气、温补脾阳作用的治法，用于脾虚证候。健脾益气常用异功散；滋脾养血常用四物汤；补脾养阴常用

spleen and boost qi. *Four Agents Decoction* (Si Wu Tang) is often used to enrich the spleen and nourish blood. *Stomach-Boosting Decoction* (Yi Wei Tang) is used to supplement the spleen and nourish yin. *Center-Rectifying Decoction* (Li Zhong Tang) is often used to warm up and supplement spleen yang.

益胃汤；温补脾阳常用理中汤等。

(12) Method to restore origin and supplement the kidney　This method is to enrich yin and replenish essence, warm up and invigorate the original yang, supplement the kidney and secure the foundation, used for kidney deficiency patterns. *Six-Ingredient Rehmannia Pill* (Liu Wei Di Huang Wan) is often used to supplement and boost kidney yin. *Placenta Great Creation Pill* (He Che Da Zao Wan) is used to enrich the kidney and replenish essence. *Right-Restoring Pill* (You Gui Wan) is often used to warm up the kidney and invigorate yang. *Tortoise Shell and Deerhorn Two Immortals Glue* (Lu Gui Er Xian Jiao) is often used to supplement both yin and yang.

(12) 扶元补肾法　具有滋阴填精、温壮元阳、补肾固本作用的治法，用于肾虚证候。补益肾阴常用六味地黄丸；滋肾填精常用河车大造丸；温肾壮阳常用右归丸；阴阳并补常用龟鹿二仙胶等。

(13) Method to rescue yin and yang　This method is to increase humor and rescue yin, benefit qi and return yang, and to stem conterflow and relieve depletion, used for patterns of exhaustion of qi, yang, yin, and humor. *Humor-Increasing Decoction* (Zeng Ye Tang) is used to increase humor and engender liquid. *Pulse-Engendering Powder* (Sheng Mai San) and *Injection of Pulse-Engendering Decoction* (Sheng Mai Yin Zhu She Ye) are often used to boost qi and rescue yin. *Yang-Returning Emergency Decoction* (Hui Yang Jiu Ji Tang) is used to boost qi and return yang. *Ginseng, Cyperus, Dragon Bone, Oyster Shell Counterflow Decoction* (Seng Fu Long Mu Jiu Ni Tang) is often used to re-

(13) 挽阴救阳法　具有增液挽阴、益气回阳、救逆固脱作用的治法，用于气阳阴津衰竭的证候。增液生津常用增液汤；益气救阴常用生脉散、生脉饮注射液；益气回阳常用回阳救急汤；回阳救逆常用参附龙牡救逆汤等。

turn yang and stem conterflow.

1.2 Decocting and administrative methods for pediatric herbal decoctions

Generally, it is similar to those used for the adults, but the dose is less in the infants than the adults. In terms of the general dose of herbal decoction, the newborns take 1/6 of adult's amount, the infants take about 1/3～1/2 of adults' amount, and the young children take about 2/3 or the same amount as that of adults. Preschool children take the same amount as adults. The decrease of the total amount is done by cutting off certain herbs or the amount of each herb.

Water used to decoct herbs shouldn't be too much. The amount is adequate when it just covers the medicinal stuffs after they are soaked. The total amount of decoction should be controlled according to age. Usually, for infants, it is about 60～100 ml, for young children and preschool children, about 150～200, for school children, about 200～250 ml. For the number of times for administration of decoction, it can be adjusted flexibly between 3 to 5 times a day according to the amount of each administration and pathological situation of the sick infants.

1.2 儿科汤剂的煎服方法

一般与成人相同。但小儿服药量需比成人小。汤剂处方用药总量，一般新生儿用成人量的 1/6，乳婴儿用成人量的 1/3～1/2，幼儿及幼童用成人量的 2/3 或用成人量，学龄儿童用成人量。用药总量的减少，可以通过减少药味和每味药的药量来达到。

汤剂煎煮前放水不要太多，一般以浸透后水能淹没药物为适宜。煎出的药液总量，要根据年龄大小来掌握，一般婴儿 60～100 毫升，幼儿及学龄前儿童 150～200 毫升，学龄儿童 200～250 毫升。每日服药次数，按照患儿每次服药量和病情特点灵活掌握，可分 3～5 次不等。

2 Common external therapies

2.1 Fumigation and wash therapy

It is a therapy to fumigate and wash the external body with medicinal decoction and steam. For instance, in hot summer when there is fever but no sweat, *Mosla Herba* (Xiang Ru) can be decocted to fumigate and wash the body, so as to promote perspiration and relieve fever. At the initial stage of

2 常用外治法

2.1 熏洗法

是利用中药的药液及蒸气熏洗人体外表的一种治法。如夏日高热无汗可用香薷煎汤熏洗，发汗退热；麻疹发疹初期，为助透疹，用麻黄、浮萍、芫荽子、西河柳煎

measles eruption, to help eruption of papules, *Ephedrae Herba* (Ma Huang), *Spirodelae Herba* (Fu Ping), *Fructus Coriandri* (Yan Sui Zi), *Tamaricis Cacumen* (Xi He Liu) are decocted, then added with rice wine, so as to rinse head and limbs. Boil the decoction indoors to moisten the air and the body can contact the herbal evaporation.

汤后，加黄酒擦洗头部和四肢，并将药液放在室内煮沸，使空气湿润，体表亦能接触药气。

2.2 Smearing therapy

It is an external therapy to pound and smash fresh herbs or to mix ground medical powder with water or vinegar, then apply the juice or mixture to the body surface. For instance, fresh *Herba Portulacae* (Ma Chi Xian), *Opuntiae Radix et Caulis* (Xian Ren Zhang), *Indigo Naturalis* (Qing Dai), *Golden Yellow Powder* (Jin Huang San), *Purple Gold Ingot* (Zi Jin Ding), any one of them, could be prepared and applied on the cheeks, for treating epidemic mumps. Take three portions of *Euodiae Fructus* (Wu Zhu Yu) powder and one portions of *Arisaema Cum Bile* (Dan Nan Xing) powder, mix them with rice vinegar and apply on Yongquan (KI 1), for treating wet cheek.

2.2 涂敷法

是将新鲜的中草药捣烂，或用药物研末加入水或醋调匀后，涂敷于体表的一种外治法。如用鲜马齿苋、仙人掌、青黛、金黄散、紫金锭等，任选一种，调敷于腮部，治疗流行性腮腺炎。用吴茱萸粉 3 份、胆南星粉 1 份，用米醋调成膏状涂敷于足底涌泉穴，治疗滞颐。

2.3 Bandage-compressing therapy

It is an external therapy to put herbal drugs on the local area of the skin, and then band and compress it. For instance, *Natrii Sulfas* (Pi Xiao) could be compressed on the umbilicus for treating food retention. *Sumac Gallnut* (Wu Bei Zi Fen) Powder could be mixed with vinegar and compressed on the umbilicus, for treating night sweating.

2.3 罨包法

是将药物置于皮肤局部，并加以包扎的一种外治法。如用皮硝包扎于脐部以消食积；用五倍子粉加食醋调填入脐内再包扎，治疗盗汗等。

2.4 Ironing therapy

It is an external therapy to heat the herbal drugs hot, and then wrap the hot herbal drugs with cloth to iron the body surface. For instance, salt

2.4 热熨法

是将药物炒热后，用布包裹以熨肌表的一种外治法。如炒热食盐熨腹部，治

can be heated and used to warm up abdomen to treat abdominal pain. Raw onion heated with salt can be used to warm up the area around umbilicus and lower abdomen to treat dribbling urinary retention.

疗腹痛；用生葱、食盐炒热，熨脐周围及少腹，治疗癃闭等。

2.5 Dressing therapy

It is an external therapy to make the herbal drugs into ointment or cake or grind the herbal drugs into powder to scatter onto the ordinary plaster. For instance, *Caryophylli Flos* (Ding Xiang) powder and *Cinnamomi Cortex* (Rou Gui) powder are scattered onto the ordinary plaster and pasted to umbilicus, for treating diarrhea of cold pattern. During three ten-day periods of dog day in summer, grind *Corydalis Rhizoma* (Yan Hu Suo), *Sinapis semenAlbae* (Bai Jie Zi), *Kansui Radix* (Gan Sui) and *Asari Radix et Rhizoma* (Xi Xin), then mix them with ginger juice and make into the medical cakes, paste on Feishu (BL 13), Gaohuang (BL 43) and Bailao (Extra) to treat wheezing and panting.

2.5 敷贴法

是将药物制成软膏、药饼，或研粉撒于普通膏药上，敷贴于局部的一种外治法。如用丁香、肉桂等药粉，撒于普通膏药上贴于脐部，治疗寒证泄泻。再如在夏季三伏天，用延胡索、白芥子、甘遂、细辛研末，以生姜汁调成药饼，敷于肺俞、膏肓、百劳穴上，治疗哮喘等。

2.6 Rubbing and wiping therapy

It is an external therapy to wipe and rub the local area with liquid medicine or powder. For instance, *Borneol and Borax Powder* (Bing Peng San) is used to wipe the oral cavity, or light salt solution, *Lonicera and Licorice Decoction* (Yin Hua Gan Cao Shui) is used to wipe and wash the oral cavity to treat thrush or mouth ulcer.

2.6 擦拭法

是用药液或药末擦拭局部的一种外治法。如冰硼散擦拭口腔，或用淡盐水、银花甘草水拭洗口腔，治疗鹅口疮、口疮等。

2.7 Medical bag therapy

It is an external therapy to grind the herbal drugs into powder and put it into bag, then hang the bag in front of infant's chest, abdomen or put it into the pillow. Commonly used herbs are aromatic ones like *Kaempferiae Rhizoma* (Shan Nai), *Atractylodes Rhizoma* (Cang Zhu), *Angelica Radix*

2.7 药袋疗法

是将药物研成粉末装入袋内，给小儿佩戴在胸前、腹部或枕头的一种外治法。药物常选用山奈、苍术、白芷、砂仁、丁香、肉桂、甘松、豆蔻、沉香、檀香、艾叶等芳香

Dahurian (Bai Zhi), *Amomi Fructus* (Sha Ren), Ding Xiang, Rou Gui, *Nardostachyos Radix et Rhizoma* (Gan Song), *Amomi Fructus Rotundus* (Dou Kou), *Aquilariae Lignum Resinatum* (Chen Xiang), *Santali Albi Lignum* (Tan Xiang), and *Artemisiae Argyi Folium* (Ai Ye). According to different conditions, the herbal drugs are selected based upon herbal formula and made into the scent bag, belly band, or scent pillow. The frequent use of them can repel foulness, resolve toxin, improve appetite, treat and prevent diseases.

药物，根据病情，选药配方，制成香袋、肚兜、香枕等。经常使用，具有辟秽解毒、增进食欲、防病治病的作用。

3 Other therapies

3 其他疗法

3.1 Tuina therapy

3.1 推拿疗法

Infantile Tuina, also known infantile massage, can promote flow of qi and blood, free the meridians and collaterals, calm down the spirit and qi, and harmonize bowels and viscera, so as to expel evils and treat disease. Clinically, in pediatric clinic, tuina can be used to treat diarrhea, abdominal pain, anorexia, wry neck, and wilting pattern in the preschool children, etc. The younger the age, the better the effects would be.

小儿推拿亦称小儿按摩，有促进气血循行、经络通畅、神气安定、脏腑调和的作用，能达到驱邪治病的目的。儿科临床常用于治疗学龄前小儿泄泻、腹痛、厌食、斜颈、痿证等疾病。年龄越小，效果越好。

Spine-pinching therapy is one common tuina method in pediatric clinics. By massaging the Governor Vessel and Bladder Meridian, this method can be used to harmonize yin and yang, free the meridians and collaterals, move qi and quicken the blood, restore functions of bowels and viscera, so as to prevent and treat diseases. The concrete operating method: After child patient lies on his face, the doctor clenches a loose fist, presses two index fingers on the spine, pinches and lifts the muscle with thumbs and index fingers, then rolls the muscle with

捏脊疗法是儿科常用的一种推拿方法，此法通过对督脉和膀胱经的按摩，调和阴阳，疏理经络，行气活血，恢复脏腑功能以防治疾病。具体操作方法：患儿俯卧，一法是医者两手半握拳，双手两食指抵于背脊上，再以两手拇指伸向食指前方，合力夹住肌肉提起，而后，食指向前，拇指向后退，作翻卷动

index fingers forward while the thumbs backward, with both hand moving forward simultaneously. Another method is that the doctor makes a pinching motion by the thumbs facing the index fingers, middle fingers and the fourth fingers, from lumbosacral area, to pinch the skin along both sides of the spine, all the way to Dazhui (GV 14), continuously for 3 to 5 times. After the third time, the doctor lifts the skin once every three pinches. This treatment can be given once every day and 6 days make one course of treatment. This therapy is prohibited for the infants with infected skin on the spine and back or with purura.

作，两手同时向前移动；另一法是医者用双手拇指与食指、中指、无名指相对，做捏物状手形，自腰骶开始，沿脊柱两侧捏起皮肤，不断向上捏至大椎穴止。如此反复3～5次，捏到第3次后，每捏3把，将皮肤提起1次。每日1次，6日为1个疗程。对有脊背皮肤感染、紫癜等疾病的患儿禁用捏脊疗法。

3.2 Acumoxatherapy

Acumoxatherapy includes acupuncture and moxibustion. Pediatric Acumoxatherapy is often used in treating infantile enuresis, wheezing and panting, diarrhea, infantile convulsion, impediment pattern, sequelae of encephalitis, etc.

To puncture Sifeng (EX-UE 10) is one common needling method in pediatric clinics. Sifeng (EX-UE 10) is an extra point, located in the middle point of crease of the middle knuckles of the index finger, middle finger, the fourth finger and the little finger. It is a point where three yin meridians of the hand pass through. To puncture this acupoint can clear away heat and eliminate vexation, free hundred meridians, and harmonize the internal organs. It is often used to treat infantile anorexia, and indigestion. Manipulation: Clean the skin, puncture the point with a three-edge needle for about 0.1 inch (a unit of length = 0.33 centimeter) deep, squeeze out a little yellowish and white sticky fluid after needling.

3.2 针灸疗法

针灸疗法包括针法与灸法。儿科针灸疗法常用于治疗遗尿、哮喘、泄泻、惊风、痹证、乙脑后遗症等病证。

刺四缝疗法是儿科针法中常用的一种。四缝是经外奇穴，位置在食指、中指、无名指及小指四指中节横纹中点，是手三阴经所经过之处。针刺四缝可以清热除烦、通畅百脉、调和脏腑，常用于治疗小儿厌食、疳证。具体操作方法：皮肤局部消毒后，用三棱针刺约1分深，刺后用手挤出黄白色黏液少许。

3.3 Cupping therapy

It is an external therapy to treat diseases by using cuplike tools to cause negative pressure in cups, and suck on the acupoints or diseased parts, causing local blood congestion. This method can increase circulation of qi and blood, speed up Ying-nutrient system and Wei-defensive system, dispel wind and disperse cold, soothe the sinews and stop the pain. It is often used to treat pneumonia, wheezing and panting, abdominal pain, and enuresis.

3.3 拔罐疗法

拔罐疗法是运用罐具，造成罐内负压，使之吸附于患处或穴位上，产生局部充血，从而达到治疗病证的一种治法，有促进气血流畅、营卫运行、祛风散寒、舒筋止痛等作用，常用于肺炎喘嗽、哮喘、腹痛、遗尿等疾病。

3.4 Dietetic therapy

This therapy, also called for short as food therapy, is a method to use the properties and components of the foodstuffs to function on the relevant organs, so as to regulate body functions, to prevent and treat diseases, to preserve the life activities and restore health, under the guidance of Chinese medical philosophy.

3.4 饮食疗法

饮食疗法，简称食疗，是在中医药学理论指导下，运用食物的性味和所含成分，作用于有关脏腑，以调节机体功能、防治疾病、养生康复的一种方法。

Specific Introduction

各 论

Chapter 1 Diseases of Respiratory System

第1章 呼吸系统疾病

Section 1 Acute Infection of Upper Respiratory Tract

第1节 急性上呼吸道感染

Acute infection of the upper respiratory tract refers to the acute infection of nose, nasopharynx, and pharynx caused by pathogens attacking the respiratory tract above throat, clinically manifested by fever, nasal obstruction and runny nose, sneezing, cough, etc, and often diagnosed as "acute nasopharyngitis, acute sore throat, and acute tonsillitis". It mostly happens at sudden change of weather or in winter and spring. The infants are more likely to catch it, and the prognosis is usually good. For those with weak physique or severe infection of evils, the secondary diseases tend to occur easily.

急性上呼吸道感染是指各种病原体侵犯喉部以上呼吸道引起的鼻、鼻咽和咽部的急性感染，以发热、鼻塞、流涕、喷嚏、咳嗽为主要临床特征，常用"急性鼻咽炎、急性咽炎、急性扁桃体炎"等诊断，简称"上感"。以气候骤变及冬春季节发病率高。婴幼儿更为多见。一般预后良好，若体质较弱或感邪重者，易继发其他疾病。

The disease belongs to "cold" and "nipple moth" in Chinese medicine. Due to infantile tender lung, deficient spleen, weak and timid spirit and qi, after contracting evils, concurrent patterns complicated with phlegm, with stagnancy and with fright tend to occur.

本病相当于中医学"感冒""乳蛾"等范畴。因小儿肺脏娇嫩，脾常不足，神气怯弱，感邪之后，易出现夹痰、夹滞、夹惊的兼证。

1 Etiology and pathogenesis

1 病因病机

The cause of disease is mainly due to infection of wind evil. Wind evil is often complicated with cold, heat, summer-heat, dampness, or dryness, etc. It tends

病因主要为感受风邪。风邪常兼杂寒、热、暑、湿、燥等，在气候变化，冷暖失常，

to occur at the time of climatic change, usually on cold or hot days, or as a result of improper care.

调护不当时易发生本病。

Wind evil invades from the mouth, nose, skin, or hair, blocking the fleshy exterior, and leading to the failure of the lung in defending and diffusing abilities and various symptoms of common cold arise. Since there are different types of evils involved, common cold can be differentiated as cold in pattern of wind cold, wind heat, or summer-heat and dampness. Due to the delicacy of the lung in the infants, after contracted with evils, the lung fails in diffusing and depurating ability, so qi dynamic is inhibited and body fluids fail to be distributed, condensing into phlegm, obstructing the airways. There are aggravating cough and gurgling with sputum in the throat. This is common cold complicated with phlegm. The infants are often deficient in the spleen and unable to control their ingestion of food and milk. After contracted with evils, the spleen fails to perform its transportation and transformation, leading to retention of food and milk, distention and pain in stomach and abdomen, no desire for milk and food, or accompanied vomiting and diarrhea. This is common cold complicated with stagnation. Since the infants are timid and weak in spirit and qi, and surplus in the heart and liver, after contracting evils, the heat would harass the heart and liver, which will easily cause restlessness of mind, unsound sleep, fright, and convulsion. This is common cold complicated with fright.

风邪由口鼻或皮毛而入,束于肌表,肺卫失宣致感冒诸症发生。由于感邪不同,故有风寒、风热、暑湿感冒之别。小儿肺脏娇嫩,感邪之后,失于宣肃,气机不利,津液不得敷布聚而为痰,痰阻气道,则咳嗽加剧,喉间痰鸣,为感冒夹痰。小儿脾常不足,乳食不知自节,感邪之后脾失健运,乳食停滞,则脘腹胀满、不思乳食,或伴呕吐泄泻,为感冒夹滞。小儿神气怯弱,心肝常有余,感邪之后热扰心肝,易致心神不宁,睡卧不实,惊惕抽风,为感冒夹惊。

2 Key to diagnosis

(1) It often occurs at a time of sudden climatic change, when cold and heat are not in harmony, or

2 诊断要点

(1) 常发于气候骤变,冷暖失调之时,或有与感冒患

after contacting other patients with common cold.

(2) The chief manifestations are fever, aversion to wind or cold, nasal congestion and runny nose, sneezing, and slight cough. There can be accompanied redness in the throat or sore throat.

(3) For common cold complicated with other patterns, there can be exacerbated cough, phlegm rale in the throat, distention and pain in the stomach and abdomen, no desire for food and drink, putrid and sour vomiting, irregular bowel movement, or restless sleep, and convulsion by fright.

者接触史。

（2）以发热、恶风寒、鼻塞流涕、喷嚏微咳为主证，可伴咽红或咽痛。

（3）感冒伴兼夹证者，可见咳嗽加剧，喉间痰鸣；或脘腹胀痛，不思饮食，呕吐酸腐，大便失调；或睡卧不宁，惊惕抽风。

3 Pattern identification and treatment

According to the nature of exogenous pathogenic evils, there can be differences in pattern of wind and cold, wind and heat, summer-heat or dampness. In the winter and spring, it is more likely to be pattern of wind and cold or wind and heat; in the summer, more likely to be pattern of summer-heat or dampness. For those with pattern of wind and cold, there are nasal congestion, clear nasal discharge, and no redness in the tongue and throat. For those with pattern of wind and heat, there are nasal congestion, turbid nasal discharge, red tongue and red throat. When there is high fever, with no sweat or little sweat, thirst, vexation, it can be abnormally exuberancy of summer-heat. When there is stuffy sensation in the chest, upwelling and nausea, heavy and tired sensation in the body, poor appetite, greasy tongue coating, it can be abnormally exuberancy of summer-heat and dampness. Influenza usually has severe symptoms and there is a history of epidemics. Clinically, it is necessary to differentiate the pattern of cold with phlegm, with

3 辨证论治

根据外感病邪的性质，有风寒、风热、暑湿之不同。冬春多为风寒、风热；夏季多为暑湿。风寒者，鼻塞涕清，舌、咽不红；风热者，鼻塞涕浊，舌红咽赤。若发热较高，无汗或少汗，口渴心烦为暑热偏盛；胸闷，泛恶，身重困倦，食少纳呆，舌苔腻为暑湿偏盛。时行感冒一般症状较重，有流行病学史。临床亦注意辨别夹痰、夹滞、夹惊的不同。

stagnation and with fright.

The basic therapeutic principle is to expel wind and relieve the exterior. In accordance with the different infecting pathogens, it is necessary to relieve the exterior by spicy and warm herbs, to relieve the exterior by spicy and cool herbs, to clear away summer-heat and relieve the exterior, or to dissipate pestilence and dissolve toxin respectively. When there are concurrent and complicated patterns, methods to dissolve phlegm, to help digestion, to remove stagnancy and to settle fright can be used respectively.

治疗以疏风解表为基本治则。根据感邪的不同分别治以辛温解表、辛凉解表、清暑解表、清瘟解毒等。若有兼夹证，分别佐以化痰、消导、镇惊之法。

3.1 Main Patterns

3.1 主证

(1) Common cold in pattern of wind and cold

(1) 风寒感冒

Manifestations: Strong aversion to cold, low-grade fever, no sweat, headache and body pain, clear snivel, sneezing and cough, no redness in the pharynx, white and thin tongue coating, tight and floating pulse, floating and red fingerprints.

证候：恶寒重，发热轻，无汗，头身疼痛，鼻流清涕，喷嚏咳嗽，咽不红，舌苔薄白，脉浮紧，指纹浮红。

Therapeutic method: To relieve the exterior with warmth and acridity.

治法：辛温解表。

Formula: *Schizonepeta and Saposhnikovia Toxin-Vanquishing Powder* (Jing Fang Bai Du San) with modification.

主方：荆防败毒散加减。

Commonly used herbs: *Schizonepetae Herba* (Jing Jie), *Ledebouriellae Radix* (Fang Feng), *Notopterygii Rhizoma seu Radix* (Qiang Huo), *Perillae Folium* (Zi Su Ye), *Platycodonis Radix* (Jie Geng), *Peucedani Radix* (Qian Hu), *Bulbus Allii Fistulosi* (Cong Bai), *Sojae Semen Praeparatum* (Dan Dou Chi), *Glycyrrhizae Radix Et Rhizoma* (Gan Cao).

常用药：荆芥、防风、羌活、紫苏叶、桔梗、前胡、葱白、淡豆豉、甘草。

Modification: For heavy headache, add *Angelicae Radix Dahuricae* (Bai Zhi), *Puerariae Radix* (Ge Geng); for cough and copious phlegm, add *Sinapis semenAlbae* (Bai Jie Zi), and *Cynanchi*

加减：头痛甚者，加白芷、葛根；咳嗽痰多者，加白芥子、白前；恶心呕吐者，加藿香、半夏；发热渐重、舌红

Stauntonii Rhizoma et Radix (Bai Qian); for nausea and vomiting, add *Pogostmonis Herba* (Huo Xiang), and *Rhizoma Pinelliae* (Ban Xia); for worsening fever, red tongue and thin coating, add *Lonicerae Flos Japonicae* (Jin Yin Hua) and *Forsythiae Fructus* (Lian Qiao).

苔薄黄者,加金银花、连翘。

(2) Common cold in pattern of wind and heat

(2) 风热感冒

Manifestations: Heavy fever, slight aversion to wind, headache, body pain, turbid snivel, sneezing and coughing, thirsty, red pharynx or red and swollen throat, thin and yellow tongue coating, rapid and floating pulse, purple and floating fingerprints.

证候:发热重,微恶风,头身疼痛,鼻流浊涕,喷嚏咳嗽,口渴,咽红或喉核赤肿,舌苔薄黄,脉浮数,指纹浮紫。

Therapeutic method: To relieve the exterior with cool and acrid herbs.

治法:辛凉解表。

Main Formula: *Lonicera and Forsythia Powder* (Yin Qiao San) with modifications.

主方:银翘散加减。

Commonly used herbs: *Japonicae* (Jin Yin Hua), *Forsythiae Fructus* (Lian Qiao), Schizonepetae Herba (Jing Jie), *Lophatheri Herba* (Dan Zhu Ye), *Isatidis Folium* (Da Qing Ye), *Menthae Haploalycis Herba* (Bo He), *Platycodonis Radix* (Jie Geng), Arctii Fructus(Niu Bang Zi).

常用药:金银花、连翘、荆芥、淡竹叶、大青叶、薄荷、桔梗、牛蒡子。

Modification: For high fever, add *Gypsum Fibrosum* (Sheng Shi Gao), *Scutellariae Radix*(Huang Qin), *Gardeniae Fructus*(Zhi Zi). For cough with copious phlegm, add *Armeniacae Semen Amarum* (Ku Xing Ren), *Peucedani Radix*(Qian Hu), *Richosanthis Fructus* (Gua Lou); for red, swollen and painful pharynx, add *Scrophulariae Radix* (Xuan Shen), *Belamcandae Rhizoma* (She Gan); for nosebleed, add *Imperatae Rhizoma* (Bai Mao Gen) and *Agrimoniae Herba* (Xian He Cao).

加减:高热者,加生石膏、黄芩、栀子;咳嗽痰多者,加苦杏仁、前胡、瓜蒌;咽红肿痛者,加玄参、射干;鼻衄者,加白茅根、仙鹤草。

(3) Common cold in pattern of summer-heat

(3) 暑邪感冒

Manifestations: Fever without sweat, heavy

证候:发热无汗,头身困

sensation in the head and body, fullness and oppression in the chest and stomach, poor appetite, vomiting, diarrhea, nasal congestion, red tongue body, greasy tongue coating, rapid pulse.

重,胸脘满闷,食欲不振,或呕吐腹泻,或鼻塞流涕,舌质红,苔腻,脉数。

Therapeutic method: To dispel summer-heat and relieve the exterior.

治法:祛暑解表。

Formula: *Newly Supplemented Mosla Decoction* (Xin Jia Xiang Ru Yin) with modification.

主方:新加香薷饮加减。

Commonly used herbs: *Moslae Herba* (Xiang Ru), *Lonicerae Flos Japonicae* (Jin Yin Hua), *Magnoliae Officinalis Cortex* (Hou Pu), *Forsythiae Fructus* (Lian Qiao), *Lablab Flos* (Bian Dou Hua), *Pogostmonis Herba* (Huo Xiang), *Eupatorii Herba* (Pei Lan).

常用药:香薷、金银花、厚朴、连翘、扁豆花、藿香、佩兰。

Modification: For high fever, vexation and thirst, no sweat, exubrance of Yangming heat, add *White Tiger Decoction* (Bai Hu Tang); for heart vexation, easy crying, add *Lophatheri Herba* (Dan Zhu Ye), *Nelumbinis Plumula* (Lian Zi Xin); for oppression in the stomach and poor appetite, thick and greasy tongue coating, add *Atractylodes Rhizoma* (Cang Zhu) and *Coicis Semen* (Yi Yi Ren).

加减:高热、烦渴、无汗,阳明热甚者合白虎汤;心烦易哭者,加淡竹叶、莲子心;脘闷纳呆、舌苔厚腻湿重者,加苍术、薏苡仁。

(4) Influenza

(4) 时行感冒

Manifestations: Rapid and sudden onset, vigorous heat, aversion to cold, no sweat or no relief of heat after sweating, headache, vexation, red eye, red pharynx, aching pain of muscles, abdominal pain, or accompanied nausea, vomiting, red tongue body, yellow tongue coating, rapid pulse.

证候:起病急骤,壮热,恶寒,无汗或汗出热不解,头痛,心烦,目赤咽红,肌肉酸痛,腹痛,或有恶心、呕吐,舌质红,苔黄,脉数。

Therapeutic method: To clear away heat and dissolve toxin, and dissipate evil out of the exterior.

治法:清热解毒,透邪出表。

Main formula: *Lonicera and Forsythia Powder* (Yin Qiao San) and *Universal Salvation Toxin-Dispersing Decoction* (Pu Ji Xiao Du Yin) with modifications.

主方:银翘散合普济消毒饮加减。

Commonly used herbs: *Lonicerae Flos Japonicae* (Jin Yin Hua), *Forsythiae Fructus* (Lian Qiao), Schizonepetae Herba (Jing Jie), *Bupleuri Radix* (Chai Hu), Arctii Fructus (Niu Bang Zi), *Menthae Haploalycis Herba* (Bo He), *Platycodonis Radix* (Jie Geng), *Scutellariae Radix* (Huang Qin), *Isatidis Radix* (Ban Lan Gen), *Paridis Rhizoma* (Chou Lou), and *Cicadae Periostracum* (Chan Tui).

常用药：金银花、连翘、荆芥、柴胡、牛蒡子、薄荷、桔梗、黄芩、板蓝根、重楼、蝉蜕。

Modification: For high fever, add *Gypsum Fibrosum* (Sheng Shi Gao), *Gardeniae Fructus* (Zhi Zi); for nausea and vomiting, add *Bumbusae Caulis in Taenis* (Zhu Ru) and *Pinelliae Rhizoma* (Ban Xia).

加减：高热者，加生石膏、栀子；恶心呕吐者，加竹茹、半夏。

3.2 Concurrent patterns

(1) Complicated with phlegm: Sometimes, concurrently there is worsening coughing, heavy and turbid coughing sound, phlegm rale in the throat, thick and greasy tongue coating, slippery pulse. For common cold in pattern of wind and cold, it is appropriate to relieve the exterior with warmth and acridity, plus the method to diffuse the lung qi and dissolve phlegm, by adding *Apricot Kernel and Perilla Powder* (Xin Su San). For complicated phlegm in common cold in pattern of wind and heat, it is appropriate to relieve the exterior with cool and acrid herbs, plus the method to clarify the lung qi and dissolve phlegm, by adding *Mori Cortex* (Sang Bai Pi), *Peucedani Radix* (Qian Hu), and *Bambusae Concretio Silicea* (Tian Zhu Huang).

3.2 兼证

（1）夹痰：兼见咳嗽加重，咳声重浊，喉间痰鸣者，舌苔厚腻，脉滑。风寒感冒夹痰者，治宜辛温解表，佐以宣肺化痰，加用杏苏散；风热感冒夹痰者，治宜辛凉解表，佐以清肺化痰，加用桑白皮、前胡、天竺黄。

(2) Complicated with stagnation: Sometimes, concurrently there is poor appetite, abdominal distention, bad breath, sour and malodorous stool or abdominal pain and diarrhea, or constipated stool, turbid and white urine, thick and greasy tongue

（2）夹滞：兼见食少纳差，腹胀口臭，呕吐酸腐，大便酸臭，或腹痛泄泻，或大便秘结，小便白浊，舌苔厚腻。治宜解表为主，佐以消食导

coating. It is appropriate to relieve the exterior principally, plus the method to digest food and remove food retention, by accordingly adding *Crataegi Fructus* (Shan Zha), *Fermentata Massa Medicata* (Liu Shen Qu), *Hordei Fructus Germinatus* (Mai Ya), *Galli Endothelium Corneum Gigerii* (Ji Nei Jin), *Raphani Semen* (Lai Fu Zi), etc. For manifestations like constipated stool, scanty brown urine, abdominal distention, thirst, yellow and turbid tongue coating, due to obstruction of the intestines by food retention turning into heat, add accordingly *Rhei Radix et Rhizoma* (Da Huang), *Aurantii Fructus Immaturus* (Zhi Shi), and *Arecae Semen* (Bing Lang).

滞,酌加山楂、六神曲、麦芽、鸡内金、莱菔子等。若症见大便秘结,小便短赤,腹满口渴,舌苔黄垢,则为食滞化热,壅塞肠道,可酌加大黄、枳实、槟榔。

(3) Complicated with fright: Sometimes, concurrently there is fright, fear, crying and screaming, restless sleep or grinding of the teeth, even convulsion due to fright, red tongue body, yellow tongue coating, string-like pulse. It is appropriate to clear away heat and relieve the exterior, plus the method to relieve convulsion and tranquilize the mind, by accordingly adding *Cicadae Periostracum* (Chan Tui), *Uncariae ramulus Cum uncis* (Gou Teng), *Bombyx Batryticatus* (Jiang Chan), or *Children's Rejuvenation Elixir* (Xiao Er Hui Chun Dan).

(3) 夹惊:兼见惊惕哭叫,睡卧不宁或齘齿,甚至惊厥,舌质红,苔黄,脉弦。治宜清热解表,佐以镇惊安神,酌加蝉蜕、钩藤、僵蚕等,或加服小儿回春丹。

4 Other therapies

(1) *Wind-cold Common Cold Granules* (Feng Han Gan Mao Ke Li) can be applied to wind-cold common cold.

(2) *Wind-heat Common Cold Granules* (Feng Re Gan Mao Ke Li) can be applied to wind-heat common cold.

4 其他疗法

(1) 风寒感冒颗粒:适用于风寒感冒。

(2) 风热感冒颗粒:适用于风热感冒。

(3) *Agastache Qi-Righting Decoction* (Huo Xiang Zhen Qi Shui) can be applied to common cold in pattern of summer-heat and dampness.

(3) 藿香正气水：适用于暑湿感冒。

(4) *Lotus flower Scourge-Clearing Capsules* (Lian Hua Qing Wen Jiao Nang) can be applied to influenza.

(4) 连花清瘟胶囊：适用于时行感冒。

(5) *Child-Fortifying Clearing and Resolving Liquid* (Jian Er Qing Jie Ye) can be applied to wind-heat common cold complicated with stagnation.

(5) 健儿清解液：适用于风热感冒夹滞。

(6) *Compound Fresh Bamboo Sap Liquid* (Fu Fang Xian Zhu Li Ye) can be applied to common cold complicated with phlegm.

(6) 复方鲜竹沥液：适用于感冒夹痰。

(7) *Child Golden Elixir Tablets* (Xiao Er Jin Dan Pian) can be used for common cold complicated with fright.

(7) 小儿金丹片：适用于感冒夹惊。

Section 2 Acute Bronchitis

第 2 节 急性支气管炎

Acute bronchitis is the acute inflammation of the endotracheal mucosa. It often affects trachea as well, so it is also called "acute tracheobronchitis". Clinically the main manifestations are coughing and expectoration. This disease is often secondary to infection of the upper respiratory tract, mostly occurs during the dry climate in winter or early spring. It is frequently seen in children under three.

It belongs to the scope of "cough" in traditional Chinese medicine, divided into dry cough and productive cough.

急性支气管炎是支气管黏膜的急性炎症，常累及气管，故又称"急性气管-支气管炎"。临床以咳嗽、咯痰为主要症状。往往继发于上呼吸道感染之后，冬季与早春气候干燥时发病较多。多见于 3 岁以内的幼儿。

本病属中医学"咳嗽"范畴。有声无痰为咳，有痰无声为嗽，通称咳嗽。

1 Etiology and pathogenesis

The disease can be caused by infection of exogenous pathogens and internal damage. The exogenous pathogens include the external evils invading the lung. The internal damage refers to internal production of turbid phlegm, lung qi depletion or insufficiency of lung yin.

The main pathogenesis is that the lung is invaded by evils and fails in its diffusing and descending ability, leading to counterflow of the lung qi.

2 Key to diagnosis

(1) This disease often occurs after common cold. Clinically the main signs are coughing and expectoration.

(2) X-ray check of the chest shows normal or with the increased bronchovascular shadows.

3 Pattern identification and treatment

It is necessary to differentiate between exogenous infection or internal damage, heat or cold, deficiency or excess. Coughing due to exogenous infection often starts suddenly, with rough breathing and loud sound, thick and tenacious sputum, accompanied by exterior symptoms. The duration is short. It belongs to excessive. Coughing due to internal damage often starts gradually, with low and weak coughing sound, thin and white sputum, long duration, often complicated with interior symptoms in varying degrees, also with coexistence of deficient and excessive pattern, but deficient patterns in majority. Coughing, thin sputum, pale tongue, slimy white or thin white tongue coating are often ascribed to cold pattern. Coughing with yellow and thick sputum, red tongue, thin yellow or slimy

1 病因病机

病因分外感与内伤，外感为外邪犯肺，痰浊内生、肺气亏虚、肺阴不足等为常见内伤病因。

主要病机为肺脏受邪，失于宣降，肺气上逆。

2 诊断要点

（1）本病常见于感冒之后，临床以咳嗽、咯痰为主要表现。

（2）X 线胸片检查无异常或可见肺纹理增粗。

3 辨证论治

主要为辨外感内伤与辨寒热虚实。外感咳嗽大多起病急，咳嗽常气粗声高，痰液稠厚，伴有表证，病程较短，多属实证。内伤咳嗽发病多缓，咳声低弱，痰稀色白，病程较长，往往兼有不同程度的里证，亦可虚实互见，但虚证居多。咳嗽，痰稀，舌淡，苔白腻或薄白，多属寒证。咳嗽痰黄稠，舌红，苔薄黄或黄腻，多属热证。

yellow tongue coating are, often ascribed to heat pattern.

The basic therapeutic principle is to diffuse and depurate the lung qi. In accorcance with symptoms and signs, it is necessary to expel wind and relieve the exterior for the patients due to exogenous infection; for those with coughing of internal damage, it is to dry up dampness and dissolve phlegm, or to clear away heat and resolve dampness, or to nourish yin and moisten the lung.

以宣肃肺气为基本治则。外感咳嗽者，佐以疏风解表；内伤咳嗽者，佐以燥湿化痰，或清热化湿，或养阴润肺等法随证施治。

(1) Wind-cold cough

(1) 风寒咳嗽

Manifestations: frequent cough, thin and white sputum, itchy throat, heavy voice, runny nose with clear snivel, aversion to cold, absence of sweating, painful head and body, thin and white tongue coating, floating and tight pulse.

证候：咳嗽频作，咳痰稀白，咽痒声重，鼻流清涕，或恶寒无汗，头身疼痛，舌苔薄白，脉浮紧。

Therapies are to expel wind and disperse cold, diffuse and depurate the lung qi.

治法：疏风散寒，宣肃肺气。

Main formula: *Apricot Kernel and Perilla Powder* (Xing Su San) with modification.

主方：杏苏散加减。

Commonly used herbs: *Armeniacae Semen Amarum*(Ku Xing Ren), *Perillae Folium* (Zi Su Ye), *Peucedani Radix*(Qian Hu), *Pinelliae Rhizoma*(Ban Xia), *Platycodonis Radix*(Jie Geng), *Citri Reticulatae Pericarpium* (Chen Pi), *Poria* (Fu Ling), *Aurantii Fructus (Zhi Qiao)*, *Glycyrrhizae Radix Et Rhizoma* (Gan Cao), *Zingiberis Rhizoma Recens* (Sheng Jiang), *Jujubae Fructs* (Da Zao).

常用药：苦杏仁、紫苏叶、前胡、半夏、桔梗、陈皮、茯苓、枳壳、甘草、生姜、大枣。

Modification: For those with heavy external cold, add *Schizonepetae Herba* (Jing Jie), *Saposhnikoviae Radix* (Fang Feng), *Ephedrae Herba* (Ma Huang). For copious clear and thin sputum, add *Inulae Herba*(Jin Fei Cao), *Perillae Fructus* (Zi Su Zi). For sore and swollen throat, hoarse voice, red

加减：外寒重者，加荆芥、防风、麻黄；痰多清稀者，加金沸草、紫苏子；咽喉肿痛，声音嘶哑，舌质红，风寒化热者，加鱼腥草、黄芩、枇杷叶。

tongue, transformation of wind and cold into heat, add *Houttuyniae Herba* (Yu Xing Cao), *Scutellariae Radix* (*Huang Qin*), *Eriobotryae Folium* (Pi Pa Ye).

(2) Wind-heat cough

(2) 风热咳嗽

Manifestations: Ungratifying cough, scanty and yellow sputum difficult to cough up, runny nose with yellow snivel, or with fever and thirst, sore throat, red tongue, thin and yellow tongue coating, rapid and floating pulse, floating and violet fingerprint.

证候:咳嗽不爽,痰黄量少,不易咯出,鼻流黄涕,或有发热口渴,咽喉疼痛,舌质红,苔薄黄,脉浮数,指纹浮紫。

Therapies are to expel wind and clear away heat, diffuse and purify the lung qi.

治法:疏风清热,宣肃肺气。

Main formula: *Mulberry Leaf and Chrysanthemum Decoction* (Sang Ju Yin) with modification.

主方:桑菊饮加减。

Commonly used herbs: *Mori Folium* (Sang Ye), *Chrysanthemi Flos* (Ju Hua), *Armeniacae Semen Amarum* (Ku Xing Ren), *Forsythiae Fructus* (Lian Qiao), *Arctii Fructus* (Niu bang zi), *Menthae Haploalycis Herba* (Bo He), *Peucedani Radix* (Qian Hu), *Platycodonis Radix* (Jie Geng), *Glycyrrhizae Radix* (Gan Cao), *Phragmitis Rhizoma* (Lu Gen).

常用药:桑叶、菊花、苦杏仁、连翘、牛蒡子、薄荷、前胡、桔梗、甘草、芦根。

Modifications: For those with severe fever, add *Gypsum Fibrosum* (Sheng Shi Gao), *Houttuyniae Herba* (Yu Xing Cao), *Scutellariae Radix* (Huang Qin); for those with severe cough and copious sputum, add *Trichosanthis Pericarpium* (Gua Lou Pi), *Bambusae Concretio Silicea* (Tian Zhu Huang), *Descurainiae Lepidii Semen* (Ting Li Zi).

加减:发热甚者,加生石膏、鱼腥草、黄芩;咳甚痰多者,酌加瓜蒌皮、天竺黄、葶苈子。

(3) Phlegm-heat cough

(3) 痰热咳嗽

Manifestations: Cough with copious yellow and thick sputum, sticky and difficult to expectorate; or accompanied by fever, thirst, vexation, agitation, scanty brown urine, dry stool, red tongue, yellow

证候:咳嗽痰多,色黄黏稠难咯,或伴发热口渴,烦躁不安,小便黄少,大便干燥,舌质红,苔黄腻,脉滑数,指

and sticky tongue coating, rapid and slippery pulse, green-blue fingerprints.

纹青紫。

Therapies are to clear away heat and dissipate the lung fire, diffuse and depurate the lung qi.

治法:清热泻肺,宣肃肺气。

Main formula: *Metal-Clearing and Phlegm-Transforming Decoction* (Qing Jin Hua Tan Tang) with modification.

主方:清金化痰汤加减。

Commonly used herbs: *Scutellariae Radix* (Huang Qin), *Gardeniae Fructus* (Zhi Zi), *Mori Cortex* (Sang Bai Pi), *Trichosanthis Semen* (Gua Lou Zi), *Fritillariae Thunbergii Bulbus* (Zhe Bei Mu), *Ophiopogonis Radix* (Mai Dong), *Citri Exocarpium Rubrum* (Ju Hong), *Poria* (Fu Ling), *Platycodonis Radix* (Jie Geng), *Glycyrrhizae Radix Et Rhizoma* (Gan Cao).

常用药:黄芩、栀子、桑白皮、瓜蒌子、浙贝母、麦冬、橘红、茯苓、桔梗、甘草。

Modification: For high fever, add *Gypsum Fibrosum* (Sheng Shi Gao), *Anemarrhenae Rhizoma* (Zhi Mu); for copious expectoration, add *Houttuyniae Herba* (Yu Xing Cao), *Descurainiae Lepidii Semen* (Ting Li Zi), and fresh *Succus Bambusae* (Zhu Li) judiciously; for severe thirst, add *Phragmitis Rhizoma* (Lu Gen), *Trichosanthis Radix (Tian Hua Fen)*; for dry stool, add *Richosanthis Fructus* (Gua Lou), *Rhei Radix Et Rhizoma* (Da Huang).

加减:高热者,加生石膏、知母;咳痰多者,酌加鱼腥草、葶苈子、鲜竹沥;口渴甚者,加芦根、天花粉;大便干结者,加瓜蒌、大黄。

(4) Phlegm-damp cough

(4) 痰湿咳嗽

Manifestations: Cough with copious sputum in white, clear and thin nature, oppression in the chest and poor appetite, fatigue and lack of strength, slight red tongue, white and glossy tongue coating, slippery pulse.

证候:咳嗽痰多,色白清稀,胸闷纳呆,困倦乏力,舌质淡红,苔白滑,脉滑。

Therapies are to dry up dampness and dissolve phlegm, diffuse and depurate the lung qi.

治法:燥湿化痰,宣肃肺气。

Main Formula: *Supplemented Two Matured*

主方:二陈汤加减。

Ingredients Decoction (Er Cheng Tang) with modifications.

Commonly used herbs: *Poria* (Fu Ling), *Citri Reticulatae Pericarpium* (Chen Pi), *Pinelliae Rhizoma* (Ban Xia), *Raphani Semen*(Lai Fu Zi), *Armeniacae Semen Amarum* (Ku Xing Ren), *Perillae Fructus* (Zi Su Zi), *Sinapis semen Albae* (Bai Jie Zi), *Glycyrrhizae Radix Et Rhizoma*(Gan Cao).

常用药:茯苓、陈皮、半夏、莱菔子、苦杏仁、紫苏子、白芥子、甘草。

Modification: For oppression in the chest and cough with ungratifying expectoration, add *Aurantii Fructus (Zhi Qiao)*, *Platycodonis Radix* (Jie Geng). For severe cold-damp, white, clear and thin sputum, white and glossy tongue coating, add *Zingiberis Rhizoma* (Gan Jiang), *Asari Radix Et Rhizoma* (Xi Xin); for poor appetite, add *Atractylodis Macrocephalae Rhizoma* (Bai Zhu), *Fermentata Massa Medicata* (Liu Shen Qu).

加减:胸闷不适,咳痰不爽者,加枳壳、桔梗;寒湿较重,痰白清稀,舌苔白滑者,加干姜、细辛;食少纳呆者,加白术、六神曲。

(5) Yin-deficiency cough

(5) 阴虚咳嗽

Manifestations: Enduring cough, dry cough with scanty sputum or sticky and difficult expectoration, dry mouth and throat, hoarse voice, feverish sensation in the chest, palms and soles, tidal feverish sensation and night sweating, red lips and tongue, scanty or peeled tongue coating, thread and rapid pulse, pale green-blue fingerprint.

证候:久咳不愈,干咳少痰或痰黏难咯,口咽干燥,声音嘶哑,手足心热或潮热盗汗,唇红,舌质红,苔少或花剥,脉细数,指纹淡紫。

Therapies are to nourish yin and moisten the lung, dissolve phlegm and suppress cough.

治法:养阴润肺,化痰止咳。

Main Formula: *Glehnia and Ophiopogon Decoction* (Sha Seng Mai Dong Tang) with modification.

主方:沙参麦冬汤加减。

Commonly used herbs: *Adenophorae Radix* (Sha Seng), *Ophiopogonis Radix* (Mai Dong), *Polygonati Rhizoma* (Huang Jing), *Polygonati Odorati Rhizoma* (Yu Zhu), *Mori Folium* (Sang Ye), *Lablab Semen Album* (Bai Bian Dou), *Trichosanthis*

常用药:沙参、麦冬、黄精、玉竹、桑叶、白扁豆、天花粉、紫菀、款冬花。

Radix (Tian Hua Fen), *Asteris Radix Et Rhizoma* (Zi Wan), *Farfarae Flos*(Kuan Dong Hua).

Modification: For unabated low-grade heat, add *Artemisiae Annuae Herba* (Qing Hao), *Lycii Cortex* (Di Gu Pi), *Picrorhizae Rhizoma* (Hu Huang Lian); for enduring cough and sticky sputum, use *Ophiopogonis Radix* (Mai Dong) in large dose; for those with insufficient stomach yin, poor appetite, add *Crataegi Fructus* (Shan Zha), *Setariae Fructus Germinatus* (Gu Ya), *Dendrobii Herba* (Shi Hu); for cough with blood-flecked sputum, add *Imperatae Rhizoma* (Bai Mao Gen), *Rehmanniae Radix Cruda* (Sheng Di Huang).

加减:低热不退者,加青蒿、地骨皮、胡黄连;久咳痰黏者,重用麦冬;兼胃阴不足,食少纳差者,加山楂、谷芽、石斛;咳痰带血丝者,加白茅根、生地黄。

4 Other therapies

4 其他疗法

4.1 Chinese Patent Medicine

4.1 中成药

(1) *Soluble Granules of Apricot Kernel and Perilla for Suppressing Cough* (Xing Su Zhi Ke Chong Ji) is used for wind-cold cough.

(1) 杏苏止咳冲剂:用于治疗风寒咳嗽。

(2) *Syrup for Acute Bronchitis* (Ji Zhi Tang Jiang) can be used for wind-heat cough.

(2) 急支糖浆:用于治疗风热咳嗽。

(3) *Gold-Vitalizing Oral Liquid* (Jin Zhen Kou Fu Ye) can be used for phlegm-heat cough.

(3) 金振口服液:用于治疗痰热咳嗽。

(4) *Liquid of Red Tangerine Peel for Phlegm-cough* (Ju Hong Tan Ke Ye) can be applied to phlegm-damp cough.

(4) 橘红痰咳液:用于治疗痰湿咳嗽。

(5) *Yin-Nourishing and Lung-Clarifying Syrup* (Yang Yin Qing Fei Tang Jiang) can be applied to yin-deficiency cough.

(5) 养阴清肺糖浆:用于治疗阴虚咳嗽。

4.2 External therapy

4.2 外治疗法

Usually, after *Sinapis semen Albae* (Bai Jie Zi), *Corydalis Rhizoma* (Yan Hu Suo), *Kansui Radix* (Gan Sui) and *Asari Radix Et Rhizoma* (Xi Xin) are ground into fine powder, add fresh ginger

常用白芥子、延胡索、甘遂、细辛,共研细末,加生姜汁调膏,分别贴在肺俞、心俞、膈俞、膻中穴。

juice and make into paste, then apply respectively on Feishu (BL 13), Xinshu (BL 15), Geshu (BL 17) and Danzhong (CV 17).

Section 3 Pneumonia

第3节 肺炎

Pneumonia is infection of the lung caused by various pathogens or other factors. Clinically the main manifestations are fever, cough, hasty breathing, difficult breathing, and pulmonary rales. It occurs mainly in the cold seasons of winter and spring and is frequently seen in children under 3 years old.

肺炎是由不同病原体或其他因素引起的肺部感染。以发热、咳嗽、气促、呼吸困难及肺部湿啰音为主要临床表现。冬春寒冷季节较多。多见于3岁以下婴幼儿。

In Chinese medicine, it is termed as "Pneumonia and panting and cough".

中医称之为"肺炎喘嗽"。

1 Etiology and pathogenesis

1 病因病机

The external factor is related to invasion of exogenous wind. The internal factor is related to delicacy of the lung in the infants.

外因责之于感受风邪，内因责之于肺脏娇嫩。

After entering through the skin and hair or mouth and nose, the wind evil blocks the lung, leading to failure of the lung in its power of governing diffusing and depurating abilities. Then there is fever, aversion to cold, and cough, etc. Wind is the chief of hundred disasters, and it is often accompanied by other evils, so there are different manifestations, like blockage of the lung by wind and cold, and blockage of the lung by wind and heat.

风邪由皮毛或口鼻而入，邪气闭肺，肺失宣发肃降之令，故可见发热、恶寒、咳嗽等证候；风为百病之长，常夹杂其他邪气致病，故有风寒闭肺与风热闭肺的不同证候。

If the evils linger in Wei-defensive qi of the lung, turn heat into the interior, condense liquid into phlegm, and mix phlegm and heat, obstructing the lung collaterals and blocking the lung qi, there will be typical clinical manifestations of this disease, such as fever, cough, hasty breathing, flaring

若邪在肺卫不解，化热入里，炼液成痰，痰热互结，闭阻肺络，肺气郁闭，则出现本病典型临床表现如发热、咳嗽、气促、鼻煽、痰鸣等。若毒热之邪郁闭于肺，肺热

nostrils, and gurgling sound with sputum, etc. If toxic heat is accumulated and blocked in the lung, the lung heat is exuberant, and humor and fluid are scorched, then there will be high fever, severe cough, vexation and agitation, and hasty panting. The lung and large intestine stand in an interior-exterior relationship. When the lung fails in its depurating and descending abilities and the large intestine qi is unable to go downward, then manifestations of bowel excess like abdominal distention and constipation will appear. If evil heat is exuberant and penetrates into Jueyin system internally, stirring up the liver wind, there would be deteriorated symptoms, like high fever, coma and convulsion. Qi is the commander of the blood. If the lung qi is obstructed and blocked, the heart will be affected, leading to inhibited blood flow and obstruction of the meridians and hence arise the symptoms of qi stagnation and blood stasis, such as cyanosis in the lips and nails, purple patches on the tongue, etc. There may even be failure of nourishment in the heart, insufficiency of heart qi, and deficiency and depletion of the heart yang, with the critical phenomena of pale face and cold limbs, quick and hasty breathing, vexation and agitation, enlarged lumps under the right ribs, and feeble and expiring pulse. For those in severely critical condition, there can be internal blockage and external prostration.

壅盛，灼津耗液，可见高热、咳剧、烦躁、喘促等。肺与大肠相表里，肺失肃降，大肠之气不得下行，则出现腹胀、便秘等腑实证候。若邪热炽盛，内陷厥阴，引动肝风，则出现高热、神昏、抽搐等邪陷厥阴之变证；气为血之帅，若肺气郁闭，影响及心，致血行不畅，脉道涩滞，则出现唇甲紫绀、舌有瘀斑等气滞血瘀证候，甚或心失所养，心气不足，心阳虚衰，而出现面白肢冷，呼吸急促，心烦不安，右胁下痞块增大，脉微欲绝等重危之象。病情严重者，可出现内闭外脱。

In the later stage of the disease, due to gradual withdrawal of pathogens and consumptive damamage of the vital energy, deficiency in the vital energy and lingering of pathogens would appear. If the residual pathogens linger, due to damage of the lung by pathogenic heat and comsumptive damage of the

本病后期，可因邪气渐退，正气耗伤，而出现正虚邪恋之象。因于邪热伤肺，肺阴耗伤，余邪留恋者，则见阴虚肺热之证候；因于素体虚弱，或久咳伤肺，肺病及脾

lung yin, there could be the clinical manifestations of heat in the lung due to yin deficiency. If the pulmonary problem involves the spleen, due to original deficiency and weakness of the body constitution, or damage of the lung by lingering cough, there would be the clinical manifestations of qi deficiency in the lung and spleen.

者,则见肺脾气虚之证候。

Generally, the pathological location of pneumonia lies mainly in the lung, but the spleen is often involved, and the heart and liver, too. Phlegm and heat are the pathological products and also the important pathogenic factors. The pathomechanism lies in the transmutation of the obstruction and blockage of the lung qi.

总之,肺炎喘嗽的病变部位主要在肺,常累及脾,亦可内窜心肝。痰热既是病理产物,也是重要的致病因素,其病理机制主要是肺气郁闭之演变。

2 Key to diagnosis

2 诊断要点

(1) Relatively sudden onset, with symptoms like fever, cough, short breath, flaring nostrils, phlegm rale, or cyanosis.

(1) 起病较急,有发热、咳嗽、气急、鼻煽、痰鸣等症,或有发绀。

(2) In severe illness, often there is hasty and fidgety panting, vexation and agitation, pale face, cyanosis in the mouth and lips, or unabated high fever.

(2) 病情严重时,常见喘促不安,烦躁不宁,面色苍白,口唇青紫发绀,或高热不退。

(3) The newborns with pneumonia are manifested by failure to take milk, listless spirit, or foaming at the mouth, without the above-mentioned typical symptoms.

(3) 新生儿患肺炎常以不乳、精神萎靡、口吐白沫等症状为主,而无上述典型表现。

(4) In auscultation of the lung, fixed and medium and fine rale can be heard.

(4) 肺部听诊可闻及固定的中细湿啰音。

(5) By X-ray, small-pieced or patchy shadows or uneven big shadows can be seen.

(5) X线检查可见小片状、斑片状阴影,或见不均匀的大片阴影。

(6) Lab examination: ① Routine blood test: In bacteria induced pneumonia, total count of white

(6) 实验室检查:①血常规检查,细菌引起的肺炎,白

cells is relatively high, and neutrophil increases. In virus induced pneumonia, total count of white cells is normal or decreases. ② Etiological test: By bacteria cultivation and virus separation, the relevant etiological diagnosis can be obtained. The inspections of etiological specific antigens or antibody are often helpful to the early diagnosis.

细胞总数较高，中性粒细胞增多；若由病毒引起，白细胞总数正常或降低。②病原学检查，细菌培养、病毒分离等，可获得相应的病原学诊断，病原特异性抗原或抗体检测常有助于早期诊断。

3 Pattern identification and treatment

Pattern identification is mainly done to differentiate if it is in pattern of wind and cold, or wind and heat, or phlegm and heat or heat, in pattern of qi deficiency or yin deficiency, in regular pattern or transmuted pattern. The early stage of pneumonia can be judged by rapid breathing and hasty panting. In pattern of blockage of the lung by wind and cold, there could be the manifestations of exogenous infection of wind and cold. In pattern of blockage of the lung by wind and heat, there could be the manifestations of exogenous infection of wind and heat. If cold and heat are difficult to be differentiated, it is advisable to refer to sore throat for making identification. In blockage of the lung by phlegm and heat, phlegm, heat, cough and panting are all severe. In blockage of the lung by toxic heat, phlegm sign is not obvious, and instead there are exuberant heat toxin, vigorous heat, severe cough, stifling panting, vexation and other manifestations of yin damage. In transmuted pattern, there can be vigorous heat, clouded spirit, convulsion in the limbs, rigidity of the neck and nape, termed as pattern of pathogens penetrating into Jueyin system, or pale face, cyanosis in the lips and nails, shallow and rapid breath, sweating forehead without warmth, weak

3 辨证论治

辨证主要为辨风寒与风热，辨痰证与热证，辨气虚与阴虚，辨常证与变证。肺炎早期以气急喘促为依据，风寒闭肺见外感风寒证候，风热闭肺有外感风热之候，若寒热难辨可借鉴是否有咽红等症以佐证；痰热闭肺者，痰、热、咳、喘均剧；毒热闭肺虽痰象不著，但热毒炽盛，壮热、咳剧、喘憋、烦躁及可见伤阴诸象。变证可见壮热，神昏，四肢抽搐，颈项强直等邪陷厥阴证或面色苍白，口唇爪甲紫绀，呼吸浅促，额汗不温，脉微弱疾数等心阳虚衰证。

and rapid pulse, termed as pattern of heart yang deficiency and debilitation.

The basic therapeutic principle is to diffuse lung qi and remove the blockage, dissolve phlegm and stop panting. For those with copious accumulation of phlegm, it is advisable to descend qi and flush phlegm; for severe stifling panting, it is advisable to stop panting and disinhibit qi; for qi stagnation and blood stasis, it is advisable to quicken blood flow and dissolve blood stasis; for vigorous and exuberant heat and constipation, it is advisable to relax the bowels and reduce heat; for those with transmuted patterns, depending upon various manifestations, it is advisable to warm up and supplement heart yang, or open the apertures and extinguish wind. For qi deficiency in the lung and spleen due to enduring illness, it is appropriate to support the body constitution dominantly by fortifying the spleen and supplementing the lung. For dryness in the lung due to yin deficiency and lingering evils, it is advisable to nourish yin, moisten the lung and dissolve phlegm, clear away and resolve residual evils as well.

以宣肺开闭、化痰平喘为基本治则。若痰多壅盛者，宜降气涤痰；喘憋严重者，治以平喘利气；气滞血瘀者，佐以活血化瘀；壮热炽盛、大便秘结者佐以通腑泻热。出现变证者，或温补心阳，或开窍息风，随证施治。病久肺脾气虚者，宜健脾补肺以扶正为主；阴虚肺燥，余邪留恋，宜养阴润肺化痰，兼清解余邪。

3.1 Regular Patterns

(1) Wind and cold blocking the lung

Manifestations: Aversion to cold, fever, no thirsty, no sweat, cough, hasty breathing, white and thin sputum, light red tongue, thin white tongue coating, tight and floating pulse.

Therapeutic method: To open the lung by spicy and warm herbs, dissolve phlegm and downbear counter flow of qi.

Main Formulas: *Three Disobedience Decoction* (San Ao Tang) plus *Scallion and Fermented Soybean*

3.1 常证

(1) 风寒闭肺

证候：恶寒发热，无汗不渴，咳嗽气促，痰稀色白，舌质淡红，苔薄白，脉浮紧。

治法：辛温开肺，化痰降逆。

主方：三拗汤合葱豉汤加减。

Decoction (Cong Chi Tang) with modifications.

Commonly used herbs: *Ephedrae Herba* (Ma Huang), *Armeniacae Semen Amarum* (Ku Xing Ren), *Glycyrrhizae Radix Et Rhizoma* (Gan Cao), *Schizonepetae Herba* (Jing Jie), *Peucedani Radix* (Qian Hu), *Perillae Folium* (Zi Su Ye), *Platycodonis Radix* (Jie Geng), *Ledebouriellae Radix* (Fang Feng).

常用药:麻黄、苦杏仁、甘草、荆芥、淡豆豉、前胡、紫苏叶、桔梗、防风。

Modification: For copious white and sticky sputum, slimy and white tongue coating, add *Citri Reticulatae Pericarpium* (Chen Pi), *Pinelliae Rhizoma* (Ban Xia), and *Raphani Semen* (Lai Fu Zi).

加减:痰多白黏,苔白腻者,加陈皮、半夏、莱菔子。

(2) Wind and heat blocking the lung

(2) 风热闭肺

Manifestations: Severe fever, slight aversion to cold, cough, yellow thick sputum, rapid and hasty breathing, red throat, red tongue, thin white or thin yellow tongue fur, rapid and floating pulse, green-blue or purple fingerprints.

证候:发热重,恶寒轻,咳嗽,痰稠色黄,呼吸急促,咽红,舌质红,苔薄白或薄黄,脉浮数,指纹青紫。

Therapies are to open the lung by acridity and coolness, descend the counterflow and dissolve phlegm.

治法:辛凉开肺,降逆化痰。

Main formula: *Lonicera and Forsythia Powder* (Yin Qiao San), *Ephedra, Apricot Kernel, Gypsum*, and *Licorice Decoction* (Ma Xing Shi Gan Tang) with modifications.

主方:银翘散合麻杏石甘汤加减。

Commonly used herbs: *Ephedrae Herba* (Ma Huang), *Armeniacae Semen Amarum* (Ku Xing Ren), *Gypsum Fibrosum* (Sheng Shi Gao), *Glycyrrhizae Radix Et Rhizoma* (Gan Cao), *Lonicerae Flos Japonicae* (Jin Yin Hua), *Forsythiae Fructus* (Lian Qiao), *Menthae Haploalycis Herba* (Bo He), *Platycodonis Radix* (Jie Geng), Arctii Fructus (Niu Bang Zi).

常用药:麻黄、苦杏仁、生石膏、甘草、金银花、连翘、薄荷、桔梗、牛蒡子。

Modification: For vigorous heat, thirst and

加减:壮热烦渴者,倍用

vexation, use *Gypsum Fibrosum* (Sheng Shi Gao) in multiple amount, add *Anemarrhenae Rhizoma* (Zhi Mu); for panting and phlegm rale, add *Descurainiae Lepidii Semen* (Ting Li Zi), *Bulbus Fritillariae Thumbergii* (Zhe Bei Mu); for sore throat, add *Belamecandae Rhizoma* (She Gan), *Cicadae Periostracum* (Chan Tui); for thirst, add *Trichosanthis Radix* (Tian Hua Fen) and *Phragmitis Rhizoma* (Lu Gen).

生石膏,加知母;喘息痰鸣者,加葶苈子、浙贝母;咽喉红肿疼痛者,加射干、蝉蜕;口渴者,加天花粉、芦根。

(3) Phlegm and heat obstructing the lung

(3) 痰热闭肺

Manifestations: Vigorous heat, vexation and agitation, phlegm rale in the throat, thick yellow sputum, hasty breathing, stifling panting, flaring nostrils, or cyanosis in the mouth and lips, red tongue, slimy and yellow tongue coating, rapid and slippery pulse.

证候:壮热烦躁,喉间痰鸣,痰稠色黄,气促喘憋,鼻翼煽动,或口唇青紫,舌质红,苔黄腻,脉滑数。

Therapies are to clear away heat and flush phlegm, diffuse the lung qi and downbear the counterflow.

治法:清热涤痰,宣肺降逆。

Main formula: *Five Tigers Decoction* (Wu Hu Tang) and *Descurainiae and Jujube Lung-Draining Decoction* (Ting Li Da Zao Xie Fei Tang) with modification.

主方:五虎汤合葶苈大枣泻肺汤加减。

Commonly used herbs: *Ephedrae Herba* (Ma Huang), *Armeniacae Semen Amarum* (Ku Xing Ren), *Gypsum Fibrosum* (Sheng Shi Gao), *Glycyrrhizae Radix Et Rhizoma* (Gan Cao), *Catechu* (Er Cha), *Mori Cortex* (Sang Bai Pi), *Descurainiae Lepidii Semen* (Ting Li Zi), *Perillae Fructus* (Zi Su Zi), *Peucedani Radix* (Qian Hu), *Scutellariae Radix* (Huang Qin), *Polygoni Cuspidati Rhizoma Et Radix* (Hu Zhang).

常用药:麻黄、苦杏仁、生石膏、甘草、儿茶、桑白皮、葶苈子、紫苏子、前胡、黄芩、虎杖。

Modification: For severe heat and dry stool, add *Rhei Radix Et Rhizoma* (Da Huang), *Natrii*

加减:热甚便干者,加大黄、玄明粉;痰多者,加天竺

Sulfas Exsiccatus (Xuan Ming Fen); for copious phlegm, add *Bambusae Concretio Silicea* (Tian Zhu Huang), *Arisaema Cum Bile* (Dan Nan Xing); for purple lips, add *Salviae Miltiorrhizae Radix Et Rhizoma* (Dan Shen), and *Paeoniae Radix Rubra* (Chi Shao).

黄、胆南星;唇紫者,加丹参、赤芍。

(4) Toxic heat blocking the lung

(4) 毒热闭肺

Manifestations: Enduring high fever, severe cough, rapid breathing and flaring nostrils, stifling panting, no tears and snivels, red face and lips, vexation and thirst, brown urine and constipation, red and dry tongue, coarse and yellow tongue coating, slippery and rapid pulse.

证候:高热持续,咳嗽剧烈,气急鼻煽,甚至喘憋,涕泪俱无,面赤唇红,烦躁口渴,溲赤便秘,舌质红而干,苔黄而糙,脉滑数。

Therapies are to clear away heat and resolve toxin, reduce the lung fire and open the blockage.

治法:清热解毒,泻肺开闭。

Main Formula: *Coptis Toxin-Resolving Decoction* (Huang Lian Jie Du Tang) and *Three Disobedience Decoction* (San Ao Tang) with modification.

主方:黄连解毒汤合三拗汤加减。

Commonly used herbs: *Honeyed Ephedrae Herba* (Mi Ma Huang), *Armeniacae Semen Amarum* (Ku Xing Ren), *Aurantii Fructus (Zhi Qiao)*, *Coptidis Rhizoma* (Huang Lian), *Scutellariae Radix* (Huang Qin), *Gardeniae Fructus* (Zhi Zi), *Gypsum Fibrosum* (Sheng Shi Gao), *Anemarrhenae Rhizoma* (Zhi Mu).

常用药:蜜麻黄、苦杏仁、枳壳、黄连、黄芩、栀子、生石膏、知母。

Modification: For severe heat toxin, add *Polygoni Cuspidati Rhizoma Et Radix* (Hu Zhang), *Taraxaci Herba* (Pu Gong Ying), and *Paridis Rhizoma* (Chong Lou); for abdominal distention, add *Rhei Radix Et Rhizoma* (Da Huang), *Natrii Sulfas Exsiccatus* (Xuan Ming Fen); for dry mouth and nose, add *Phragmitis Rhizoma* (Lu Gen), *Scrophulariae Radix* (Xuan Shen), *Ophiopogonis Radix* (Mai Dong); for severe cough, add *Bulbus Fritillariae*

加减:热毒重者,加虎杖、蒲公英、重楼;便秘腹胀者,加大黄、玄明粉;口干鼻燥者,加芦根、玄参、麦冬;咳重者,加浙贝母、款冬花;烦躁不宁者,加淡竹叶、钩藤。

Thumbergii (Zhe Bei Mu), *Farfarae Flos* (Kuan Dong Hua); for vexation and agitation, add *Lophatheri Herba* (Dan Zhu Ye), *Uncariae ramulus Cum uncis* (Gou Teng).

(5) Lung heat due to yin deficiency

(5) 阴虚肺热

Manifestations: Relatively long course of illness, low-grade fever, night sweating, cough with scanty or no sputum, dry mouth and thirst, tidal flushed cheeks, red tongue, scanty or patchy tongue coating, thready and rapid pulse, purple fingerprints.

证候:病程较长,低热盗汗,咳嗽少痰或无痰,口干口渴,面色潮红,舌质红,苔少或花剥,脉细数,指纹紫。

Therapies are to nourish yin and clear away heat, moisten the lung and dissolve phlegm.

治法:养阴清热,润肺化痰。

Main Formula: *Glehnia and Ophiopogon Decoction* (Sha Shen Mai Dong Tang).

主方:沙参麦冬汤。

Commonly used herbs: *Adenophorae Radix* (Sha Seng), *Ophiopogonis Radix* (Mai Dong), *Polygonati Odorati Rhizoma* (Yu Zhu), *Trichosanthis Radix* (Tian Hua Fen), *Mori Cortex* (Sang Bai Pi), *Farfarae Flos* (Kuan Dong Hua), *Lablab Semen Album* (Bai Bian Dou), *Glycyrrhizae Radix Et Rhizoma* (Gan Cao).

常用药:沙参、麦冬、玉竹、天花粉、桑白皮、款冬花、白扁豆、甘草。

Modification: For unbated low fever, add *Artemisiae Annuae Herba* (Qing Hao), *Lycii Cortex* (Di Gu Pi); for enduring cough and sticky sputum, add *Phragmitis Rhizoma* (Lu Gen), *Stemonae Radix* (Bai Bu); for reduced and poor food intake, add *Crataegi Fructus* (Shan Zha), *Setariae Fructus Germinatus* (Gu Ya), *Dendrobii Herba* (Shi Hu).

加减:低热不退者,加青蒿、地骨皮;久咳痰黏者,加芦根、百部;食少纳差者,加山楂、谷芽、石斛。

(6) Qi deficiency in the lung and spleen

(6) 肺脾气虚

Manifestations: Fluctuating low fever, lusterless complexion, cough, lack of strength, copious sputum, low spirit and fatigue, sweating by exertion, poor appetite, sloppy stool, pale tongue, thin

证候:低热起伏不定,面色少华,咳嗽无力,痰多,神疲倦怠,动则汗出,纳差便溏,舌质淡,苔薄白或腻,脉

white or sticky tongue coating, thready and feeble pulse, slight red fingerprints.

细弱无力，指纹淡红。

Therapies are to fortify the spleen and boost qi, dissolve phlegm and suppress cough.

治法：健脾益气，化痰止咳。

Main formula: *Ginseng and Schisandra Decoction* (Ren Shen Wu Wei Zi Tang) with modification.

主方：人参五味子汤加减。

Commonly used herbs: *Codonopsis Radix* (Dang Shen), *Atractylodis Macrocephalae Rhizoma* (Bai Zhu), *Poria* (Fu Ling), *Schisandrae Fructus Chinensis* (Wu Wei Zi), *Ophiopogonis Radix* (Mai Dong), *Citri Reticulatae Pericarpium* (Chen Pi), *Pinelliae Rhizoma* (Ban Xia), *Asteris Radix Et Rhizoma* (Zi Wan), *Glycyrrhizae Radix Et Rhizoma* (Gan Cao).

常用药：党参、白术、茯苓、五味子、麦冬、陈皮、半夏、紫菀、甘草。

Modification: For cough with copious sputum, add *Raphani Semen* (Lai Fu Zi), *Trichosanthis Pericarpium* (Gua Lou Pi); for sloppy stool, add *Dioscoreae Rhizoma* (Shan Yao), *Atractylodis Rhizoma* (Cang Zhu); for poor appetite, abdominal distention, add *Crataegi Fructus* (Shan Zha), *Fermentata Massa Medicata* (Liu Shen Qu), *Aucklandiae Radix* (Mu Xiang); for copious sweating and easy affection, add *Astragali Radix* (Huang Qi), *Ledebouriellae Radix* (Fang Feng), *Tritici Levis Fructus* (Fu Xiao Mai).

加减：咳嗽痰多者，加莱菔子、瓜蒌皮；大便稀溏者，加山药、苍术；食欲不振，腹部胀满者，加山楂、六神曲、木香；汗多易感者，加黄芪、防风、浮小麦。

3.2 Transmuted patterns

3.2 变证

(1) Heart yang deficiency and debilitation

(1) 心阳虚衰

Manifestations: Sudden rapid and hasty breathing, palpitation and flusteredness, vexations and agitations, pale face, cyanosis in the mouth and lips, extreme cold sensation in the limbs, palpable lump in the rib-side, dark and purple tongue, white tongue coating, feeble and slight rapid pulse.

证候：突然呼吸急促，心悸心慌，烦躁不安，面色苍白，口唇发绀，四肢厥冷，胁下痞块，舌质紫暗，苔白，脉微急促。

Therapies are to boost qi and warm up yang, stem counterflow and desertion.

治法：益气温阳，救逆固脱。

Main formula: *Ginseng, Aconite, Dragon Bone, and Oyster Shell Counterflow-Steming Decoction* (Shen Fu Long Mu Jiu Ni Tang) with modification.

主方：参附龙牡救逆汤加减。

Commonly used herbs: *Ginseng Radix* (Ren Shen), *Aconiti Lateralis Radix Praeparata* (Fu Zi), *Os Draconis* (Long Gu), *Ostreae Concha* (Mu Li), *Paeoniae Radix Albae* (Bai Shao), *Glycyrrhizae Radix Et Rhizoma* (Gan Cao)

常用药：人参、附子、龙骨、牡蛎、白芍、甘草。

Modification: For rapid breathing and pulse, cyanosis in the mouth and lips, lack of warmth in the limbs, add judiciously *Ginseng Radix Et Rhizoma Rubra* (Hong Shen); for fatigued spirit and lack of strength, red lips and tongue, scanty tongue coating, add *Pulse-Engendering Powder* (Shen Fu San); for palpable lump in the rib-side, cyanosis in the mouth and lips, add *Salviae Miltiorrhizae Radix Et Rhizoma* (Dan Shen), *Chuanxiong Rhizoma* (Chuan Xiong), *Carthami Flos* (Hong Hua).

加减：若呼吸、脉率偏快，口唇发绀，四肢不温者，佐加红参；神疲乏力，唇红舌红，少苔者，加生脉散；胁下痞块，口唇发绀者，加丹参、川芎、红花。

For those with qi and yang deficiency and debilitation, take *Pure Ginseng Decoction* (Du Shen Tang) or *Ginseng and Aconite Decoction* (Shen Fu Tang) frequently in small dose to meet emergency needs; use *Ginseng and Aconite Injection Fluid* (Shen Fu Zhu She Ye) by intravenous infusion. If both qi and yin are exhausted, use *Pulse-engendering Injection* (Sheng Mai Zhu She Ye) by intravenous infusion. If this pattern occurs, it indicates that the condition is critical and severe, and it is necessary to give emergent treatment by integrated therapy of traditional and western medicine. For emergent treatment, please refer to the related sections of

气阳虚衰者亦可用独参汤或参附汤少量频服以急救，还可用参附注射液静脉滴注。若气阴两竭，可加用生脉注射液静脉滴注。出现本证，病情危重，应予中西医结合抢救治疗，参照"急性心功能不全"节应急处理。

"Acute Cardiac Insufficiency".

(2) Evils penetrating into Jueyin system

Manifestations: Lingering high fever, convulsion of the limbs, clouded spirit and delirious speech, rigidity of the neck and nape, upward staring eyes, red tongue, yellow tongue coating, and rapid pulse.

Therapies are to tranqulize the liver and extinguish wind, clarify the heart and open orifices.

Main formula: *Antelope Horn and Uncaria Decoction* (Ling Jiao Gou Teng Tang) plus *Bovine Bezoar Heart-Clearing Pill* (Niu Huang Qing Xin Wan) with modification.

Commonly used herbs: *Antelopis Tataricae Cornu* (Ling Yang Jiao), *Uncariae ramulus Cum uncis* (Gou Teng), *Poria Cum Ligno Hospite* (Fu Shen), *Rehmanniae Radix Cruda* (Sheng Di Huang), *Gardeniae Fructus* (Zhi Zi), *Scutellariae Radix* (Huang Qin), *Chrysanthemi Flos* (Ju Hua), *Bulbus Fritillariae Thumbergii* (Zhe Bei Mu), *Paeoniae Radix Albae* (Bai Shao), *Glycyrrhizae Radix Et Rhizoma* (Gan Cao).

Modification: For lingering high fever, add *Gypsum Fibrosum* (Sheng Shi Gao), *Bubali Cornu* (Shui Niu Jiao); for convulsion of the limbs, add *Margaritifera Concha* (Zhen Zhu Mu), *Bombyx Batryticatus* (Jiang Can), *Scorpio* (Quan Xie); for clouded spirit and copious sputum, add *Arisaema Cum Bile* (Dan Nan Xing), *Curcumae Radix* (Yu Jin), *Bambusae Concretio Silicea* (Tian Zhu Huang); when the condition is critical and severe, it is necessary to give emergent treatment by integrated therapy of traditional and western medicine. For emergent treatment, please refer to the related

(2) 邪陷厥阴

证候：壮热不退，四肢抽搐，神昏谵语，颈项强直，两目上视，舌质红，苔黄，脉数。

治法：平肝息风，清心开窍。

主方：羚角钩藤汤合牛黄清心丸加味。

常用药：羚羊角、钩藤、茯神、生地黄、栀子、黄芩、菊花、浙贝母、白芍、甘草。

加减：壮热不退者，加生石膏、水牛角；四肢抽搐者，加珍珠母、僵蚕、全蝎；神昏痰多者，加胆南星、郁金、天竺黄；病情危重，应予中西医结合抢救治疗，参照"高热"及"惊厥"等相关章节应急处理。

sections of "Fever" and "Convulsion due to Fright".

4 Other therapies

4.1 Chinese Patent Medicine

(1) *Oral Liquid for Children with Lung-heat Cough and Panting* (Xiao Er Fei Re Ke Chuan Kou Fu Ye) is used for pattern of wind and heat blocking the lung and of phlegm and heat blocking the lung.

(2) *Gold-Vitalizing Oral Liquid* (Jin Zhen Kou Fu Ye) is used for pattern of phlegm and heat blocking the lung

(3) *Heat Toxin Quieting Injection* (Re Du Ning Zhu She Ye) is used for patterns of wind and heat blocking the lung or of phlegm and heat blocking the lung.

(4) *Glad Inflammation-Subsiding Injection* (Xi Yan Ping Zhu She Ye) is used for pattern of wind and heat blocking the lung or of phlegm and heat blocking the lung.

4.2 External therapy

Mix *Rhei Radix Et Rhizoma* (Da Huang) powder, *Natrii Sulfas* (Mang Xiao) powder, mushed garlic by the proportion of 4 : 1 : 4, make paste with water, spread the paste evenly on the dressing, and then apply it on the scapular region or the region with dense rale of the lung by auscultation. The dressing time depends on the age of the patient, once every day, 7 days as a course of treatment. It is applied to those with pneumonia manifested by cough, panting and rale in the lung.

4 其他疗法

4.1 中成药

（1）小儿肺热咳喘口服液：用于治疗风热闭肺与痰热闭肺证。

（2）金振口服液：用于治疗痰热闭肺证。

（3）热毒宁注射液：用于治疗风热闭肺与痰热闭肺证。

（4）喜炎平注射液：用于治疗风热闭肺与痰热闭肺证。

4.2 外治疗法

大黄粉、芒硝粉、蒜泥，按 4 ∶ 1 ∶ 4 比例配伍，以清水调成糊状，将上药调好均匀平摊于敷料上，敷在背部肩胛间区及肺部听诊湿啰音密集处。根据不同年龄选择敷药时间，每日 1 次，7 日为 1 个疗程。用于肺炎喘嗽肺部有啰音者。

Chapter 2 Diseases of Digestive System

第2章 消化系统疾病

Section 1 Stomatitis

第1节 口炎

Stomatitis refers to inflammation of the oral mucosa, induced by various infections. If the pathological changes are limited locally to the tongue, gums, or corner of the mouth, the disease can also be called inflammation of the tongue, of the gums or of the corner of the mouth, etc. Commonly seen diseases are thrush and herpetic stomatitis.

口炎是指口腔黏膜由于各种感染引起的炎症，若病变限于局部如舌、齿龈、口角亦可称为舌炎，齿龈炎或口角炎等。常见者有鹅口疮、疱疹性口炎。

Thrush

鹅口疮

This disease is caused by infection of Candida albicans, and belongs to oral candidiasis, characterised by scattered or suffused white flakes over the mouth or tongue. The white flakes look like goose mouth, and the color is like snow flakes, so it is described as "goose mouth" in Chinese language. It often appears in the newborns or premature infants, or infants who are weak, suffer malnutrition, enduring illnesses or diarrhea, or who take broad-spectrum antibiotics or immunosuppressor for a long time. The symptoms usually are not serious, and after careful treatment, the prognosis is good.

鹅口疮是由感染白色念珠菌所致，属口腔念珠菌病。以口腔、舌上散在或满布白色屑状物为特征。因其白屑状如鹅口、色白如雪片，故又称"鹅口"。多见于新生儿、早产儿，以及体质虚弱、营养不良、久病久泻、长期使用广谱抗生素或免疫抑制剂的小儿。症状一般较轻，经积极治疗，预后良好。

1 Etiology and pathogenesis

1 病因病机

It is mainly related to internal accumulation of fetal heat, or weak body constitution, or improper

主要由胎热内蕴，或体质虚弱，或调护不当，口腔不

care and nursing, which result in unclean oral cavity and infection of foul toxins.

洁,感受秽毒之邪所致。

If a pregnant woman likes eating acrid, hot, or fried food, the heat will stay in the spleen or stomach, and then the fetus will be infected with heat toxin from mother, resulting in its accumulation in the heart and spleen. Or because of invasion of the foul toxins during the delivery, or improper feeding of sweet and greasy food, resulting in accumulation of heat in the spleen and stomach, or because of unclean oral cavity due to improper nursing, the evils of foul toxins would take the chance to mix with the internal evils and external evils together, leading to accumulation of heat toxins in the heart and spleen. The tongue is a mirror of the heart, and the mouth is an orifice of the spleen. When fire and heat attack upward along the meridians, they would scorch the mouth and tongue, thus thrush is caused. When there is constitutional yin deficiency, or damage of yin body fluid by heat disease, or damage of yin by enduring diarrhea which results in kidney yin depletion and yang hyperactivity due to yin deficiency, the water would fail to control fire and heat. Vacuity fire would float upward, scorching and steaming the mouth and tongue, and hence spread white flakes.

孕妇平素喜食辛热炙煿之品,热留脾胃;患儿胎中禀受其母热毒,蕴积心脾;或出生时孕母产道秽毒侵入;或喂养不当,嗜食肥甘厚味,脾胃蕴热;或护理不当口腔不洁,秽毒之邪乘虚而入,内外合邪,热毒蕴积心脾。舌为心之苗,口为脾之窍,火热循经上攻,熏灼口舌,发为鹅口疮。素体阴虚;或热病之后灼伤阴津;或久泻伤阴,以致肾阴亏虚,阴虚阳亢,水不制火,虚火上浮,熏蒸口舌而散布白屑。

The pathological location mainly lies in the heart and spleen. Clinically there are deficiency and excess patterns. Excess patterns mostly are caused by accumulated heat in the heart and spleen, which flows through the meridians and scorches the mouth and tongue. The deficiency patterns are caused by vacuity fire flaming upward.

病位主要在心脾,临床上有虚实之分:实证多由心脾积热循经熏灼口舌而起;虚证则因虚火上炎所致。

2 Key to diagnosis

(1) It mostly occurs in the new-born infants, weak infants suffering enduring disease, or infants who have taken antibiotics, hormone, or immunosuppressor for a long time.

(2) White flakes can be scattered over the tongue, inside the cheeks, on the gums or upper lips, or in large patchs. In serious conditions, the patchs can extend to other places like throat, influencing milk sucking or breathing.

(3) Spores and hypha of Candida albicans can be seen in smear microscopic exam of a few white flakes.

3 Pattern identification and treatment

The key point is to identify deficiency and excess, and the severity. The excess pattern often happens to the infants with strong constitution, characterized by sudden onset and short duration, many or patched white flakes in the oral cavity, reddened surrounding mucous membrane, and accompanied by the symptoms of fever, flushed cheeks, vexation, thirst, brown urine, or constipation, etc, with thick and slimy tongue coating. The deficiency pattern often happens to the premature infants, weak infants after enduring illness or serious illness, characterized by gradual onset, long duration and lingering and repteated duration. There are sparsely scattered white flakes, pale surrounding mucous membrane, and often accompanied symptoms like emaciation, fatigued spirit, vexation due to deficiency, pale face, flushed cheeks, low fever, etc. In mild cases, there are relatively fewer white flakes, and the symptoms of the whole body are

2 诊断要点

（1）多见于新生儿、久病体弱儿，或有长期使用抗生素、激素及免疫抑制剂史。

（2）舌上、颊内、牙龈或上唇、上腭散布白屑，可融合成片。重者可向咽喉等处蔓延，影响吮乳或呼吸。

（3）取白屑少许涂片镜检，可见白色念珠菌芽孢及菌丝。

3 辨证论治

重在辨明虚实及轻重。实证多见于体壮儿，起病急，病程短，口腔白屑较多甚至堆积成块，周围黏膜红赤，可伴发热、面赤、心烦口渴、尿赤、便秘等症，舌苔较为厚腻；虚证多见于早产、久病体弱儿，或大病之后，起病缓，病程长，常迁延反复，口腔白屑稀散，周围黏膜色淡，常伴消瘦、神疲虚烦、面白颧红或低热等症状。轻证白屑较少，全身症状轻微或无，饮食睡眠尚可；重证白屑堆积，甚或蔓延到鼻腔、咽喉、气道、胃肠，可伴高热、烦躁、吐泻、气促及吮乳困难等，极重者可危及生命。

mild or do not appear, with normal diet and sleep. In severe cases, the white flakes may pile up and accumulate, even spread to nasal cavity, throat, airway, or stomach and intestines, accompanied by the symptoms of high fever, vexation, vomiting and diarrhea, and difficult sucking. The extremely critical cases may threaten life.

The excess patterns should be treated by clearing away and drain the accumulated heat from the heart and spleen. The deficiency patterns should be treated by nourishing yin and downbearing fire. For local focus in the mouth, besides oral administration of the medicine, the external therapies are often combined.

实证治疗宜清泻心脾积热，虚证宜滋肾养阴降火。病灶在口腔局部，除内服药物外，常配合外治疗法。

(1) Accumulated heat in the heart and spleen

(1) 心脾积热

Manifestations: White flakes over the whole oral cavity and tongue, extreme red color in the surrounding areas, flushed cheeks, red lips, vexation and agitation, crying while sucking milk, dry mouth or thirst, or accompanied by fever, dry stool, yellow and brown urine, red tongue body, thick yellow tongue coating, slippery and rapid pulse, purple stagnant fingerprint.

证候：口腔舌面满布白屑，周围焮红较甚，面赤，唇红，烦躁不宁，吮乳多啼，口干或渴，或伴发热，大便干结，小便黄赤，舌质红，苔黄厚，脉滑数，指纹紫滞。

Therapeutic method: To clarify the heart and drain the spleen fire.

治法：清心泻脾。

Main formula: *Heat-Clearing Away and Spleen Fire-Draining Powder* (Qing Re Xie Pi San) with modification.

主方：清热泻脾散加减。

Commonly used herbs: *Coptidis Rhizoma* (Huang Lian), *Gardeniae Fructus*(Zhi Zi), *Scutellariae Radix*(Huang Qin), *Gypsum Fibrosum* (Sheng Shi Gao), *Rehmanniae Radix Cruda* (Sheng Di Huang), *Poria* (Fu Ling), *Junci Medulla* (Deng Xin Cao), *Glycyrrhizae Radix Et Rhizoma* (Gan

常用药：黄连、栀子、黄芩、生石膏、生地黄、茯苓、灯心草、甘草。

Cao).

Modification: For constipation, add *Rhei Radix Et Rhizoma* (Da Huang); for mild heat, with white, thick and slimy tongue coating, add *Pogostmonis Herba* (Huo Xiang), *Eupatorii Herba* (Pei Lan); for thirst with desire to drink water, add *Phragmitis Rhizoma* (Lu Gen), *Ophiopogonis Radix* (Mai Dong); for abdominal retention and poor appetite, add *Crataegi Fructus Ustus* (Jiao Shan Zha), *Hordei Fructus Germinatus* (Mai Ya) and *Arecae Semen* (Bing Lang).

加减:大便秘结者,加大黄;热象不盛,舌苔白厚腻者,加藿香、佩兰;口干喜饮者,加芦根、麦冬;腹胀纳呆者,加焦山楂、麦芽、槟榔。

(2) Upward flaming of deficient fire

(2) 虚火上炎

Manifestations: Scarce white flakes over oral cavity and tongue, slight red surrounding areas, weak and timid constitution, flushed cheeks and night sweating, feverish sensation in the chest, palms and soles, accompanied by symptoms of low fever, vexation and agitation due to deficiency, tender and red tongue body, scanty tongue coating, thread and rapid pulse, slight purple fingerprints.

证候:口腔舌上白屑稀散,周围焮红不甚,形体怯弱,颧红盗汗,手足心热,可伴低热,虚烦不安,舌质嫩红,苔少,脉细数,指纹淡紫。

Therapeutic method: To enrich yin and downbear fire.

治法:滋阴降火。

Main formula: *Anemarrhena, Phellodendron, and Rehmannia Pill* (Zhi Bo Di Huang Wan) with modification.

主方:知柏地黄丸加减。

Commonly used herbs: *Arecae Semen* (Bing Lang), *Corni Fructus* (Shan Zhu Yu), *Dioscoreae Rhizoma* (Shan Yao), *Poria* (Fu Ling), *Alismatis Rhizoma* (Ze Xie), *Moutan Cortex Radicis* (Mu Dan Pi), *Anemarrhenae Rhizoma* (Zhi Mu), *Phellodendri Cortex Chinensis(Huang Bo)*, *Cinnamomi Cortex* (Rou Gui).

常用药:熟地黄、山茱萸、山药、茯苓、泽泻、牡丹皮、知母、黄柏、肉桂。

Modification: For thirst with desire to drink water, add *Dendrobii Herba* (Shi Hu), *Polygonati*

加减:口干欲饮者,加石斛、玉竹;低热者,加地骨皮、

Odorati Rhizoma(Yu Zhu); for low fever, add *Lycii Cortex* (Di Gu Pi), and *Cynanchi Atrati Radix Et Rhizoma* (Bai Wei); for poor appetite, add *Mume Fructus* (Wu Mei), *Chaenomelis Fructus*(Mu Gua), and *Hordei Fructus Germinatus* (Mai Ya); for constipation, add *Cannabis Fructus*(Huo Ma Ren).

白薇；食欲不振者，加乌梅、木瓜、麦芽；大便秘结者，加火麻仁。

4 Other therapies

4 其他疗法

4.1 Chinese Patent medicine

4.1 中成药

(1) *Red-Abducting Pill* (Dao Chi Wan) is used for pattern of accumulated heat in heart and spleen in treating thrush.

（1）导赤丸：用于治疗鹅口疮心脾积热证。

(2) *Anemarrhena, Phellodendron, and Rehmannia Pill* (Zhi Bo Di Huang Wan) is used for upward flaming of deficiency fire.

（2）知柏地黄丸：用于治疗鹅口疮虚火上炎证。

4.2 External therapy

4.2 外治疗法

(1) *Boneol and Borax Powder* (Bing Peng San), *Indigo Powder* (Qing Dai San), *Pearl and Bezoar Powde*(Zhu Huang San), *Mirabilitum Praeparatum Spray* (Xi Gua Shuang Peng Ji). Choose one of these, spread adequate amount to the affected area, for treating thrush in pattern of accumulated heat in the heart and spleen.

（1）冰硼散、青黛散、珠黄散、西瓜霜喷剂，任选 1 种，每次适量，涂敷患处。用于治疗鹅口疮心脾积热证。

(2) *Euodia Fructus* (Wu Zhu Yu) 10g, Grind it to fine powder, mix with mature vinegar into paste, and apply to Yongquan (KI 1) on the foot, for thrush in pattern of upward flaming of deficiency fire.

（2）吴茱萸 10 克，研为细末，以陈醋适量调成糊状，敷于两足涌泉穴。用于治疗鹅口疮虚火上炎证。

Herpetic Stomatitis

疱疹性口炎

Herpetic stomatitis is an inflammation of the oral cavity, clinically characterized by single herpes or cluster of small herpes in the oral cavity, and by yellowish and white ulcer over the gums, tongue body, cheeks, and palate, pain, or accompanied by

疱疹性口炎是以口腔内出现单个或成簇小疱疹为主要临床特征的口腔炎症。以齿龈、舌体、两颊、上腭等处出现黄白色溃疡，疼痛，或伴

fever and salivation. It is often seen in the infants aged from 1 to 3 years old. It may happen in any season.

发热、流涎为特征。多见于1～3岁小儿，发病无明显季节差异。

In Chinese medicine, it is termed as oral ulcers. If the ulcerating sore is big or spreads to the whole mouth, it is called oral ulceration. If the ulcerating sore occurs at both sides of the mouth and lips, it is called swallow-mouth sore in Chinese language.

中医称之为"口疮"，若溃疡面积较大，甚至满口糜烂者，称为口糜。溃疡发生在口唇两侧，称为燕口疮。

1　Etiology and pathogenesis

1　病因病机

The causative reasons are mainly related to infection of exogenous evils, overaction of the spleen by wind and heat, invasion of foul toxins by improper care, accumulation of heat in the heart and spleen, or upward floating of deficienct fire due to weak body after enduring illness. The heart opens into the tongue. The spleen opens into the mouth. The stomach meridian communicates with the teeth and gums, and the kidney meridian is connected to the tongue root. Therefore, the diseased location of oral ulcer mainly lies in the heart, spleen, stomach, and kidney.

病因主要有感受外邪，风热乘脾，或调护不当，秽毒内侵，心脾积热，或久病体弱，虚火上浮等。心开窍开舌，脾开窍于口，胃经络齿龈，肾脉连舌本，故口疮的病位主要在心脾胃肾。

The excess pattern is mainly caused by overaction of the spleen by wind and heat or accumulation of heat in the heart and spleen. Those caused by weak body constitution and upward floating of deficiency fire belong to deficiency pattern.

实证多为风热乘脾或心脾积热，而体质虚弱，虚火上浮者则为虚证。

2　Key to diagnosis

2　诊断要点

(1) There is a history of improper feeding, overeating of fried and greasy food, or fever by external infection.

（1）有喂养不当，过食炙煿厚味，或外感发热病史。

(2) Yellowish and white ulcerating sores, in varying size, are present on the mucosa of the gums, tongue body, cheeks, and palate, and even

（2）齿龈、舌体、两颊、上腭等黏膜处出现黄白色溃疡点，大小不等，甚则满口糜

erosion in the whole mouth, pain and salivation, probably accompanied by fever or swollen and painful lymph node below the jaw.

3 Pattern identification and treatment

Pattern identification is to differentiate between excess and deficiency and to see which organ is involved. Excess patterns are mostly caused by infection of exogenous wind, heat or internal damage by milk feeding, characterized by short duration and sudden onset, many oral ulcers, red surrounding mucous membrane, local scorching hot and painful sensation, foul breathing, salivation, or accompanied by fever and vexation. The diseased location mainly lies in the heart and spleen. Deficiency pattern is mainly characterized by gradual onset, long duration, relatively fewer ulcers, and repeated occurrence, slight red surrounding mucous membrane, slight pain, or low fever, flushed cheeks, and night sweating. The diseased location mainly lies in the liver and kidney. When the diseased location lies in the heart, oral ulcers would often appear at the sides or tip of the tongue, accompanied by vexation, crying and screaming, restless night sleep, brown urine, etc. If the diseased location lies in the spleen and stomach, oral ulcers often occur on lips and cheeks, palate and gums, often accompanied by foul breathing, salivation, distention in the epigastric region and abdomen, and constipation.

The excess pattern is predominantly treated by clearing away heat and resolving toxin, discharging accumulated heat from the heart and spleen. The deficiency pattern is predominantly treated by enriching yin and downbearing fire, and returning fire

腐，疼痛流涎，可伴发热或常有颌下臀核肿大、疼痛。

3 辨证论治

辨证应分实虚及脏腑：实证多由外感风热或乳食内伤所致，起病急，病程短，口腔溃疡数目多，周围黏膜红赤，局部灼热疼痛，口臭流涎，或伴发热烦躁，其病位多在心脾。虚证口疮起病缓，病程长，口腔溃疡相对较少，反复发作，周围黏膜淡红，疼痛轻微，或伴低热、颧红盗汗，其病位多在肝肾。病变部位在心者，口疮常发生于舌边、尖部，并伴烦躁叫扰啼哭，夜眠不安，尿赤等；在脾胃者，口疮每以唇颊、上腭、齿龈处居多，并伴口臭流涎，脘腹胀满，大便秘结等。

治疗实证以清热解毒，泻心脾积热为主；虚证则以滋阴降火，引火归元为法。

to the origin.

(1) Wind and heat overacting the spleen

Manifestations: Ulcers in the mouth, lips, inside cheeks, palate, gums, scorching redness in the margins, scorching pain, drooling, refusal to take food, accompanied by fever, sore and swollen painful throat, scanty brown urine, dry stool, red tongue, thin and yellow tongue coating, rapid and floating pulse, floating and purple fingerprints.

Therapeutic method: To expel wind, discharge fire, clear away heat and resolve toxin.

Main formula: *Diaphragm-cooling Powder* (Liang Ge San) with modification.

Commonly used herbs: *Scutellariae Radix* (Huang Qin), *Lonicerae Flos Japonicae* (Jin Yin Hua), *Forsythiae Fructus* (Lian Qiao), *Gardeniae Fructus* (Zhi Zi), *Rhei Radix Et Rhizoma* (Da Huang), *Lophatheri Herba* (Dan Zhu Ye), *Menthae Haploalycis Herba* (Bo He), *Glycyrrhizae Radix Et Rhizoma* (Gan Cao).

Modification: For fever, add *Bupleuri Radix* (Chai Hu), and *Gypsum Fibrosum* (Sheng Shi Gao); for vomiting, add *Bambusae Caulis in Taenias* (Zhu Ru); for swollen and sore throat, add *Belamecandae Rhizoma* (She Gan), and *Scrophulariae Radix* (Xuan Shen); for dry mouth with little body fluid, add *Phragmitis Rhizoma* (Lu Gen), *Trichosanthis Radix* (Tian Hua Fen).

(2) Accumulated heat in the heart and spleen

Manifestations: Ulcers or erosions in the mouth and tongue, mainly on the surface and tip of tongue, in red color and pain, foul breathing, drooling, vexation, crying, flushed cheeks, thirst, or accompanied by fever, constipation, scanty brown

（1）风热乘脾

证候：口唇、颊内、上腭、齿龈等处溃疡，周围焮红，灼热疼痛，流涎拒食，伴发热，咽喉红肿疼痛，小便短赤，大便秘结，舌质红，苔薄黄，脉浮数，指纹浮紫。

治法：疏风泻火，清热解毒。

主方：凉膈散加减。

常用药：黄芩、金银花、连翘、栀子、大黄、淡竹叶、薄荷、甘草。

加减：发热者，加柴胡、生石膏；呕吐者，加竹茹；咽喉肿痛者，加射干、玄参；口干少津者，加芦根、天花粉。

（2）心脾积热

证候：口舌溃疡或糜烂，舌面、尖边较多，色红疼痛，口臭流涎，烦躁啼哭，面赤口渴，或伴发热，大便秘结，小便短赤，舌尖红，苔薄黄，脉

urine, red tongue tip, thin yellow tongue coating, rapid pulse, purple and stagnant fingerprints.

数,指纹紫滞。

Therapeutic method: To clarify the heart and discharge the spleen heat.

治法:清心泻脾。

Main formula: *Red-Abducting Powder* (Dao Chi San) and *Yellow-Draining Powder* (Xie Huang San) with modification.

主方:导赤散合泻黄散加减。

Commonly used herbs: *Rehmanniae Radix Cruda* (Sheng Di Huang), *Lophatheri Herba* (Dan Zhu Ye), *Tetrapanacis Medulla* (Tong Cao), *Pogostmonis Herba* (Huo Xiang), *Gardeniae Fructus* (Zhi Zi), *Coptidis Rhizoma* (Huang Lian), *Gypsum Fibrosum* (Sheng Shi Gao), *Ledebouriellae Radix* (Fang Feng), *Glycyrrhizae Radix Et Rhizoma* (Gan Cao).

常用药:生地黄、淡竹叶、通草、藿香、栀子、黄连、生石膏、防风、甘草。

Modification: For scanty urine, add Plantaginis Semen(Che Qian Zi), *Talcum* (Hua Shi); for severe thirst, add *Phragmitis Rhizoma* (Lu Gen), *Trichosanthis Radix* (Tian Hua Fen); for constipation, add *Rhei Radix Et Rhizoma* (Da Huang).

加减:尿少者,加车前子,滑石;口渴甚者,加芦根、天花粉;大便秘结者,加大黄。

(3) Upward floating of deficient fire

(3) 虚火上浮

Manifestations: Oral ulceration, no redness or slight redness in the surrounding parts, mild pain in recurrent or prolonged nature, fatigued spirit, flushed cheeks, dry mouth without thirst, red tongue, scanty or partially peeled tongue coating.

证候:口腔溃烂,周围色不红或微红,疼痛不甚,反复发作或迁延不愈,神疲颧红,口干不渴,舌质红,苔少或花剥。

Therapeutic method: To enrich yin and downbear fire, return fire to the origin.

治法:滋阴降火,引火归元。

Main formula: *Six-Ingredient Rehmannia Pill* (Liu Wei Di Huang Wan) with supplementation.

主方:六味地黄丸加味。

Commonly used herbs: *Rehmanniae Radix Cruda* (Sheng Di Huang), *Dioscoreae Rhizoma* (Shan Yao), *Corni Fructus* (Shan Zhu Yu), *Alismatis Rhizoma* (Ze Xie), *Moutan Cortex Radicis* (Mu Dan Pi), *Poria* (Fu Ling), *Cinnamomi Cortex*

常用药:生地黄、山药、山茱萸、泽泻、牡丹皮、茯苓、肉桂、牛膝。

(Rou Gui), *Achyranthis Bidentatae Radix* (Niu Xi).

Modification: For exuberant deficiency fire, add *Anemarrhenae Rhizoma* (Zhi Mu), *Phellodendri Cortex Chinensis (Huang Bo)*; for constipation, add honey, *Cannabis Fructus* (Huo Ma Ren); for enduring illness plus vomiting and diarrhea, or depletion of the spleen yang and failure of the clear yang in ascending due to over administration of cold and cool stuffs, use *Seven-Ingredient and Atractylodes Powder* (Qi Wei Bai Zhu San), and *Puerariae Radix* (Ge Gen) in a large dose. For upward floating of rootless fire due to severe depletion of the spleen and kidney, manifested by ulcers occurring in the mouth and tongue, fatigued spirit, pale face, thin and loose stool, pale tongue, white tongue coating, use *Center-rectifying Decoction* (Li Zhong Tang) plus *Cinnamomi Cortex* (Rou Gui).

加减：虚火盛者，加知母、黄柏；大便秘结者，加蜂蜜、火麻仁。若久病吐泻，或过服寒凉，脾阳亏虚，清阳不升者，可用七味白术散，重用葛根；若脾肾大虚，无根之火上浮而见口舌生疮，神疲面白，大便溏薄，舌淡苔白者，可用理中汤加肉桂。

4　Other therapies

4.1　Chinese Patent medicine

(1) *Bovine Bezoar Toxin Resolving Pills* (Niu Huang Jie Du Pian) is used for patterns of wind and heat overacting the spleen, and upward flaring of the heart fire.

(2) *Anemarrhena, Phellodendron, and Rehmannia Pill* (Zhi Bo Di Huang Wan) is used for patterns of upward floating of deficiency fire.

4.2　Tuina Therapy

(1) Push Pt. Tianzhugu, knead Tiantu (CV 22), clarify Pt. Wei and Pt. Banmen. For fever, push Pt. Liufu, Pt. and push Pt. Ershanmen by the method of "fishing for the moon from the bottom of water", used for pattern of wind and heat overact-

4　其他疗法

4.1　中成药

（1）牛黄解毒片：用于治疗口疮风热乘脾证、心火上炎证。

（2）知柏地黄丸：用于治疗口疮虚火上浮证。

4.2　推拿疗法

（1）推天柱骨，揉天突，清胃，清板门。发热加退六腑，水底捞明月，二扇门。用于治疗口疮风热乘脾证。

ing the spleen.

(2) Clarify the heart and tranquilize the liver. Clarify Pt. Tianheshui, clarify Pt. Xiaochang, and knead Pt. Xiaotianxin, used for oral ulcer in pattern of accumulated heat in the heart and spleen.

（2）清心平肝，清天河水，清小肠，捣小天心。用于治疗口疮心脾积热证。

(3) Supplement Pt. Shen, rub Pt. Erma, divide hand yin and yang, clarify Pt. Tianheshui, push Yongquan (KI 1), used for oral ulcer in pattern of upward floating of deficiency fire.

（3）补肾，揉二马，分手阴阳，清天河水，推涌泉穴。用于治疗口疮虚火上浮证。

4.3 External therapy

(1) Choose one of these: *Boneol and Borax Powder* (Bing Peng San), *Indigo Powder* (Qing Dai San), *Pearl and Bezoar Powder* (Zhu Huang San), *Mirabilitum Praeparatum* (Xi Gua Shuang), and spread adequate amount to the affected area, for oral ulcer of excess pattern.

(2) Choose *Tin-like Powder* (Xi Lei San) or *Nourishing Yin and Engendering Flesh Powder* (Yang Yin Sheng Ji San), and spread adequate amount to the affected area, for pattern of upward floating of deficiency fire.

4.3 外治疗法

（1）冰硼散、青黛散、西瓜霜、珠黄散，任选一种，取适量涂敷患处。适用于实证口疮。

（2）锡类散、养阴生肌散，任选一种，取适量涂敷患处。用于治疗口疮虚火上浮证。

Section 2 Gastritis

Gastritis refers to an inflammatory change of gastric wall or gastric mucous membrane, caused by various physical, chemical or biological injurious factors. Gastritis is a common disease of the digestive system in pediatric clinics. According to its duration, it can be divided into acute gastritis and chronic gastritis. The latter is high in incidence.

In Chinese medicine, it belongs to scope of "epigastric pain", "gastric distention", and "vomiting".

第2节 胃炎

胃炎是指由各种物理性、化学性或生物性有害因子引起的胃黏膜或胃壁炎性改变的一种疾病。胃炎是儿科消化系统的常见病。根据病程分急性和慢性两种，后者发病率高。

本病属中医学"胃脘痛""胃胀""呕吐"等范畴。

1 Etiology and pathogenesis

Mostly, it is caused by retention of milk food, invasion of cold evil or liver qi. It may also be caused by constitutional accumulation of heat in the stomach, and deficiency and cold of the spleen and stomach.

Improper food ingestion, over ingestion of drinks and food, or indigestible food, would injure the spleen and stomach, leading to pain. The invasion of cold and wind, or over ingestion of cold and raw melons and fruits, would result in congelation of cold and qi stagnation. Once qi and blood are obstructed and fail to flow, pain would occur. If the nursing mother likes roast, sour and spicy food, the infants who drink mother's milk would have heat accumulated in stomach. If older children over-eat acrid and spicy food, heat will be accumulated in the stomach. When dampness and heat in summer and autumn are affected, they may be accumulated in the Middle Energizer, resulting in transformation of dampness and food into fire, qi stagnation and pain. If the emotional disorder and inhibited liver qi attack the stomach transversely, pain would be induced in the epigastric region. If the spleen and stomach are invaded by cold, or the infants eat too much cold food or fruits, or take too much attacking herbs in bitter and cold property in the treatment of diseases, yang in the Middle Energizer may fail to function and qi dynamic may be inhibited, leading to pain.

1 病因病机

多由乳食积滞，寒邪、肝气侵犯，或素体胃有积热、脾胃虚寒所引起。

小儿饮食不节，或暴饮暴食，或过食不易消化的食物，以致脾胃损伤而痛。风冷寒气所侵，或过食生冷瓜果之品，寒凝则气滞，气血壅阻不行而痛。乳母喜嗜炙煿、辛辣之品，儿食母乳热积于胃；或较大儿童过食辛热之品，热积胃中；或感受夏秋湿热，蕴于中焦，皆可致湿食化火，气滞不畅而痛。情志不舒肝气不畅，横逆犯胃，发为胃脘痛。脾胃受寒，或小儿过食瓜果生冷，或病程中过服苦寒攻伐之剂，中阳不运，气机不畅而痛。

2 Key to diagnosis

(1) There is a history of pain in the epigastric region.

2 诊断要点

（1）胃脘痛病史。

(2) Clinical manifestations: Acute gastritis is characterized by sudden and quick onset; for mild cases, only poor appetite, abdominal pain, nausea and vomiting; for severe cases, spitting of blood, black stool and often accompanied by general poisoning like fever in those with infection. Chronic gastritis is characterized by the symptoms of recurrent abdominal pain, pain during eating or after meal, at the upper abdomen and around the umbilicus in most cases, and manifested by intermittent dull pain in mild cases, and severe colic pain in severe cases. It is often accompanied by poor appetite, nausea, vomiting, and abdominal distention.

(2) 临床表现:急性胃炎:发病急骤,轻者仅有食欲不振、腹痛、恶心、呕吐,严重者可出现呕血、黑便,有感染者常伴有发热等全身中毒症状。慢性胃炎:常见症状为反复发作性腹痛,疼痛经常出现于进食过程中或餐后,多数位于上腹部、脐周,轻者为间歇性隐痛或钝痛,严重者为剧烈绞痛。常伴有食欲不振、恶心、呕吐、腹胀。

(3) Gastroscopy: As the most valuable, safest, and most reliable diagnostic method, it is to directly observe the pathological change of the gastric mucosa and its severity, to see extensive congestion, edema, erosion, or bleeding of the gastric mucosa, and to observe the mucous patches or reflux bile of the mucous surface.

(3) 胃镜检查:为最有价值、安全、可靠的诊断手段。可直接观察胃黏膜病变及其程度,可见黏膜广泛充血、水肿、糜烂、出血,有时可见黏膜表面的黏液斑或反流的胆汁。

3 Pattern identification and treatment

3 辨证论治

It is necessary to identify the causes of the disease and the pattern of cold or heat, excess or depletion. If injured by food ingestion, there may be symptoms of accumulation and stagnation. If the liver qi attacks the stomach, there will be manifestations of belching and acid regurgitation. Only by knowing the causative reason, can it be possible to treat its underlying reason. Preference for pressure belongs to deficiency and refusal of pressure belongs to excess. The lingering conditions are mostly attributed to deficient pattern and the new conditions are mostly attributed to excessive pattern. If pain

辨别病因及寒热虚实:如饮食所伤,可有积滞的症状;肝气犯胃,可有嗳气泛酸之症,知其所因,方能治其根本。喜按为虚,拒按为实;久病多虚,新病多实;得食痛减为虚,食后疼痛加剧为实;痛处不移者为实,反则为虚。实证多热,虚证多寒。但也有寒热错杂,虚实互见的。

Galli Endothelium Corneum Gigerii (Ji Nei Jin).

(3) Pattern of accumulated heat in the stomach

Manifestations: Oppressive pain in the epigastric region, distention and fullness in the epigastric region and abdomen, bitter taste in the mouth, sticky sensation in the mouth and poor appetite, vomiting in severe condition, putrid and sour vomitus, heavy sensation in the body and head, dry mouth and brown urine, red tongue, yellow and slimy tongue coating, rapid and slippery pulse.

Therapeutic method: to clear away heat and dissolve accumulation, regulate qi and relieve pain.

Formula: *Diaphragm-cooling powde*r (Liang Ge San) with modification.

Commonly used herbs: *Rhei Radix Et Rhizoma Sichuan* (Dai Huang), *Mirabilitum Depuratum* (Pu Xiao), *Glycyrrhizae Radix Et Rhizoma* (Gan Cao), *Semen Gardeniae* (Zhi Zi Ren), *Menthae haplocalycis herba* (Bo He Ye).

Modification: For severe pain in the epigastric region, add *Corydalis Rhizoma* (Yan Hu Suo), *Aurantii Fructus* (Zhi Qiao); for vigorous heat, add *Coptidis Rhizoma* (Huang Lian), *Taraxaci Herba* (Pu Gong Ying); for sticky mouth and poor appetite, add *Pogostmonis Herba* (Huo Xiang), *Eupatorii Herba* (Pei Lan), *Massa Medicata Fermentata* (Jaio Shen Qu).

(4) Pattern of liver qi invading the stomach

Manifestations: Distention and pain in the epigastric region and rib side, oppression in the chest and belching, sour and bitter vomiting in severe conditions, difficult defecation, relieved with belching or flatus, pain happening or aggravated by vexation, depression or anger, red tongue margins,

(3) 胃有积热

证候:胃脘闷痛,脘腹痞满,口苦、口黏纳呆,甚者呕吐,吐物酸臭,头身重着,口干尿赤,舌质红,苔黄腻,脉滑数。

治法:清热化积,理气止痛。

主方:凉膈散加减。

常用药:大黄、朴硝、甘草、栀子仁、薄荷叶。

加减:胃脘痛甚者,加延胡索、枳壳;热偏盛者,加黄连、蒲公英;口黏纳呆者,加藿香、佩兰、焦神曲。

(4) 肝气犯胃

证候:胃脘胀痛连胁,胸闷嗳气,甚者呕吐酸苦,大便不畅,得嗳气、矢气则舒,遇烦恼郁怒则痛作或痛甚,舌边红,苔白腻,脉弦。

white and slimy tongue coating, string-taut pulse.

Therapeutic method: To soothe the liver and regulate qi, harmonize the stomach and relieve pain.

治法:疏肝理气,和胃止痛。

Formula: *Bupleurum Liver-Soothing Powder* (Chai Hu Su Gan Tang) with modification.

主方:柴胡疏肝散加减。

Commonly used herbs: *Citri Reticulatae Pericarpium* (Chen Pi), *Bupleuri Radix* (Chai Hu), *Chuanxiong Rhizoma* (Chuan Xiong), *Aurantii Fructus* (Zhi Qiao), *Paeoniae Radix* (Shao Yao), *Radix Glycyrrhizae* (Gan Cao), *Cyperi Rhizoma* (Xiang Fu).

常用药:陈皮、柴胡、川芎、枳壳、芍药、甘草、香附。

Modification: For severe distention, add *Citri Reticulatae Pericarpium Viride* (Qing Pi), *Cur Cumae Radix*(Yu Jin), *Aucklandiae Radix* (Mu Xiang); for severe pain, add *Toosendan Fructus* (Chuan Lian Zi), *Corydalis Rhizoma* (Yan Hu Suo); for frequent belching, add *Pinelliae Rhizoma* (Ban Xia), *Perillae Caulis* (Zi Su Geng).

加减:若胀重者,可加青皮、郁金、木香;若痛甚者,可加川楝子、延胡索;嗳气频作者,可加半夏、紫苏梗。

(5) Pattern of deficiency and cold in the spleen and stomach

(5) 脾胃虚寒

Manifestations: Enduring and insidious pain in the epigastric region, relieved by warmth and pressure and after meals, occasional vomiting of clear water, lusterless complexion, fatigued spirit and lack of strength, lack of warmth in hand and foot, thin and sloppy stool, even blood stool, pale tongue, white tongue coating, thready and weak pulse or slow and deep pulse.

证候:胃脘隐隐作痛,绵绵不断,喜暖喜按,得食则减,时吐清水,面色无华,神疲乏力,手足欠温,大便溏薄,甚则便血。舌质淡,苔白,脉细弱或沉缓。

Therapeutic method: To warm up yang, fortify the Middle Energizer, boost qi and harmonize the stomach.

治法:温阳建中,益气和胃。

Formula: *Astragali Center-Fortifying Decoction* (Huang Qi Jian Zhong Tang) with modification.

主方:黄芪建中汤加减。

Commonly used herbs: *Maltosum* (Yi Tang), *Cinnamomi Ramulus* (Gui Zhi), *Radix Paeoniae* (Shao Yao), *Zingiberis Rhizoma Recens* (Sheng Jiang), *Jujubae Fructus* (Da Zao), *Astragali Radix* (Huang Qi), *Glycyrrhizae Radix Et Rhizoma Praeparata* (Zhi Gan Cao).

常用药:饴糖、桂枝、芍药、生姜、大枣、黄芪、炙甘草。

Modification: For vomiting of clear water, add *Citri Reticulatae Pericarpium* (Chen Pi), *Pinelliae Rhizoma* (Ban Xia), *Poria* (Fu Ling); for acid regurgitation, remove *Maltosum* (Yi Tang) and *Astragali Radix* (Huang Qi), add *Sepiae Endoconcha* (Wu Zei Gu).

加减:若呕吐清水者,加陈皮、半夏、茯苓;泛酸者,去饴糖、黄芪,加乌贼骨。

(6) Pattern of stomach yin insufficiency

(6) 胃阴不足

Manifestations: Insidious scorching pain in the epigastric region, hungry sensation without appetite, dry mouth and throat, feverish sensation in the chest, palms and soles, emaciation and lack of strength, thirst with desire for water, dry stool, red tongue and lack of fluid, thready and rapid pulse.

证候:胃脘隐隐灼痛,似饥而不欲食,口燥咽干,五心烦热,消瘦乏力,口渴思饮,大便干结,舌红少津,脉细数。

Therapeutic method: To nourish yin and boost the stomach, harmonize the Middle Energizer and relieve pain.

治法:养阴益胃,和中止痛。

Formula: *An Ever Effective Decoction for Nourishing Liver and Kidney* (Yi Guan Jian) and *Peony and Licorice Decoction* (Shao Yao Gan Cao Tang) with modification.

主方:一贯煎合芍药甘草汤加减。

Commonly used herbs: *Glehniae Radix* (Bei Sha Shen), *Ophiopogonis Radix* (Mai Dong), *Rehmanniae Radix Cruda* (Sheng Di Huang), *Lycii Fructus* (Gou Qi Zi), *Toosendan Fructus* (Chuan Lian Zi), *Paeoniae Radix* (Shao Yao), *Glycyrrhizae Radix Et Rhizoma* (Gan Cao).

常用药:北沙参、麦冬、生地黄、枸杞子、川楝子、芍药、甘草。

4 Other therapies

4.1 Acumoxatherapy

Select Zhongwan (CV 12), Neiguan (PC 6), Gongsun (SP 4), and Zusanli (ST 36), puncture the acupoints by routine needling method. It is advisable to apply moxibustion, or ginger-insulated moxibustion.

4.2 Tuina therapy

Push and rub Zhongwan (CV 12), Qihai (CV 6), Tianshu (ST 25), Zusanli (ST 36), Pishu (BL 20), Weishu (BL 21), Sanjiaoshu (BL 22). Pinch the Spine.

4 其他疗法

4.1 针灸疗法

取中脘、内关、公孙、足三里，常规针刺，可行灸法或隔姜灸。

4.2 推拿疗法

按揉中脘、气海、天枢、足三里、脾俞、胃俞、三焦俞，捏脊。

Section 3 Diarrhea

Infantile diarrhea is a complex syndrome of the digestive tract, caused by multiple pathogens and factors and characterized by increased defecation and change in nature and form of stool. It often occurs in the summer and autumn and mostly in the infants aged from 6 months old to two years old. It is one of the main causes to cause malnutrition, retardation of growth and development, and death in the infants.

It belongs to the scope of "diarrhea" in traditional Chinese medicine. In mild cases, the prognosis is good. In serious cases, body fluids are easily damaged and consumed, causing injury in qi and yin, and even resulting in critical condition of exhaustion of yin and desertion of yang. In those with enduring diarrhea, there can be infantile malnutrition, or chronic infantile convulsion.

第3节 腹泻

小儿腹泻是一组由多病原、多因素引起的以大便次数增多和大便性状改变为特点的消化道综合征。夏秋季节多见。6 个月～2 岁婴幼儿发病率高，是造成小儿营养不良、生长发育障碍和死亡的主要原因之一。

本病属中医学“泄泻”范畴。轻者预后良好，重者极易伤津耗液，导致气阴两伤，甚至出现阴竭阳脱之危候；若久泻迁延不愈者，常可导致疳证，或慢惊风。

1 Etiology and pathogenesis

The common causes are infection of external evils, food damage, weak spleen and stomach, yang deficiency of the spleen and kidney. The diseased location lies in the spleen and stomach. When the infants are damaged in the spleen and stomach, water and food cannot be digested, the essentials cannot be distributed, the clear cannot be separated from the turbid, come down with the dirty and leading to diarrhea.

The basic pathogenesis is exuberance of dampness due to spleen deficiency. Because the tender yang has not fully developed and the tender yin has not fully grown in the infants, their yang and yin are easily injured after diarrhea than the adults, leading to transmuted patterns. If the sick child suffers from serious diarrhea, yin will be easily damaged and qi is exhuased, presenting the damage of both qi and yin, and even injury of yang due to yin demage, leading to critical condition of yin exhaustion and yang desertion. If the prolonged diarrhea continues, causing deficiency of the spleen qi, the liver qi would be exuberant to produce the internal wind, leading to chronic infantile convulsion. If the spleen is deficient and fails to perform its transformation, resulting in lack of resources for transformation, qi and blood would not be sufficient to nourish the viscera, muscles and skin, causing infantile malnutrition after a long period of time.

1 病因病机

常见原因有感受外邪、伤于饮食、脾胃虚弱与脾肾阳虚，病位在脾胃。小儿脾胃受伤，水谷不化，精微不布，清浊不分，合污而下，而成泄泻。

基本病机为脾虚湿盛。由于小儿稚阳未充、稚阴未长，患泄泻后较成人更易于损阴伤阳发生变证。重症患儿，泻下过度，易于伤阴耗气，出现气阴两伤，甚则阴伤及阳，导致阴竭阳脱的危重变证。若久泻不止，脾气虚弱，肝旺而生内风，可成慢惊风；脾虚失运，生化乏源，气血不足以荣养脏腑肌肤，久则形成疳证。

2 Key to diagnosis

(1) A history of improper food ingestion, or ingestion of unclean food, and infection of contraction of seasonal evils.

2 诊断要点

(1) 有乳食不节、饮食不洁，或感受时邪的病史。

(2) Increased defecation and thin stool.

(2) 大便次数增多,粪质稀薄。

(3) Serious diarrhea is presented with scanty urine, high fever, vexation and thirst, listlessness of spirit, dry skin, depressed fontanel, sunken eyes, crying without tears, cherry-red mouth and lips, long and deep breathing, abdominal distention, etc.

(3) 重症泄泻,可见小便短少,高热,烦渴,神萎,皮肤干瘪,囟门凹陷,目眶下陷,啼哭无泪,口唇樱红,呼吸深长,腹胀等症。

3 Pattern identification and treatment

3 辨证论治

Predominantly, based upon the eight principles, it is necessary to differentiate cold, heat, deficiency and excess for ordinary patterns, and to differntiate yin and yang for transmuted patterns. In accordance with the onset and duration, the ordinary patterns can be divided into fulminant diarrhea and prolonged diarrhea. The fulminant diarrhea is mostly in pattern of excess, and the prolonged diarrhea is mostly in pattern of deficiency or deficiency mixed with excess. The transmuted pattern often starts with non-stop diarrhea, present with pattern of qi and yin damage, and even pattern of yin exhaustion and yang desertion, belonging to the critical condition.

以八纲辨证为主,常证重在辨寒、热、虚、实;变证重在辨阴、阳。常证按起病缓急、病程长短分为暴泻、久泻,暴泻多属实,久泻多属虚或虚中夹实;变证起于泻下不止,可出现气阴两伤证,甚则导致阴竭阳脱证,属危重症。

Based upon the therapeutic principle to strengthen the spleen and dissolve dampness, the excess patterns could mainly be treated by expelling evils and could be treated respectively by the method to clear away heat and dissolve dampness, to promote digestion and abduct stagnation, and to expel wind and relieve the exterior, in accordance with different pathogenic factors. The deficiency patterns could mainly be treated by supporting the vital energy, and could be treated by the method to fortify the spleen and boost qi, warm up and supple-

以运脾化湿为基本治则。实证以祛邪为主,针对病因不同,分别给予清热利湿,消食导滞,疏风解表等法。虚证以扶正为主,根据脏腑虚损的不同,进行健脾益气,温补脾肾,固涩止泻治疗。泄泻变证,气阴两伤者,治以益气养阴、酸甘敛阴;阴竭阳脱者,当即挽阴回阳、救逆固脱。

ment the spleen and kidney, induce astringency and stop diarrhea, in accordance with different severity of deficiency and depletion in the organs. The transmuted pattern of diarrhea, with injury of both qi and yin, should be treated by boosting qi and nourishing yin, and constraining yin with sweet and sour herbs; the transmuted pattern of diarrhea, with yin exhaustion and yang desertion, should be treated immediately by rescuing yin and returning yang, and rectifying counterflow and prostration.

3.1 Ordinary patterns

(1) Wind-cold diarrhea

Manifestations: Clear and thin stool, with light color and bubbles, slight foul smell, abdominal pain and borborygmus before defecation, often accompanied by aversion to cold, fever, nasal obstruction and running nose, slight red tongue, white tongue coating, floating pulse, slight red fingerprints.

Therapeutic method: To expel wind, disperse cold, strengthen the spleen and dissolve dampness.

Main formula: *Agastache Qi-Normalizing Powder* (Huo Xiang Zheng Qi San) with modification.

Commonly used herbs: *Pogostmonis Herba*(Huo Xiang), *Puerariae Radix* (Ge Gen), *Perillae Folium* (Zi Su Ye), *Angelicae Radix Dahuricae* (Bai Zhi), *Pinelliae Rhizoma* (Ban Xia), *Citri Reticulatae Pericarpium* (Chen Pi), *Poria* (Fu Ling), *Atractylodis Rhizoma* (Cang Zhu), *Magnoliae Officinalis Cortex* (Hou Pu), *Arecae Pericarpium*(Da Fu Pi), *Glycyrrhizae Radix Et Rhizoma*(Gan Cao).

Modification: For abdominal distention, add *Aucklandiae Radix* (Mu Xiang), and *Aurantii Fructus* (Zhi Qiao); for abdominal pain, add *Paeoniae Radix Albae* (Bai Shao), and *Corydalis*

3.1 常证

(1)风寒泻

证候:大便清稀,色淡夹泡沫,臭味不甚,便前腹痛肠鸣,常伴恶寒发热,鼻塞流涕。舌淡红苔白,脉浮,指纹淡红。

治法:疏风散寒,运脾化湿。

主方:藿香正气散加减。

常用药:藿香、葛根、紫苏叶、白芷、半夏、陈皮、茯苓、苍术、厚朴、大腹皮、甘草。

加减:腹胀者,加木香、枳壳;腹痛者,加白芍、延胡索;纳呆食少者,加六神曲、山楂;尿少者,加车前子、泽泻。

Rhizoma (Yan Hu Suo); for poor appetite, add *Massa Medicata Fermentata* (Liu Shen Qu), *Crataegi Fructus* (Shan Zha); for scanty urine, add *Plantaginis Semen* (Che Qian Zi), *Alismatis Rhizoma* (Ze Xie).

(2) Damp-heat diarrhea

(2) 湿热泻

Manifestations: Water-like stool, urgent in defecation, frequent and copious in quantity, foul smell, paroxysmal abdominal pain, or stool with mucus, red anus, fever, vexation, thirst, nausea, vomiting, scanty and brown urine, red tongue, yellow and slimy tongue coating, rapid and slippery pulse, purple fingerprint.

证候:大便水样,泻势急迫,量多次频,气味秽臭,腹痛阵作,或大便夹有黏液、肛门红赤、发热,烦躁口渴,恶心呕吐,小便短黄。舌质红,苔黄腻,脉滑数,指纹紫。

Therapeutic method: To clear heat and disinhibit dampness.

治法:清热利湿。

Main formula: *Pueraria, Scutellaria, and Coptis Decoction* (Ge Geng Huang Qin Huang Lian Tang)with modification.

主方:葛根黄芩黄连汤加味。

Commonly used herbs: *Puerariae Radix* (Ge Gen), *Scutellariae Radix* (Huang Qin), *Coptidis Rhizoma* (Huang Lian), *Portulacae Herba* (Ma Chi Xian), *Euphorbiae Humifusae Herba* (Di Jin Cao), *Glycyrrhizae Radix Et Rhizoma* (Gan Cao).

常用药:葛根、黄芩、黄连、马齿苋、地锦草、甘草。

Modification: For heat more severe than dampness, add *Pulsatillae Radix* (Bai Tou Wen), *Forsythiae Fructus* (Lian Qiao); for dampness severe than heat, add *Coicis Semen* (Yi Yi Ren), *Plantaginis Semen* (Che Qian Zi); for abdominal distention and fullness, add *Magnoliae Officinalis Cortex* (Hou Pu), and *Aucklandiae Radix* (Mu Xiang); for vomiting, add *Pogostmonis Herba* (Huo Xiang), and *Pinelliae Rhizoma* (Ban Xia).

加减:热重于湿者,加白头翁、连翘;湿重于热者,加薏苡仁、车前子;腹胀满者,加厚朴、木香;呕吐者,加藿香、半夏。

(3) Diarrhea by food damage

(3) 伤食泻

Manifestations: Increased defecation, mixed

证候:大便次数增多,夹

with milk-like lumps or undigested food, abdominal pain with desire for diarrhea, pain lessened after defecation, sour and malodorous like bad egg, sour belching, little or refusal of food intake, frequent foul flatus, restless night sleep, thick and slimy or yellow and grimy tongue coating, rapid and slippery pulse, purple and stagnant fingerprint.

有乳块或不消化的食物残渣，腹痛欲泻，泻后痛减，大便酸臭或如败卵，嗳气酸馊，食少或拒食，矢气频频臭秽，夜寐欠安，舌苔厚腻或黄垢，脉滑数，指纹紫滞。

Therapeutic method: To promote digestion and remove stagnation, strengthen the spleen and check diarrhea.

治法: 消食化滞，运脾止泻。

Main formula: *Harmony-Preserving pills* (Bao He Wan) with modification.

主方: 保和丸加减。

Commonly used herbs: *Crataegi Fructus* (Shan Zha), *Massa Medicinalis Fermentata* (Liu Shen Qu), *Raphani Semen* (Lai Fu Zi), *Pinelliae Rhizoma* (Ban Xia), *Poria* (Fu Ling), *Citri Reticulatae Pericarpium* (Chen Pi), *Forsythiae Fructus* (Lian Qiao), *Galli Endothelium Corneum Gigerii* (Ji Nei Jin).

常用药: 山楂、六神曲、莱菔子、半夏、茯苓、陈皮、连翘、鸡内金。

Modification: For vomiting, add *Bambusae Caulis in Taenias* (Zhu Ru), and *Amomi Fructus* (Sha Ren); for sloppy and water-like stool, add *Atractylodis Rhizoma* (Cang Zhu) and *Plantaginis Semen* (Che Qian Zi); for ungratifying defecation, add *Magnoliae Officinalis Cortex* (Hou Pu) and *Aurantii Fructus* (Zhi Qiao); for severe abdominal pain, add *Paeoniae Radix Albae* (Bai Shao) and *Aucklandiae Radix* (Mu Xiang).

加减: 呕吐者，加竹茹、砂仁；大便稀水样者，加苍术、车前子；大便不爽者，加厚朴、枳壳；腹痛较重者，加白芍、木香。

(4) Diarrhea due to spleen deficiency

(4) 脾虚泻

Manifestations: Thin and sloppy stool in light color with no stink, defecation after food intake, recurrent attack with intermittent severity, withered complexion, poor appetite, fatigued and tired spirit, pale tongue, white tongue coating, thready

证候: 大便稀溏，多于食后作泻，色淡不臭，反复发作，时轻时重，面色萎黄，食欲不振，神疲倦怠，舌淡苔白，脉细弱，指纹淡。

and weak pulse, pale fingerprints.

Therapeutic method: To fortify the spleen and disinhibit qi, strengthen the spleen and check diarrhea.

治法:健脾益气,运脾止泻。

Main formula: *Seven-Ingredient White Atractyodest Powder* (Qi Wei Bai Zhu San) with modification.

主方:七味白术散加味。

Commonly used herbs: *Codonopsis Radix* (Dang Shen), *Poria* (Fu Ling), *Atractylodis Macrocephalae Rhizoma* (Bai Zhu), *Pogostmonis Herba* (Huo Xiang), *Aucklandiae Radix* (Mu Xiang), *Puerariae Radix* (Ge Gen), *Dioscoreae Rhizoma* (Shan Yao), *Glycyrrhizae Radix Et Rhizoma* (Gan Cao).

常用药:党参、茯苓、白术、藿香、木香、葛根、山药、甘草。

Modification: For slimy tongue coating, add *Eupatorii Herba* (Pei Lan) and *Coicis Semen* (Yi Yi Ren); for poor appetite and abdominal distention, add *Massa Medicinalis Fermentata* (Liu Shen Qu), *Hordei Fructus Germinatus* (Mai Ya), and *Magnoliae Officinalis Cortex* (Hou Pu).

加减:苔腻者,加佩兰、薏苡仁;食少腹胀者,加六神曲、麦芽、厚朴。

(5) Diarrhea due to yang deficiency in the spleen and kidney

(5) 脾肾阳虚泻

Manifestations: Enduring diarrhea, thin stool, in clear and cold nature, with undigested food, or accompanied by prolapse of the rectum, cold body shape and cold limbs, lustreless complexion, listlessness, sleeping with the eyes half-closed, pale tongue and white tongue coating, deep pulse and pale fingerprints.

证候:久泻不愈,大便清稀,澄澈清冷,完谷不化,或伴脱肛,形寒,肢冷,面白无华,精神萎靡,睡时露睛,舌淡苔白,脉沉细,指纹色淡。

Therapeutic method: to fortify the spleen and warm up the kidney, induce astringenc and check diarrhea.

治法:健脾温肾,固涩止泻。

Main formula: *Aconite Center-Rectifying Decoction* (Fu Zi Li Zhong Tang) and *Four Spirits Pills* (Si Shen Wan) with modification.

主方:附子理中汤合四神丸加减。

Commonly used herbs: *Aconiti Lateralis Radix*

常用药:附子、人参、白

Praeparata (Fu Zi), *Ginseng Radix* (Ren Shen), *Atractylodis Macrocephalae Rhizoma* (Bai Zhu), *Zingiberis Rhizoma* (Gan Jiang), *Psoraleae Fructus* (Bu Gu Zhi), *Amomi Fructus Rotundus* (Bai Dou Kou), *Chebulae Fructus* (He Zi), *Schisandrae Fructus Chinensis* (Wu Wei Zi), *Glycyrrhizae Radix Et Rhizoma*(Gan Cao).

术、干姜、补骨脂、肉豆蔻、诃子、五味子、甘草。

Modification: For prolapse of the rectum, add *Astragali Radix* (Huang Qi), and *Cimicifugae Rhizoma* (Sheng Ma); for enduring diarrhea, add *Granati Pericarpium* (Shi Liu Pi), and *Halloysitum Rubrum* (Chi Shi Zhi), and *Limonitum* (Yu Yu Liang).

加减:脱肛者,加黄芪、升麻;久泻不止者,加石榴皮、赤石脂、禹余粮。

3.2 Transmuted Patterns

3.2 变证

(1) Both damage of qi and yin

(1) 气阴两伤

Manifestations: Intractable diarrhea, listlessness, lack of strength in four limbs, depression in the orbit and fontanel, dry skin, vexation, crying without tears, thirst with desire for drinks, scanty urine, or no urine, dry red lips, red tongue with little liquid, little or no tongue coating, thready and rapid pulse.

证候:泻下无度,神萎不振,四肢乏力,眼眶、囟门凹陷,皮肤干燥,心烦不安,啼哭无泪,口渴引饮,小便短少,甚则无尿,唇红而干。舌红少津,苔少或无苔,脉细数。

Therapeutic method: To boost qi and nourish yin.

治法:益气养阴。

Main formula: *Ginseng and Mume Decoction* (Ren Shen Wu Mei Tang) with modification.

主方:人参乌梅汤加减。

Commonly used herbs: *Pseudostellariae Radix* (Tai Zi Shen), *Poria* (Fu Ling), *Mume Fructus* (Wu Mei), *Nelumbinis Semen* (Lian Zi), *Dioscoreae Rhizoma* (Shan Yao), *Glycyrrhizae Radix Et Rhizoma*(Gan Cao).

常用药:太子参、茯苓、乌梅、莲子、山药、甘草。

Modification: For enduring diarrhea, add *Chebulae Fructus* (He Zi) and *Limonitum* (Yu Yu Liang); for thirst with desire for drinks, add

加减:久泻不止者,加诃子、禹余粮;口渴引饮者,加天花粉、石斛。

Trichosanthis Radix (Tian Hua Fen) and *Dendrobii Herba* (Shi Hu).

(2) Yin exhaustion and yang desertion

Manifestations: Intractable diarrhea, thin and waterlike stool, frequent defecation in large amount, listlessness, dull expression, blue and grey face or pale face, extreme cold sensation of the limbs, weak crying, low and weak breathing, pale tongue, thin and white tongue coating, thready and fine pulse.

Therapeutic method: To return yang and stop prostration.

Main formula: *Ginseng, Aconite, Dragon Bone, Oyster Shell Counterflow Decoction* (Shen Fu Long Mu Jiu Ni Tang) with modification.

Commonly used herbs: *Ginseng Radix Et Rhizoma Rubra* (Hong Shen), *Aconiti Lateralis Radix Praeparata* (Fu Zi), *Os Draconis* (Long Gu), *Ostreae Concha* (Mu Li), *Zingiberis Rhizoma* (Gan Jiang), *Atractylodis Macrocephalae Rhizoma* (Bai Zhu), and *Glycyrrhizae Radix Et Rhizoma*(Gan Cao).

Modification: For scanty urine and no tears, add *Ophiopogonis Radix* (Mai Dong) and *Schisandrae Fructus Chinensis* (Wu Wei Zi); for extreme cold sensation of the limbs and profuse sweating, immediately use *Ginseng and Aconite Injection* (Shen Fu Zhu She Ye) through intravenous drip. This disease is rather critical and must be treated by integrated therapy of traditional Chinese medicine and Western medicine.

4 Other therapies

4.1 Chinese Patent medicine

(1) *Agastache Qi-Normalizing Liquid* (Huo

(2) 阴竭阳脱

证候:泻下不止,便稀如水,次频量多,精神萎靡,表情淡漠,面色青灰或苍白,四肢厥冷,哭声微弱,气息低微,舌淡,苔薄白,脉细微欲绝。

治法:回阳固脱。

主方:参附龙牡救逆汤加减。

常用药:红参、附子、龙骨、牡蛎、干姜、白术、甘草。

加减:尿少无泪者,加麦冬、五味子;四肢厥冷,大汗淋漓者,即予参附注射液静脉滴注。本证病情危重,应中西医结合治疗。

4 其他疗法

4.1 中成药

(1) 藿香正气水:适用于

Xiang Zheng Qi Shui) is used for diahhrea in pattern of wind and cold.

风寒泻。

(2) *Puerariae, Scutellariae and Coptis Pills* (Ge Gen Qin Lian Wan) is used for diarrhea in pattern of dampness and heat.

(2) 葛根芩连丸:适用于湿热泻。

(3) *Salvation-Preserving Oral liquid* (Bao Ji Kou Fu Ye) is used for diarrhea in pattern of food damage.

(3) 保济口服液:适用于伤食泻。

(4) *Aconite Center-Rectifying Pills* (Fu Zi Li Zhong Wan) is appropriate for diarrhea in pattern of yang deficiency in the spleen and kidney.

(4) 附子理中丸:适用于脾肾阳虚泻。

4.2 Acumoxatherapy

4.2 针灸疗法

(1) Body acupuncture: Select Zusanli (ST 36), Zhongwan (CV 12), Tianshu (ST 25) and Pishu (BL 20) as main acupoints, Neiting (ST 44), Qihai (CV 6) and Quchi (LI 11) as additional acupoints. For vomiting, add Neiguan (PC 6) and Shangwan (CV 13); for abdominal distention, add Xiawan (CV 10). For excess pattern, use the reducing needling technique; for deficiency pattern, use the tonifying needling technique.

(1) 体针:主穴取足三里、中脘、天枢、脾俞。配穴取内庭、气海、曲池。呕吐者,加内关、上脘;腹胀者,加下脘。实证用泻法,虚证用补法。

(2) Moxibustion: Choose Zusanli (ST 36), Zhongwan (CV 12), Shenque (CV 8) for moxibustion, or ginger-insulated moxibustion, for diarrhea due to spleen deficiency, and diarrhea in pattern of yang deficiency in the spleen and kidney.

(2) 灸法:取足三里、中脘、神阙。艾灸或隔姜灸。适用于脾虚泻、脾肾阳虚泻。

4.3 Tuina therapy

4.3 推拿疗法

(1) Clarify Pt. Dachang, Pt. Banmen and clarify and supplement Pt. Pitu, clarify Pt. Liufu, grasp Pt. Dujiao, push Pt. Shangqijiegu, press and knead Zusanli (ST 36), for diarrhea in excessive pattern.

(1) 清大肠、清板门、清补脾土、退六腑、拿肚角、推上七节骨、按揉足三里,治疗实证泄泻。

(2) Supplement Pt. Pitu and Pt. Dachang, push Pt. Shangsanguan, rub the abdomen, push Pt.

(2) 补脾土、补大肠、推上三关、摩腹、推上七节骨、

Shangqijiegu, and pinch the spine, for diarrhea in pattern of deficiency.

捏脊,治疗虚证泄泻。

4.4 External therapy

4.4 外治疗法

(1) Grind *Galla Chinensis* (Wu Bei Zi) and *Zingiberis Rhizoma* (Gan Jiang), 10g each, plus *Euodiae Fructus* (Wu Zhu Yu) and *Caryophylli Flos* (Ding Xiang) 5g each, into fine powder, mix it with white liquor, and apply it on Shenque (CV 8), and fix and cover it with gauze, for diarrhea in pattern of deficiency and cold.

(1) 用五倍子、干姜各10克,吴茱萸、丁香各5克,共研细末,用白酒调和,贴敷神阙穴,纱布敷盖固定。适用于虚寒泄泻。

(2) Grind *Caryophylli Flos* (Ding Xiang) in one portion, *Cinnamomi Cortex* (Rou Gui) in two portions, into fine powder, and take 1～2g, each time, or make paste with ginger juice, apply on Shenque (CV 8) and cover it with gauze, for wind cold diarrhea in pattern of wind and cold, diarrhea due to spleen deficiency, and yang deficiency in the spleen and kidney.

(2) 丁香1份,肉桂2份,共研细末。每次1～2克,姜汁调成糊状,敷于神阙穴,外用胶布固定。适用于风寒泻、脾虚泻、脾肾阳虚泻。

Chapter 3 Dystrophy

第 3 章 营养障碍性疾病

Section 1 Protein-Energy Malnutrition

第 1 节 蛋白质-能量营养不良

Protein-Energy malnutrition is a deficiency disease in relation to deficiency of protein or energy due to various causes, often accompanied by functional disorders of various organs and deficiency of other nutrients. It often occurs in children under 3 years old. Clinically, it is divided into three types: emaciation type, mainly due to insufficient supply of energy, manifested by obvious reduced body weight and reduced intradermal fat; edema type, mainly due to insufficient supply of protein and manifested by edema; and emaciation-edema type, a type between the previous two types.

蛋白质-能量营养不良是由于各种原因致能量和(或)蛋白质缺乏的一种营养缺乏症,常伴有各种器官功能紊乱和其他营养素缺乏。多见于 3 岁以下婴幼儿,临床上常分为三个类型:以能量供应不足为主,表现为体重明显减轻、皮下脂肪减少者称为消瘦型;以蛋白质供应不足为主,表现为水肿者称为水肿型;介于两者之间者为消瘦-水肿型。

It belongs to the scope of "Infantile Malnutrition" in traditional Chinese medicine, clinically characterized by emaciation, lusterless face, dry and withered hair, listless spirit, vexation, and abnormal food ingestion. In ancient literature, Chinese character, "疳", for malnutrition, contains two meanings: firstly, "it is equivalent to sweet", denoting the cause of the disease, implying that children eat too much fatty, rich, sweet and heavy

本病属中医学"疳证"范畴。临床以形体消瘦,面色无华,毛发干枯,精神萎靡或烦躁不安,饮食异常为特征。古籍文献认为"疳"有两种含义:一是"疳者甘也",言其病因,指小儿因恣食肥甘厚味,损伤脾胃,形成疳证,二是"疳者干也",言其病机和主

food, damaging the spleen and stomach, and resulting in infantile malnutrition; secondly, "it means dryness", implying the pathogenesis and main patterns. In terms of duration and pathologic condition, this pattern can be divided into three types of symdromes, termed respectively as infantile malnutrition due to qi deficiency, infantile malnutrition due to accumulation, and infantile malnutrition in sign of dryness. There are other transmuted patterns.

症。结合病程和病情，可将疳证分为疳气、疳积、干疳三类证候及其他兼证。

1 Etiology and pathogenesis

It is mainly caused by improper feeding, influence of illness, or insufficiency of natural endowment, leading to damage in the spleen and stomach, exhaustion and injury of qi and body fluid, lack of resource for qi and blood formation, and lack of nourishment for organs, muscles, limbs and hundred bones.

At the beginning, the pathologic condition is not serious and emaciation is not obvious, manifested by disharmony between the spleen and stomach. This is termed as infantile malnutrition due to qi deficiency. In the middle stage, when the spleen and stomach are seriously damaged, the accumulation and stagnation, internal retention, and lack of resource for qi and blood transformation are induced, manifested by symptoms of spleen deficiency combined with accumulation, named as infantile malnutrition due to accumulation. In the late stage, when the spleen and stomach decline, the resource for qi and blood transformation is exhausted, leading to drying up of qi, blood, and body fluid and extreme deficiency and emaciation in the the whole body, named as infantile malnutrition in sign of dryness. The lingering duration of infantile malnutrition and

1 病因病机

因喂养不当、疾病影响或先天禀赋不足，导致脾胃受损，气液耗伤，气血生化无源，脏腑肌肉、四肢百骸失于濡养而成。

初起病情尚轻，形体消瘦不著，表现脾胃失和之证，称为疳气；中期脾胃受损严重，积滞内停，生化乏源，表现脾虚夹积证候，称为疳积；后期脾胃衰败，化源枯竭，气血津液干涸，全身极度虚羸，称为干疳。疳证日久，气血虚衰，必累及其他脏腑而出现诸多兼证。

deficiency and weakness in qi and blood will surely affect other organs, presenting many accompanying symptoms.

2 Key to diagnosis

(1) There is a history of insufficiency of natural endowment, longtime improper feeding or lack of care after illness.

(2) There are emaciation, lusterless face, sparse and withered hair, abnormal food ingestion, irregular defecation, distention in the epigastric region and abdomen, vexation, agitation and irascibility, devitalized spirit, with a desire to rub eyebrows and eyes, or to suck fingers and grind teeth.

(3) Body weight is 15% lower than those of the same age.

(4) Lab examination: reduced count of hemoglobin and red cells. In those accompanied by swelling, the total serum protein mostly is below 45g/L, blood albumin is below 20g/L;

(5) Grading of illness: Mild degree (malnutrition degree I), body weight is 15%～25% lower than normal value; moderate degree (malnutrition degree II), body weight is 25%～40% lower than normal value; severe degree (malnutrition degree III), body weight is over 40% lower than normal value.

3 Pattern identification and treatment

It is advisable to identify the different stages of main patterns, and to identify bowels and viscera for concurrent patterns.

At the early stage, when there is withered complexion, sparse hair, poor appetite, slightly emaci-

2 诊断要点

(1) 有先天禀赋不足，长期喂养不当或病后失调等病史。

(2) 形体消瘦，面色不华，毛发稀疏枯黄，饮食异常，大便不调，或脘腹膨胀，烦躁易怒，或精神不振，或喜揉眉擦眼，或吮指磨牙。

(3) 体重低于正常同龄儿平均值15%以上。

(4) 实验室检查：血红蛋白及红细胞减少；疳肿胀者，血清总蛋白大多在45克/升以下，血清白蛋白常在20克/升以下。

(5) 病情分级：轻度(即Ⅰ度营养不良)，体重低于正常值15%～25%；中度(即Ⅱ度营养不良)，体重低于正常值25%～40%；重度(即Ⅲ度营养不良)，体重低于正常值40%以上。

3 辨证论治

主证应辨分期，兼证辨脏腑。

初期症见面黄发疏，食欲欠佳，形体略瘦，大便不

ated body, irregular defecation, irascibility, the condition is mild and the organs are not affected, termed as infantile malnutrition due to qi deficiency. With illness going on, when there are obvious emaciation, inflated abdomen, vexation, more crying, and restless night sleep, this indicates a pattern with mixture of deficiency and excess in infantile malnutrition due to accumulation, caused by accumulation, stagnation and internal retention due to weakness and deficiency of the spleen and stomach. With further development of the pathologic condition, when manifested by extreme emaciation, old-man-like countenance, no desire for food, abdomen depressed like a boat, listless spirit, it is infantile malnutrition in sign of dryness in relation to decline of the spleen and stomach, leading to extinction of body fluid. At this stage, collapse pattern could easily occur and endanger the life.

调，易发脾气，此时病尚轻浅，未涉他脏，称为疳气；病情进展，形体明显消瘦，肚腹膨隆，烦躁多啼，夜卧不宁，此为脾胃虚弱、积滞内停、虚实夹杂之疳积；病情进一步发展，形体极度消瘦，貌似老人，杳不思食，腹凹如舟，精神萎靡，为脾胃衰败，津液消亡之干疳，此期极易发生脱证，危及生命。

If accompanied by ulcers in the mouth and tongue, feverish sensation in the chest, palms and soles, or spitting and wagging of the tongue, it is called infantile malnutrition in relation to the heart. If accompanied by nebula, dry eyes and night blindness, fear of light and tears, red eyes with much gum, it is called infantile malnutrition in relation to the liver. If accompanied by tidal feverish sensation, cough, panting and phlegm rale, enduring cough, it is called infantile malnutrition in relation to the lung. If accompanied by developmental retardness, chicken chest and turtle back, metopism and soft limbs, it is called infantile malnutrition in relation to the kidney.

若伴口舌生疮，五心烦热，或吐舌弄舌等症者，称为心疳；伴目生云翳，干涩夜盲，畏光流泪，目赤多眵等症者，称为肝疳；伴潮热咳嗽，气喘痰鸣，久咳不愈等症者，称为肺疳；伴发育迟缓，鸡胸龟背，解颅肢软等症者，称为肾疳。

The basic therapeutic principle is to fortify the spleen and boost qi. The different therapies should

以健脾益气为基本治则，根据疳证的不同阶段，采

be applied at the different stages of infantile malnutrition. For infantile malnutrition in relation to qi deficiency, it is necessary to use the harmonizing technique. For infantile malnutrition due to accumulation, it is necessary to use the dispersing technique mainly or the dispersing and supplementing techniques together. For infantile malnutrition in sign of dryness, it is necessary to use the supplementing technique. For those with concurrent symptoms, it is necessary to treat the symptoms accordingly in consideration of the main pattern. Moreover, there is a need to supplement nutrients reasonably, correct bad diet habits, and treat various primary diseases positively.

取不同的治法。疳气以和为主，疳积以消为主，或消补兼施，干疳以补为主。出现兼证者，则应结合主证，随症治之。此外，合理补充营养，纠正不良饮食习惯，积极治疗各种原发疾病。

3.1 Main patterns

(1) Infantile malnutrition due to qi deficiency

Manifestations: Slight emaciation, lusterless complexion, sparse hair, poor appetite, agitated and irascible, sloppy stool or constipation, pale tongue, thin, slightly slimy tongue coating, thready pulse, pale and purple fingerprints.

Therapeutic method: To arouse the spleen and facilitate transformation, dissolve dampness and harmonize the Middle Energizer.

Main formula: *Life-Promoting and Spleen-Fortifying Pill* (Zi Sheng Jian Pi Wan) with modification.

Commonly used herbs: *Ginseng Radix* (Ren Shen), *Atractylodis Macrocephalae Rhizoma* (Bai Zhu), *Poria* (Fu Ling), *Dioscoreae Rhizoma* (Shan Yao), *Coicis Semen* (Yi Yi Ren), *Pogostmonis Herba* (Huo Xiang), *Citri Reticulatae Pericarpium* (Chen Pi), *Amomi Fructus* (Sha Ren), *Coptidis Rhizoma* (Huang Lian), *Crataegi Fructus* (Shan

3.1 主证

（1）疳气

证候：形体略瘦，面色少华，毛发稀疏，食欲不振，精神欠佳，急躁易怒，大便或溏或秘，舌质淡，苔薄微腻，脉细，指纹淡紫。

治法：启脾助运，化湿和中。

主方：资生健脾丸加减。

常用药：人参、白术、茯苓、山药、薏苡仁、藿香、陈皮、砂仁、黄连、山楂、麦芽、豆蔻。

Zha), *Hordei Fructus Germinatus* (Mai Ya), *Amomi Fructus Rotundus* (Dou Kou).

Modification: For obvious abdominal distention, add *Aurantii Fructus Immaturus* (Zhi Shi), and *Aucklandiae Radix* (Mu Xiang); for agitation and restless sleep, add *Nelumbinis Plumula* (Lian Zi Xin), and *Picrorhizae Rhizoma* (Hu Huang Lian); for thin sloppy stool, add *Baked Zingiberis Rhizoma Recens* (Sheng Jiang), *Amomi Fructus Rotundus* (Bai Dou Kou); for constipated stool, add *Cannabis Fructus*(Huo Ma Ren) and *Cassiae Semen* (Jue Ming Zi).

加减:腹胀明显者,加枳实、木香;性情急躁,夜卧不宁者,加莲子心、胡黄连;大便稀溏者,加炮姜、肉豆蔻;大便秘结者,加火麻仁、决明子。

(2) Infantile malnutrition due to accumulation

(2) 疳积

Manifestations: Obvious emaciation, withered facial complexion, lack of luster, withered and thin limbs, abdominal distention, even with prominent green-blue veins, scanty hair like wheat ears, devitalized spirit or being irritable, agitated, restless night sleep, finger sucking, teeth grinding, eyebrow rubbing, nose picking, poor appetite, or large portion of food intake with frequent defecation, sour and foul stool, slight red tongue, slimy tongue coating, thready and deep pulse, purple and stagnant fingerprints.

证候:形体明显消瘦,面色萎黄无华,四肢枯细,肚腹膨胀,甚则青筋暴露,毛发稀疏如穗,精神不振或易烦躁激动,夜卧不宁,或伴吮指磨牙,揉眉挖鼻,食欲不振或多食多便,大便酸臭,舌质淡红,苔腻,脉沉细,指纹紫滞。

Therapeutic method: To disperse accumulation, rectify the spleen; digest food and remove accumulation.

治法:消积理脾,消食导滞。

Main formula: *Chubby Child Pill* (Fei Er Wan) with modification.

主方:肥儿丸加减。

Commonly used herbs: *Ginseng Radix* (Ren Shen), *Poria* (Fu Ling), *Atractylodis Macrocephalae Rhizoma* (Bai Zhu), *Picrorhizae Rhizoma* (Hu Huang Lian), *Coptidis Rhizoma* (Huang Lian), *Hordei Fructus Germinatus* (Mai Ya), *Massa

常用药:人参、茯苓、白术、胡黄连、黄连、麦芽、六神曲、山楂、芦荟、使君子、甘草。

Medicinalis Fermentata (Liu Shen Qu), *Crataegi Fructus* (Shan Zha), *Aloes* (Lu Hui), *Baked Zingiberis Rhizoma Recens* (Sheng Jiang), *Quisqualis Fructus* (Shi Jun Zi), *Glycyrrhizae Radix Et Rhizoma* (Gan Cao).

Modification: For obvious abdominal distention, add *Aurantii Fructus Immaturus* (Zhi Shi), *Aucklandiae Radix (Mu Xiang)*; for constipation, add *Cannabis Fructus* (Huo Ma Ren), *Pruni Semen* (Yu Li Ren); for irritability and restlessness, add *Gardeniae Fructus* (Zhi Zi) and *Nelumbinis Plumula* (Lian Zi Xin); for hyperorexia with easy hunger, add *Forsythiae Fructus* (Lian Qiao), and *Scutellariae Radix* (Huang Qin); for thirst with desire for drinking, add *Dendrobii Herba* (Shi Hu)and *Trichosanthis Radix* (Tian Hua Fen); for predilection for strange food, rubbing eyebrow, picking nose, or sucking fingers and grinding teeth, or stool with worm, add *Meliae Cortex* (Ku Lian Pi), *Torreyae Semen* (Fei Zi); for abdomen with prominent green-blue veins, and lumps at rid side, add *Salviae Miltiorrhizae Radix Et Rhizoma* (Dan Shen), and *Manis Squama* (Chuan Shan Jia).

加减：腹胀明显者，加枳实、木香；大便秘结者，加火麻仁、郁李仁；烦躁不安者，加栀子、莲子心；多食易饥者，加连翘、黄芩；口渴喜饮者，加石斛、天花粉；嗜食异物，揉眉挖鼻，或吮指磨牙，或大便下虫者，加苦楝皮、榧子；腹部青筋暴露，胁下痞块者，加丹参、穿山甲。

(3) Infantile malnutrition in sign of dryness

Manifestations: Extreme emaciation, old-man-like countenance, dry and withered skin with wrinkles, lusterless complexion, dry hair, disvitalized spirit, weak crying, depressed abdomen like a boat, no thought of food, sloppy stool or constipation, pale and tender tongue, little tongue coating, thready and weak pulse, slight red fingerprints.

Therapeutic method: To supplement qi and blood, restore the resource for transformation.

Main formula: *Eight-Gem Decoction* (Ba Zhen

(3) 干疳

证候：形体极度消瘦，面呈老人貌，皮肤干瘪起皱，面色无华，毛发干枯，精神萎靡，啼哭无力，腹凹如舟，杳不思食，大便稀溏或便秘，舌质淡嫩，苔少，脉细弱，指纹淡红。

治法：补益气血，以复化源。

主方：八珍汤加减。

Tang) with modification.

Commonly used herbs: *Angelicae Sinensis Radix* (Dang Gui), *Chuanxiong Rhizoma* (Chuan Xiong), *Arecae Semen* (Bing Lang), *Paeoniae Radix Albae* (Bai Shao), *Ginseng Radix* (Ren Shen), *Atractylodis Macrocephalae Rhizoma* (Bai Zhu), *Poria* (Fu Ling), *Glycyrrhizae Radix Et Rhizoma* (Gan Cao).

常用药:当归、川芎、熟地黄、白芍、人参、白术、茯苓、甘草。

Modification: For bright pale facial complexion, cold sensation in the four limbs, sloppy stool, remove *Rehmanniae Radix Praeparata* (Shu Di Huang) and *Angelicae Sinensis Radix* (Dang Gui), add *Cinnamomi Cortex* (Rou Gui) and *Baked Zingiberis Rhizoma Recens* (Sheng Jiang); for restless night sleep, add *Schisandrae Fructus Chinensis* (Wu Wei Zi), and *Polygoni Multiflori* Caulis (Shou Wu Teng); for dry and red tongue, no tongue coating, add *Mume Fructus* (Wu Mei), *Dendrobii Herba* (Shi Hu); for no thought of food, add *Citri Reticulatae Pericarpium* (Chen Pi), and *Amomi Fructus* (Sha Ren); for bright pale facial complexion, weak breathing, extreme cold limbs, and weak pulse likely to disappear, take *Ginseng, Aconite, Dragon Bone, and Oyster Shell Counterflow Stemming Decoction* (Shen Fu Long Mu Jiu Ni Tang) immediately for emergency, and transfer for treatment by integrated therapy of Western medicine and Chinese medicine.

加减:面色皖白,四肢欠温,大便溏薄者,去熟地黄、当归,加肉桂、炮姜;夜寐不安者,加五味子、首乌藤;舌干红,无苔者,加乌梅、石斛;杳不思食者,加陈皮、砂仁;面色苍白,呼吸微弱,四肢厥冷,脉微欲绝者,应急服参附龙牡救逆汤,并采取中西医结合抢救。

3.2 Transmuted Patterns

3.2 兼证

(1) Infantile malnutrition in relation to the eyes

(1) 眼疳

Manifestations: Dry eyes, fear of light, red and putrifying eye corners, nebula, even turbid eyeballs, acute conjunctivitis, and blurred vision at night.

证候:两目干涩,畏光羞明,眼角赤烂,目睛失泽,甚至黑睛混浊,白睛生翳,夜间视物不清。

Therapeutic method: To nourish the blood and emolliate the liver, enrich yin and brighten the eyes.

治法:养血柔肝,滋阴明目。

Main formula: *Dendrobium Night Vision Pill* (Shi Hu Ye Guang Wan) with modification.

主方:石斛夜光丸加减。

Commonly used herbs: *Dendrobii Herba* (Shi Hu), *Ginseng Radix* (Ren Shen), *Poria* (Fu Ling), *Ophiopogonis Radix* (Mai Dong), *Rehmanniae Radix Praeparata* (Shu Di Huang), *Lycii Fructus* (Gou Qi Zi), *Cuscutae Semen* (Tu Si Zi), *Chrysanthemi Flos* (Ju Hua), *Cassiae Semen* (Jue Ming Zi).

常用药:石斛、人参、茯苓、麦冬、熟地黄、生地黄、枸杞子、菟丝子、菊花、决明子。

Modification: For night blindness, add *Goat's Liver Pill* (Yang Gan Wan).

加减:夜盲者,加服羊肝丸。

(2) Infantile malnutrition in relation the mouth

(2) 口疳

Manifestations: Ulceration in the mouth and tongue, even erosion in the oral cavity, in foul smell, flushed face and lips, vexation and crying, restless fright and fear, restless night sleep, scanty and yellow urine, or spitting and wagging of tongue.

证候:口舌生疮,甚或口腔糜烂,秽臭难闻,面赤唇红,烦躁哭闹,惊惕不安,夜卧不宁,小便短黄,或吐舌、弄舌。

Therapeutic method: To clarify the heart and drain fire, enrich yin and engender body fluid.

治法:清心泻火,滋阴生津。

Main formula: *Heart-Draining and Red-Abducting Powder* (Xie Xin Dao Chi San) with modification.

主方:泻心导赤散加减。

Commonly used herbs: *Coptidis Rhizoma* (Huang Lian), *Lophatheri Herba* (Dan Zhu Ye), *Rehmanniae Radix Cruda* (Sheng Di Huang), *Talcum* (Hua Shi), *Polygonati Odorati Rhizoma* (Yu Zhu), *Dendrobii Herba* (Shi Hu), *Glycyrrhizae Radix Et Rhizoma* (Gan Cao).

常用药:黄连、淡竹叶、生地黄、滑石、玉竹、石斛、甘草。

(3) Tumefaction in infantile malnutrition

(3) 疳肿胀

Manifestations: Edema in foot and ankle, even in the whole body, depressed edema, lack of

证候:足踝浮肿,甚则全身浮肿,按之凹陷难起,四肢

warmth in the four limbs, inhibited urination.

欠温，小便不利。

Therapeutic method: To warm up yang and strengthen the spleen, disinhibit water and disperse swelling.

治法：温阳运脾，利水消肿。

Main formula: *True Warrior Decoction* (Zhen Wu Tang) with modification.

主方：真武汤加减。

Commonly used herbs: *Aconiti Lateralis Radix Praeparata* (Fu Zi), *Atractylodis Macrocephalae Rhizoma* (Bai Zhu), *Poria* (Fu Ling), *Paeoniae Radix Albae* (Bai Shao), *Zingiberis Rhizoma Recens* (Sheng Jiang).

常用药：附子、白术、茯苓、白芍、生姜。

Modification: For obvious swelling, add *Stephaniae Tetrandrae Radix* (Fang Ji), *Alismatis Rhizoma* (Ze Xie), and *Astragali Radix* (Huang Qi).

加减：水肿明显者，加防己、泽泻、黄芪。

4 Other therapies

4 其他疗法

4.1 Chinese Patent medicine

4.1 中成药

(1) *Chubby Child Pills* (Fei Er Wan) is used for patterns of infantile malnutrition and mild cases of infantile malnutrition due to accumulation.

（1）肥儿丸：适用于疳气证及疳积轻证。

(2) *Child Tangarine Elixir* (Xiao Er Xiang Ju Dan) is used for pattern of infantile malnutrition due to accumulation.

（2）小儿香橘丹：适用于疳积证。

(3) *Perfect Major Supplementation Pills* (Shi Quan Da Bu Wan) is used for infantile malnutrition in sign of dryness.

（3）十全大补丸：适用于干疳证。

(4) *Borneol and Borax Powder* (Bing Peng San) is used for infantile malnutrition in relation to the mouth.

（4）冰硼散：适用于口疳证。

4.2 External therapy

4.2 外治疗法

(1) Grind *Natrii Sulfas* (Mang Xiao), *Rhei Radix Et Rhizoma* (Da Huang), *Gardeniae Fructus* (Zhi Zi), *Armeniacae Semen Amarum* (Ku Xing

（1）芒硝、大黄、栀子、苦杏仁、桃仁各 6 克。共为细末，加面粉适量，用鸡蛋清、

Ren), *Persicae Semen* (Tao Ren) 6g each, together into fine powder, add adequate flour, mix with a little of each of the followings: egg white, Bulbus Allii Fistulosi (Cong Bai) juice, vinegar, white liquor. Make paste, and apply to the umbilicus, once every day, for 3 to 5 days, suitable for pattern of infantile malnutrition due to accumulation.

葱白汁、醋、白酒各少许，调成糊状，敷于脐部。每日1次，连用3～5日。用于疳积证。

(2) Grind moderate quantity of *Raphani Semen* (Lai Fu Zi) into powder, mix with water, and apply to Shenque (CV 8), once every day, 7 days as one course, for pattern of infantile malnutrition due to accumulation.

(2) 莱菔子适量研末，用水调和，外敷于神阙，每日1次，7日为1个疗程。用于疳积证。

4.3 Tuina Therapy

4.3 推拿疗法

(1) Supplement Pt. Pijing, tonify Pt. Shenjing, push Pt. Bagua, knead Pt. Banmen, Zusanli (ST 36), Weishu (BL 21), and rub abdomen, for pattern of infantile malnutrition due to qi deficiency.

(1) 补脾经，补肾经，运八卦，揉板门、足三里、胃俞，摩腹。适用于疳气证。

(2) Supplement Pt. Pijing, clarify Pt. Weijing, Pt. Xinjing and Pt. Ganjing, knead Pt. Xiaotianxin, rub Zhongwan (CV 12), push hand yin and hand yang divergently, for pattern of infantile malnutrition due to accumulation.

(2) 补脾经，清胃经、心经、肝经，捣小天心，揉中脘，分推手阴阳。适用于疳积证。

(3) Supplement Pt. Pijing, tonify Pt. Shenjing, rub Pt. Banmen, push the four transverse creases, rub Zhongwan (CV 12), rub abdomen, rub Pt. Erma, rub and press Zusanli (ST 36), for pattern of infantile malnutrition in sign of dryness.

(3) 补脾经、肾经，揉板门，推四横纹，揉中脘，摩腹，揉二马，按揉足三里。适用于干疳证。

The above-mentioned methods are applied once every day, for 20-30 min every day, 7-10 days as one course.

上述方法，每日1次，每次20～30分钟，7～10日为1个疗程。

4.4 Spine-Pinching therapy

4.4 捏脊疗法

The sick child lies down in prone position, with back bare, both sides along the spine and the spine will be pinched. The doctor puts the radial sides of

患儿俯卧，裸露背部。捏脊部位为脊柱及其两侧，医者用两拇指桡侧面置尾骶

both thumbs on the skin of the sacrococcygeal region and pinches up the skin with the index and middle finger together with the thumb forcefully to roll up the skin forward by the both hands to Dazhui (GV 14). After doing this for three times, pull up the skin once after every 3 pinches all the way to Dazhui (GV 14). Repeat this three times. It is done once every day, used for pattern of infantile malnutrition due to qi deficiency, and pattern of infantile malnutrition due to accumulation.

部皮肤，食、中指前与拇指相对用力捏起皮肤，双手分别捻动向前推移到大椎穴止。重复 3 遍后，再每捏 3 把，将皮肤提起 1 次，直至大椎穴，如此反复 3 遍。每日 1 次。可用于治疗疳气证、疳积证。

4.5 Acumoxatherapy

Select Zhongwan (CV 12), Zusanli (ST 36), and Sifeng (EX-UE10) as major acupoints, and Pishu (BL 20) and Weishu (BL 21) as additional acupoints. For distention and fullness in the epigastric region and abdomen, add Sifeng (EX-UE10). For vexation and agitation, and restless night sleep, add Shenmen (HT 7) and Neiguan (PC 6). Puncture the acupoints with moderate stimulation by in-and-out needling technique, once every day, 7 days as one course. It is used for pattern of infantile malnutrition due to qi deficiency, and mild cases of infantile malnutrition due to accumulation.

4.5 针灸疗法

主穴取中脘、足三里、四缝；配穴取脾俞、胃俞。脘腹胀满者，加刺四缝；烦躁不安，夜眠不宁者，加神门、内关。中等刺激，不留针。每日 1 次，7 日为 1 个疗程。适用于疳气证、疳积轻证。

4.6 Prick Sifeng (EX-UE10)

Sifeng (EX-UE10) is located in the middle sections of index finger, middle finger, ring finger and little finger. After local disinfection, prick Sifeng (EX-UE 10) for about 0.1 inch with a three-edged needle or thick filiform needle, and squeeze yellowish and white mucus, once every day, till no more mucus. It is used for pattern of infantile malnutrition due to qi deficiency, and pattern of infantile malnutrition due to accumulation.

4.6 刺四缝疗法

四缝穴位于食、中、无名及小指四指中节。局部消毒后，用三棱针或粗毫针针刺四缝穴约一分深，刺后用手挤出黄白色黏液，每日 1 次，直到针刺后不再有黄白色黏液挤出为止。用于疳气证、疳积证。

Section 2 Nutritional Iron Deficiency Anemia

第 2 节　营养性缺铁性贫血

Nutritional iron deficiency anemia is a microcytic hypochromic anemia caused by iron deficiency, resulting in reduced hemoglobin synthesis. Clinically differences are manifestated by different severity of anemia. There are no subjective symptoms in the mild cases, In the medium cases, there are dizziness, lack of strength, poor appetite, vexation, etc, plus pallor in facial complexion, nails, mouth, lips, and palpebral conjunctiva in varying degrees.

It often happens in the infants, especially in those between 6 months old and 2 years old. Generally the prognosis is good, but enduring anemia, lack of nourishment in the internal organs and poor anti-pathogenic ability would result in other diseases. It belongs to the scope of "blood deficiency" in traditional Chinese medicine.

营养性缺铁性贫血，是由于体内铁元素缺乏致使血红蛋白合成减少而引起的一种小细胞低色素性贫血。临床表现因贫血程度不同而异，轻者可无自觉症状，中度以上者可出现头晕乏力、纳呆、烦躁等症，并有不同程度的面色、指甲口唇和睑结膜苍白。

多见于婴幼儿，尤以 6 个月～2 岁最常见。一般预后较好，但长期贫血，脏腑失养，抗病力弱，易生他疾。本病属于中医学"血虚"范畴。

1 Etiology and pathogenesis

The cause is mainly related to prenatal natural endowment, improper feeding, and influence from other diseases.

Weak body constitution of the pregnant mother, plus deficiency in qi and blood, improper care in pregnancy or premature delivery, multiple fetuses, and injury of fetal origin would impact the growth and development of the fetus, leading to prenatal insufficiency of the kidney essence deficiency and deficiency of qi and blood, and hence anemia. If breast milk is insufficient, or the supplementary

1 病因病机

病因主要有先天禀赋不足、后天喂养不当及他病影响。

孕母体弱，气血不足，或孕期调护不当，或早产、多胎，胎元受损等，均可影响胎儿生长发育，导致先天肾精不足、气血匮乏而发生本病。若母乳不足，或未及时添加辅食，或偏食少食，则致精微乏源，无以化生气血，而成贫

food is not added in time, or particular foods are indulged or no enough portion of food is ingested, there will be a lack of resource of the essences for transformation of qi and blood, which leads to anemia. The disease could also happen due to injury and consumption of qi and blood after severe and lingering illness, or deficiency and weakness of the spleen and stomach due to lack of recuperation after illness, or profuse loss of blood after traumatic injury or prolonged loss of small quantity of blood, leading to no transformation of essence, blood and body fluid.

血。大病久病之后,气血耗伤,或病后失调,脾胃虚弱,或外伤失血过多或长期小量失血,皆致精血津液无以化生,而成本病。

The diseased location is in the spleen and kidney, involving the heart and liver. The main pathological foundation lies in that the spleen is deficient and fails to transform and produe qi and blood, the kidney is deficient and fails to replenish essence and produce blood and that blood is deficient and fails to perform its nourishing ability.

病位主要在脾肾,可涉心肝,脾虚不能化生气血,肾虚不能填精生血,血虚不荣为其主要病理基础。

2 Key to diagnosis

(1) There is a history of insufficient supply and poor absorption of iron, or chronic blood loss.

(2) It is characterized by gradual onset, gradual pallor or pallor and yellow color in the skin mucus, more obvious in the mouth, lips, mucous membrane of the oral cavity and nail bed, and low spirit, lack of strength, and loss of appetite, and dizziness in the elderly children, and probably hepatosplenomegaly in some sick children.

(3) Lab test

1) Routine test of peripheral blood: hemoglobin< 110g/L, mean cell hemoglobin concentration (MCHC) < 0.31%, mean corpuscular volume (MCV) < 80fl,

2 诊断要点

(1) 铁供给不足、吸收障碍或慢性失血等病史。

(2) 发病缓慢,皮肤黏膜逐渐苍白或苍黄,以口唇、口腔黏膜及甲床最为明显,神疲乏力,食欲减退。年长儿有头晕等症状。部分患儿可有肝脾肿大。

(3) 实验室检查

1) 外周血常规:血红蛋白<110 g/L,平均血红蛋白浓度<0.31%,红细胞平均体

mean cell hemoglobin (MCH)<26pg. The reticulocyto count is normal or slightly reduced.

2) Myelogram: Erythron hyerplasia is active, mainly intermediate or late erythroblast. The red blood cells volume is relatively small at various stages, with less cytoplasm and blue dye. The granulocyte and megakaryocytic series usually are normal.

3) Iron metabolism: serum ferritin<12μg/L, free erythrocyte protoporphyrin>0.9mol/L, serum iron<10.7μmol/L, total iron binding capacity>62.7μmol/L, transferrin saturation<15%.

(4) Effective iron treatment.

(5) Degree of conditions

1) Mild: hemoglobin in 90～110g/L in those from 6 months old to 6 years old, 90～120g/L in those above 6 years old, red blood cell in (3～4)×10^{12}/L

2) Medium: hemoglobin in 60～90g/L, red blood cell in (2～3)×10^{12}/L

3) Severe: hemoglobin in 30～60g/L, red blood cell in (1～2)×10^{12}/L

4) Very severe: hemoglobin in <30g/L, red blood cell in <1×10^{12}/L

3　Pattern identification and treatment

Pattern identification by the theory of bowels and viscera: Poor appetite, fatigue, lack of strength, and irregular defecation show the involve-

积<80 fl，平均血红蛋白<26 pg。网红细胞数正常或轻度减少。

2）骨髓象：红细胞系增生活跃，以中、晚幼红细胞为主，各期红细胞体积均较小，胞质少，染色偏蓝；粒细胞系及巨核细胞系一般正常。

3）铁代谢：血清铁蛋白<12 μg/L，红细胞游离原卟啉>0.9 μmol/L，血清铁<10.7 μmol/L，总铁结合力>62.7 μmol/L，转铁蛋白饱和度<15%。

（4）铁剂治疗有效。

（5）病情分度

1）轻度：血红蛋白 6 个月～6 岁，90～110 g/L；6 岁以上 90～120 g/L。红细胞(3～4)×10^{12}/L。

2）中度：血红蛋白 60～90 g/L；红细胞(2～3)×10^{12}/L。

3）重度：血红蛋白 30～60 g/L；红细胞(1～2)×10^{12}/L。

4）极重度：血红蛋白<30 g/L；红细胞<1×10^{12}/L。

3　辨证论治

脏腑辨证为主：食少纳呆，体倦乏力，大便不调，病位在脾；腰腿酸软，畏寒肢

ment of the spleen pathologically. Soreness and weakness in the lumbus and legs, aversion to cold and cold limbs, and retarded development show the involment of the kidney pathologically. Palpitation, flusteredness, restless night sleep, and weak voice show the involvement of the heart pathologically. Dizziness and dry eyes, tidal feverish sensation, night sweating, dry and crisp nails show the involvement of the liver pathologically.

冷,发育迟缓,病位在肾;心悸心慌,夜寐欠安,语声不振,病及于心;头晕目涩,潮热盗汗,爪甲枯脆,病及于肝。

The disease is mainly deficient. Therefore, the basic treatment principle is to rectify insufficiency and develop the spleen and kidney, transform and engender qi and blood. For patterns of weak spleen and stomach, the focus is to fortify the spleen and engender blood. In treating other patterns, it is necessary to take care of the spleen and stomach and to offer supplementation without inducing stagnation, instead of blind tonification. Besides, it is necessary to correct bad diet habits, regulate diet properly, and avoid the causative factors positively.

病以虚为主,因此,补其不足,培其脾肾,化生气血是基本治则。脾胃虚弱证当以健脾生血为主;其他各证也要注意顾护脾胃,补而不滞,不可一味滋补。同时,要纠正不良饮食习惯,合理安排饮食,积极消除病因。

(1) Deficiency and weakness of the spleen and stomach

(1) 脾胃虚弱

Manifestations: Sallow complexion, pale lips and white nails, fatigued spirit and lack of strength, poor appetite, slack muscles, irregualr defecation, pale tongue, white tongue coating, thready and weak pulse, slight red fingerprints.

证候:面色苍黄,唇淡甲白,神疲乏力,食欲不振,肌肉松弛,大便不调,舌质淡,苔白,脉细无力,指纹淡红。

Therapeutic method: To fortify and strengthen the spleen and stomach, boost qi and nourish blood.

治法:健运脾胃,益气养血。

Main formula: *Six Gentlemen Decoction* (Liu Jun Zi Tang) with modification.

主方:六君子汤加减。

Commonly used herbs: *Codonopsis Radix* (Dang Shen), *Atractylodis Macrocephalae Rhizoma* (Bai Zhu), *Poria* (Fu Ling), *Citri Reticulatae*

常用药:党参、白术、茯苓、陈皮、半夏、大枣、甘草。

Pericarpium (Chen Pi), *Pinelliae Rhizoma* (Ban xia), *Jujubae Fructus* (Da Zao), *Glycyrrhizae Radix Et Rhizoma*(Gan Cao).

Modification: For poor appetite, add *Crataegi Fructus* (Shan Zha), *Fructus Oryzae Germinatus* (Gu Ya), and *Galli Endothelium Corneum Gigerii* (Ji Nei Jin); for constipation, add *Angelicae Sinensis Radix* (Dang Gui), *Semen Platycladi* (Bai Zi Ren), and *Cannabis Fructus*(Huo Ma Ren); for sloppy stool with undigested food, add *Zingiberis Rhizoma* (Gan Jiang), *Euodiae Fructus* (Wu Zhu Yu), and *Dioscoreae Rhizoma* (Shan Yao); for abdominal distention, add *Arecae Semen* (Bin Lang), and *Aucklandiae Radix* (Mu Xiang); for recurrent infection of exogenous pathogens, add *Jade Wind-Barrier Powder* (Yu Ping Feng San).

加减:纳呆者,加山楂、谷芽、鸡内金;便秘者,加当归、柏子仁、火麻仁;便溏食物不化者,加干姜、吴茱萸、山药;腹胀者,加槟榔、木香;反复外感者,合玉屏风散。

(2) Deficiency in both the heart and spleen

(2) 心脾两虚

Manifestations: Withered or pale complexion, pale lips and nails, yellow and scanty hair, occasional dizziness and palpitation, restless night sleep, short breathing and no desire to speak, fatigue and lack of strength, poor appetite, lack of concentration, slight red tongue, thready and weak pulse, slight red fingerprints.

证候:面色萎黄或苍白,唇淡甲白,发黄稀疏,时有头晕,心悸,夜寐不安,气短懒言,体倦乏力,食欲不振,注意力涣散,舌质淡红,脉细弱,指纹淡红。

Therapeutic method: To supplement the spleen and nourish the heart, boost qi and engender blood.

治法:补脾养心,益气生血。

Main formula: *Spleen-Returning Decoction* (Gui Pi Tang) with modification.

主方:归脾汤加减。

Commonly used herbs: *Atractylodis Macrocephalae Rhizoma* (Bai Zhu), *Angelicae Sinensis Radix* (Dang Gui), *Poria* (Fu Ling), *Astragali Radix* (Huang Qi), *Longan Arillus* (Long Yan Rou), *Polygalae Radix* (Yuan Zhi), *Ziziphi Spinosi Semen* (Suan Zao Ren), *Aucklandiae Radix* (Mu Xiang),

常用药:白术、当归、茯苓、黄芪、龙眼肉、远志、酸枣仁、木香、甘草、人参。

Glycyrrhizae Radix Et Rhizoma (Gan Cao), *Ginseng Radix* (Ren Shen).

Modification: For obvious blood deficiency, add *Spatholobi Caulis* (Ji Xue Teng), and *Paeoniae Radix Albae* (Bai Shao); for poor appetite and sloppy stool, remove *Angelicae Sinensis Radix* (Dang Gui) and add *Atractylodis Rhizoma* (Cang Zhu), *Citri Reticulatae Pericarpium* (Chen Pi) *Crataegi Fructus Ustus* (Jiao Shan Zha); for palpitation and restless night sleep, add *Semen Platycladi* (Bai Zi Ren), and *Ziziphi Spinosi Semen* (Suan Zao Ren); for copious sweating by exertion, add *Tritici Levis Fructus* (Fu Xiao Mai), *Ostreae Concha Calcinata* (Duan Mu Li).

加减:血虚明显者,加鸡血藤、白芍;纳呆便溏者,去当归,加苍术、陈皮、焦山楂;心悸、夜寐不安者,加柏子仁、酸枣仁;活动后多汗者,加浮小麦、煅牡蛎。

(3) Yin deficiency in the liver and kidney

(3) 肝肾阴虚

Manifestation: Pale complexion, white and crisp nails, withered hair, retarded development, dizziness and dry eyes, night sweating, vexation, sleeplessness, tremor in the four limbs, pale tongue, little or peeled tongue coating, thready and rapid pulse, slight purple fingerprints.

证候:面色苍白,爪甲色白易脆,毛发枯黄,发育迟缓,头晕目涩,盗汗,烦躁失眠,四肢震颤,舌质淡,苔少或光剥,脉细数,指纹淡紫。

Therapeutic method: To nourish the kidney and liver, adjust and supplement essence and blood.

治法:滋养肝肾,调补精血。

Main formula: *Kidney Pills* (Zuo Gui Wan) with modification.

主方:左归丸加减。

Commonly used herbs: *Rehmanniae Radix Praeparata* (Shu Di Huang), *Dioscoreae Rhizoma* (Shan Yao), *Lycii Fructus* (Gou Qi Zi), *Corni Fructus* (Shan Zhu Yu), *Achyranthis Bidentatae Radix* (Niu Xi), *Cuscutae Semen* (Tu Si Zi), Cervi Cornu Colla (Lu Jiao Jiao), *Testudinis Carapacis Et Plastri Colla* (Gui Jia Jiao).

常用药:熟地黄、山药、枸杞子、山茱萸、牛膝、菟丝子、鹿角胶、龟甲胶。

Modification: For tidal feverish sensaiton and night sweating, add *Lycii Cortex* (Di Gu Pi),

加减:潮热盗汗者,加地骨皮、鳖甲、白薇;发育迟缓

Trionycis Carapax Et Rhizoma (Bie Jia) and *Cynanchi Atrati Radix Et Rhizoma* (Bai Wei); for retarded development, add *Placenta Hominis* (Zi He Che), *Alpiniae Oxyphyllae Fructus* (Yi Zhi); for dry eyes, add *Dendrobii Herba* (Shi Hu), and *Vespertilionis Faeces* (Ye Ming Sha); for tremor in the four limbs, add *Paeoniae Radix Albae* (Bai Shao), *Uncariae ramulus Cum uncis* (Gou Teng), *Lumbricus* (Di Long).

者,加紫河车、益智仁;眼目干涩者,加石斛、夜明砂;四肢震颤者,加白芍、钩藤、地龙。

(4) Yang deficiency of the spleen and kidney

(4) 脾肾阳虚

Manifestations: Bright pale complexion, pale nails, scanty and yellow hair, listlessness, aversion to cold, cold limbs, shortness of breathing and reluctance to move, poor appetite, sloppy stool, or undigested food, emaciation, swollen body, retarded development, pale tongue, white tongue coating, flabby and tender tongue, deep, thready and forceless pulse, pale fingerprints.

证候:面色㿠白,爪甲苍白,发黄稀少,精神萎靡,畏寒肢冷,气少懒动,纳呆便溏,或完谷不化,形体消瘦或浮肿,发育迟缓,舌质淡,苔白,舌体胖嫩,脉沉细无力,指纹淡。

Therapeutic method: To warm up and supplement the spleen and kidney, replenish essence and nourish blood.

治法:温补脾肾,填精养血。

Main formula: *Vital Gate Pills* (You Gui Wan) with modification

主方:右归丸加减。

Commonly used herbs: *Rehmanniae Radix Praeparata* (Shu Di Huang), *Dioscoreae Rhizoma* (Shan Yao), *Corni Fructus* (Shan Zhu Yu), *Lycii Fructus* (Gou Qi Zi), Cervi Cornu Colla (Lu Jiao Jiao), *Cuscutae Semen* (Tu Si Zi), *Eucommiae Cortex* (Du Zhong), *Angelicae Sinensis Radix* (Dang Gui), *Cinnamomi Cortex* (Rou Gui), *Aconiti Lateralis Radix Praeparata* (Fu Zi).

常用药:熟地黄、山药、山茱萸、枸杞子、鹿角胶、菟丝子、杜仲、当归、肉桂、附子。

Modification: For sloppy stool and diarrhea, remove *Rehmanniae Radix Praeparata* (Shu Di Huang), add *Atractylodis Macrocephalae Rhizoma*

加减:大便溏泄者,去熟地黄,加白术、炮姜、肉豆蔻;下肢浮肿者,加薏苡仁、茯

(Bai Zhu), *Zingiberis Rhizoma Praeparatum* (Pao Jiang), and *Amomi Fructus Rotundus* (Rou Dou Kou); for edema in the lower limbs, add *Coicis Semen* (Yi Yi Ren), *Poria* (Fu Ling), and *Polyporus* (Zhu Ling); for cold sweating, extreme cold limbs and fine pulse, and progressive desertion of yang qi, take *Ginseng, Aconite, Dragon Bone, Oyster Shell Counterflow Decoction* (Shen Fu Long Mu Jiu Ni Tang) immediately.

苓、猪苓。若冷汗肢厥脉微，阳气欲脱则急予参附龙牡救逆汤。

4 Other therapies

4.1 Chinese Patent medicine

(1) *Child Blood Engendering Syrup* (Xiao Er Sheng Xue Tang Jiang) is appropriate for various patterns of anemia.

(2) *Spleen-Fortifying and Blood-Engendering Granule* (Jian Pi Sheng Xue Ke Li) is appropriate for pattern of deficiency and weakness in the spleen, and pattern of deficiency in the heart and spleen.

(3) *Children Blood-Enhancing Granules* (Xiao Er Sheng Xue Ling) is appropriate for pattern of deficiency and weakness in the spleen, and pattern of deficiency in the heart and spleen.

(4) *Compound Donkey-Hide Glue Liquid* (Fu Fang E Jiao Jiang) is appropriate for pattern of deficiency in the heart and spleen.

4.2 Tuina Therapy

Push and supplement Pt. Pijing, push Pt. Sanguan, tonify Pt. Xinjing, knead yin and yang of hand divergently, press Pt. Neibagua, rub Zusanli (ST 36), rub abdomen, rub Xuehai (CV 4), pinch up the spine, once every day, 10 days as one course, rest three to five days after each session and before

4 其他疗法

4.1 中成药

(1) 小儿生血糖浆:适用于贫血各证。

(2) 健脾生血颗粒:适用于贫血脾胃虚弱证、心脾两虚证。

(3) 小儿升血灵:适用于贫血脾胃虚弱证、心脾两虚证。

(4) 复方阿胶浆:适用于贫血心脾两虚证。

4.2 推拿疗法

推补脾经，推三关，补心经，分手阴阳，运内八卦，揉足三里，摩腹，揉血海，捏脊。每日 1 次，10 日为 1 个疗程，每个疗程后休息 3～5 日继续治疗。

next session.

4.3 Acumoxatherapy

Select Geshu (BL 17), Zusanli (ST 36), Yinbai (SF 1), and Sanyinjiao (SP 6) as the main acupoints, and Qihai (CV 4) and Mingmen (GV 4) as additional acupoints, and puncture by supplementing method, once every day, plus moxibustion after acupuncture, for 10 days as one course. Moxibustion can be applied alone.

4.3 针灸疗法

取膈俞、足三里、隐白、三阴交为主穴，配气海、命门。采用补法，每日针1次，针后加灸。10日为1个疗程。亦可单用灸法。

Section 3 Vitamin D Deficiency Rickets

第3节 维生素D缺乏性佝偻病

Vitamin D deficiency rickets is characterized by general chronic deficiency due to insufficiency of vitamin D in children, resulting in metabolic disorder of calcium and phosphorus, which further leads to failed calcification of the growes epiphyseal cartilage plate, and hence causes epiphysis lesions.

维生素D缺乏性佝偻病是由于儿童体内维生素D不足，致使钙磷代谢失常，以致正在生长的骨骺端软骨板不能正常钙化，造成骨骺病变为特征的全身慢性营养性疾病。

The infants under 2 years old, especially under one year old, because of quick growth of the phyqiues and lack of outdoor activities, are the high risk population prone to the disease. Because the winter lasts long, and time of sunshine is short in northern regions, the incidence rate there is obviously higher than that in the southern regions. Most children are mild in their problem, and the proper treatment will produce a good prognosis. The severe condition could leave over skeleton deformity, affecting normal development of children.

2岁以下婴幼儿、特别是1岁以内小婴儿，体格生长快，户外活动少，是易发本病的高危人群。北方地区冬季长，日照短，发病率明显高于南方。多数患儿属轻症，治疗得当，一般预后良好。重者可遗留骨骼畸形，影响儿童正常发育。

This disease is related to many problems in Chinese medicine, "like five types of retardation",

本病与中医学"五迟""五软""夜啼""汗证""龟背"

"five types of flaccidity", "night crying", "sweating pattern", "turtle back" and "chicken chest".

"鸡胸"等多种病证相关。

1 Etiology and pathogenesis

The main cause is related to prenatal insufficiency of natural endowment and inappropriate postnatal care. The pathogenesis lies in the spleen and kidney deficiency, involving the heart, lung, and liver. Insufficient kidney qi and unfirm bones will result in soft bones and retarded growth, delayed closing of fontanel, slow growing of teeth, deformed chest and back, curled limbs and body. The failure of the spleen in performing the healthy transportation and the failure of the earth in engendering the metal would induce deficiency and depletion of the lung qi, leading to soft and weak muscles, scanty and sparse hair, and copious sweating. When yin blood of liver is insufficient and liver yang is effulgent, there would be vexation and night crying. When the tendons and meridians are not fully nourished, it will lead to lack of strength for sitting, standing, and walking, and there may even be tremor. When the heart qi is insufficient, it will lead to poor intelligence and delayed speech.

1 病因病机

病因主要为先天禀赋不足，或后天调护失宜，病机责之脾肾两虚，常累及心肺肝。肾气不足，骨髓不坚而致生长发育迟缓，囟门迟闭，牙齿晚出，胸背变形，肢体弯曲；脾不健运，土不生金，致肺气虚损，肌肉软弱，毛发稀疏，多汗；肝之阴血不足，肝阳偏旺，则烦躁夜啼；筋脉失养，致坐立、行走无力甚至抽搐；心气不足则智力低下，语言迟缓。

2 Key to diagnosis

(1) There is a history of vitamin D deficiency, mostly in the infants, from 3 months old to two years old, for lack of outdoor activities.

(2) Clinical manifestations are divided into 4 stages: the early stage, the active stage, the recovering stage and the sequela stage.

At the early stage, there are profuse sweating, vexation, restless sleep, fright and crying at night, pillow baldness, circular hair loss, delayed closure

2 诊断要点

(1) 维生素 D 缺乏史，多见于 3 个月～2 岁户外活动少的婴幼儿。

(2) 临床表现分四期：初期、活动期(激期)、恢复期、后遗症期。

初期多汗、烦躁、睡眠不安、夜间惊啼。有枕秃、脱发圈、囟门迟闭、牙齿迟出等。

of fontanel, delayed growing of teeth, etc. At the active stage, besides aggravation of the symptoms in the early stage, it is mainly manifested by the skeleton change in mild and medium degree, accompanied by the pathological changes of bones, such as ping-pang ball head, square skull, rachitic rosary, rib ecstrophy, chicken chest, funnel chest, turtle back, hand-foot bracelet, curling lower limbs, etc.

活动期除早期证候加重外，以轻中度骨骼改变为主，可见乒乓头、方颅、肋串珠、肋外翻、鸡胸、漏斗胸、龟背、手脚镯、下肢弯曲等骨骼病变。

In sick children at the recovering stage, the symptoms are lessened. X-ray shows the temporary calcification zone reappears, and blood biochemistry returns to be normal, but skeleton deformity still exist.

恢复期患儿症状改善，体征减轻，X 线示临时钙化带重现，血生化恢复正常，但可遗留骨骼畸形。

In sick children at the sequela stage, skeleton deformity in varying degree is often left over in severe condition, but without other clinical symptoms and abnormality in lab test.

后遗症期患儿因症重常残留不同程度的骨骼畸形，无其他临床症状，实验室检查亦无异常。

(3) Other manifestations: Slack muscles, slow sitting, standing and walking, dull expression, indifferent expression, pale facial complexion, frequent and repeated infection of exogenous pathogens

（3）其他证候：肌肉松弛，坐、立、行迟，表情淡漠、呆滞，面色苍白，常反复发生外感疾病。

(4) Accessory Examinations

（4）辅助检查

1) Blood biochemistry test: Serum calcium slightly decreases, and serum phosphate obviously decreases. The calcium-phosphorus product is smaller than 30, and serum alkaline phosphatase obviously increases.

1）血液生化检查：血清钙稍降低，血磷明显降低，钙磷乘积小于 30；血清碱性磷酸酶明显增高。

2) X-ray examination: It is often done at the wrist, present with obscure metaphyses, with a change of brush-like shape or cup-mouth shape, and with osteoporosis and thinning skin.

2）X 线摄片检查：常摄手腕部。可见干骺端模糊，呈毛刷状或杯口状改变，并可见骨质疏松，皮质变薄。

3　Pattern identifications and treatment

3　辨证论治

It is necessary to identify the stages, bowels

主要辨病期、脏腑及轻

and viscera, and the severity of the disease. In identification of stages, the early stage is often manifested by vexation, profuse sweating, pillow baldness, night fright and crying, no change in the skeleton. At the active stage, the above symptoms are aggravated, with obvious change in the skeleton and weak walking. After the treatment, the clinical symptoms are relieved or disappear, and this is the recovery stage. If the skeleton deformity in varying degrees is left over, it is in the sequela stage. The diseased organs include the heart, liver, lung, spleen and kidney. The early stage involves the lung and spleen, manifested by slack muscles, body puffiness due to deficiency, poor appetite, sloppy stool, scanty and dry hair, profuse sweating, and susceptability to cold. The active stage involves the heart, liver and kidney, manifested by vexation, night crying, change in skeleton, and slow sitting, slow standing, weak walking, and even convulsion. The mild condition only causes change in skeleton like slight craniomalacia, squared skull, rachitic rosary, and enlarged fontanel, etc. The severe condition will cause typical rachitic rosary, hand-foot bracelet, delayed closure of fontanel, delayed tooth growth, even chicken chest, funnel chest, spinal deformity, X-shape or O-shape leg, and pathologic fracture, etc.

重。初期症见烦躁、多汗、枕秃、夜间惊啼，无骨骼改变症状；活动期以上症状加重，并出现明显骨骼改变和行走无力；经治疗后，临床证候减轻或消失，为恢复期；若留有不同程度的骨骼畸形，为后遗症期。病变脏腑涉及心肝肺脾肾，初期病变脏腑以肺脾为主，表现肌肉松弛，形体虚浮，纳呆便溏，毛发稀疏而枯，多汗易感冒；活动期累及心肝肾，可见精神烦躁、夜啼不安，骨骼改变，以及坐迟、立迟，行走无力甚至抽搐等症。轻症仅有轻度颅骨软化、方颅、肋骨串珠、囟门增大等骨骼改变；重症有典型肋骨串珠及手、脚镯、囟门晚闭、出牙迟缓，甚至鸡胸、漏斗胸、脊柱畸形、“X”形或“O”形腿，病理性骨折等。

The basic principle is to fortify the spleen and boost qi, supplement the kidney and replenish essence. For the early stage, it is necessary to fortify the spleen, boost qi and supplement the lung in predominance. For the active stage, it is appropriate to fortify the spleen and calm the liver. For the severe condition, it is appropriate to supplement the kid-

以健脾益气，补肾填精为基本治则。初期以健脾益气补肺为主，活动期宜健脾平肝，重则补肾填精。

ney and replenish essence.

(1) Qi deficiency of the lung and spleen

Manifestations: Profuse sweating, restless sleep, delayed closure of fontanel, scanty hair and pillow baldness, lusterless complexion, slack muscles, poor appetite, irregular defecation, recurrent cold, pale tongue, thin and white tongue coating, light fingerprints, thready, soft and forceless pulse.

Therapeutic method: To fortify the spleen, supplement the lung, boost qi and secure the exterior.

Main formula is *Jade Wind-barrier Powder* (Yu Pin Feng San) and *Ginseng and Schisandra Decoction* (Ren Shen Wu Wei Zi Tang) with modification.

Commonly used herbs: *Astragali Radix* (Huang Qi), *Ledebouriellae Radix* (Fang Feng), *Atractylodis Macrocephalae Rhizoma* (Bai Zhu), *Ginseng Radix* (Ren Shen), *Schisandrae Fructus Chinensis* (Wu Wei Zi), *Poria* (Fu Ling), *Ophiopogonis Radix* (Mai Dong), *Glycyrrhizae Radix Et Rhizoma-preparata* (Zhi Gan Cao).

Modification: For profuse sweating, add *Os Draconis* (Long Gu) and *Ostreae Concha* (Mu Li); for loose stool, add *Dioscoreae Rhizoma* (Shan Yao), *Lablab Semen Album* (Bai Bian Dou) and *Nelumbinis Semen* (Lian Zi); for restless sleep, add *Radix* (*Polygalae* Yuan Zhi), and *Polygoni Multiflori Caulis* (Shou Wu Teng).

(2) Spleen deficiency and liver hyperactivity.

Manifestations: Lusterless complexion, profuse sweating, night fright and crying, even convulsion, fatigued spirit, poor appetite, lack of strength in sitting, standing and walking, pale tongue, thin tongue coating, light fingerprints, thready and

(1) 肺脾气虚

证候:多汗,睡眠不宁,囟门晚闭,头发稀疏枕秃,面色少华,肌肉松弛,纳呆,大便不调,反复感冒,舌质淡,苔薄白,指纹淡,脉细软无力。

治法:健脾补肺,益气固表。

主方:玉屏风散合人参五味子汤加减。

常用药:黄芪、防风、白术、人参、五味子、茯苓、麦冬、炙甘草。

加减:汗多者,加龙骨、牡蛎;大便不实者,加山药、白扁豆、莲子;睡眠不安者,加远志、首乌藤。

(2) 脾虚肝旺

证候:面色少华,多汗,夜惊啼哭,甚至抽搐,神疲纳呆,坐立行走无力,舌质淡,苔薄,指纹淡,脉细弦。

string-taut pulse.

Therapeutic method: To fortify the spleen and calm the liver.

治法:健脾平肝。

Main formula: *Spleen-Boosting Fright-Settling Powder* (Yi Pi Zhen Jing San) with modification.

主方:益脾镇惊散加减。

Commonly used herbs: *Ginseng Radix* (Ren Shen), *Atractylodis Macrocephalae Rhizoma* (Bai Zhu), *Poria* (Fu Ling), *Glycyrrhizae Radix Et Rhizoma* (Gan Cao), *Uncariae ramulus Cum uncis* (Gou Teng), *Junci Medulla* (Deng Xin Cao), *Curcumae Radix* (Yu Jin)

常用药:人参、白术、茯苓、甘草、钩藤、灯心草、郁金。

Modification: For copious sweating, add *Schisandrae Fructus Chinensis* (Wu Wei Zi), *Os Draconis Calcinata* (Long Gu), *Ostreae Concha* (Mu Li); for restless night sleep, add *Polygalae Radix* (Yuan Zhi), and Polygoni Multiflori Caulis (Shou Wu Teng).

加减:多汗者,加五味子、煅龙骨、煅牡蛎;夜卧不安者,加远志、首乌藤。

(3) Depletion of the spleen and kidney

(3) 脾肾亏损

Manifestations: Pale and lusterless complexion, dripping sweating of head, soft and weak limbs, dull and indifferent expression, delayed teeth, delayed standing, delayed sitting, delayed walking, no closure of fontanel, square and big skull, chicken chest, turtle back, or funnel chest, rachitic rosary, curled lower limbs, pale tongue, little tongue coating, light fingerprint, thready and forceless.

证候:面色苍白无华,头汗淋漓,肢软乏力,神情淡漠呆滞,出牙、坐立、行走迟缓,囟门不闭,头颅方大,鸡胸,龟背,或见漏斗胸,肋外翻,下肢弯曲,舌质淡,苔少,指纹淡,脉细无力。

Therapeutic method: To supplement the kidney and replenish essence.

治法:补肾填精。

Main formula: *Heaven-mending Great Creation Pills* (Bu Tian Da Zao Wan) with modification.

主方:补天大造丸加减。

Commonly used herbs: *Placenta Hominis* (Zi He Che), *Cervi Cornu* (Lu Jiao), *Testudinis Carapax Et Plastrum* (Gui Jia), *Angelicae Sinensis Radix*

常用药:紫河车、鹿角、龟甲、当归、枸杞子、茯苓、山药、生地黄、山茱萸、麦冬、五

(Dang Gui), *Lycii Fructus* (Gou Qi Zi), *Poria* (Fu Ling), *Dioscoreae Rhizoma* (Shan Yao), *Rehmanniae Radix Cruda* (Sheng Di Huang), *Corni Fructus* (Shan Zhu Yu), *Ophiopogonis Radix* (Mai Dong), *Schisandrae Fructus Chinensis* (Wu Wei Zi), *Cuscutae Semen* (Tu Si Zi), *Achyranthis Bidentatae Radix* (Niu Xi), *Eucommiae Cortex* (Du Zhong).

味子、菟丝子、牛膝、杜仲。

Modification: For copious sweating, add *Os Draconis* (Long Gu), and *Ostreae Concha* (Mu Li); for poor appetite, add *Amomi Fructus* (Sha Ren), and *Citri Reticulatae Pericarpium* (Chen Pi); for retarded intelligence, add *Acori Rhizoma Tatarinowii* (Shi Chang Pu), and *Curcumae Radix* (Yu Jin).

加减:汗多者,加龙骨、牡蛎;纳呆食少者,加砂仁、陈皮;智力落后者,加石菖蒲、郁金。

4 Other therapies

4 其他疗法

(1) *Dragon Bone and Oyster Shell Bone-Strengthening Soluble Granules* (Long Mu Zhuang Gu Chong Ji) is appropritate for qi deficiency in the lung and spleen and depletion of the spleen and kidney.

(1) 龙牡壮骨冲剂:适用于维生素 D 缺乏性佝偻病肺脾气虚及脾肾亏损证。

(2) *Jade Wind-Barrier Granules* (Yu Ping Feng) is appropritate for qi deficiency in the lung and spleen.

(2) 玉屏风颗粒:适用于维生素 D 缺乏性佝偻病肺脾气虚证。

(3) *Six-Ingredient Rehmannia Pill* (Liu Wei Di Huang Wan) is appropritate for depletion pattern of the spleen and kidney.

(3) 六味地黄丸:适用于维生素 D 缺乏性佝偻病脾肾亏损证。

Section 4 Simple Obesity

第 4 节 单纯性肥胖

Infantile simple obesity is a chronic dystrophy

小儿单纯性肥胖是由于

disorder due to prolonged excessive ingestion of energy beyond consumption in the body, which leads to excessive accumulation of fat and body weight beyond certain limit. Obesity not only affects health of children and also increases the risks of sickness and death from obesity, angiocardiopathy, type 2 diabetes, hypertension, and hyperlipemia in the adulthood.

能量摄入长期超过人体的消耗,使体内脂肪过度积聚,体重超过一定范围的一种慢性营养障碍性疾病。肥胖不仅影响小儿健康,并且增加了成年时期肥胖及心血管疾病、2 型糖尿病、高脂血症等疾病的患病和死亡的风险。

In traditional Chinese medicine, "fatty physique" is used to describe obesity nowadays.

中医学有关于脂膏形体即今之肥胖的描述。

1 Etiology and pathogenesis

1 病因病机

The etiological causes are related to prenatal natural endowment, accumulation and retention of dampness due to deficiency of vital energy, and over food ingestion and lack of physical exercises, etc.

病因有先天禀赋、正虚湿蕴、多食少动等。

Obesity is genetic. If the parents are obese, two thirds of their children would tend to be obese. It is usually caused by the constitutional deficiency in the spleen or injury of the spleen by food intake, resulting in strong function in the stomach and weak function in the spleen, quick digestion and easy hunger, and internal production of dampness and turbidity. Or there is constitutional yin deficiency or injury of body fluid after heat disease, which lead to yin deficiency and yang hyperactivity, scorching body fluid into phlegm which retain in the skin and flesh. Or there is infection of exogenous dampness, internally accumulating in the spleen. Or there is internal production of dampness due to spleen deficiency. The combination of internal dampness and external dampness turns into phlegm and turbidity. If children take too much greasy,

肥胖具有遗传性,父母肥胖者,其子女中 2/3 也有肥胖的倾向。素体脾虚,或饮食伤脾,致胃强脾弱,消谷善饥,湿浊内生,发为肥胖;素体阴虚,或热病后伤津,阴虚阳亢,灼津为痰,蕴于肌肤,而为肥胖。或外感湿邪,内蕴于脾,或因脾虚,湿自内生,内外相合,化为痰浊,而生肥胖。小儿过多进食油腻肥甘之品,加重肥胖,形成多食少动的恶性循环。

rich, heavy and sweet food, it will exacerbate obesity, resulting in a vicious cycle of overeat and decrease in physical exercises.

The obesity is characterized by deficiency in the constitution and excess in the symptoms, namely, constitutional deficiency and weakness in the spleen and kidney and dysfunction of body fluids being causative reason, and accumulation of phlegm and dampness and fat in the body being excessive symptoms. In severe obesity, the invasion of enduring dampness into meridians, leading to obstruction of blood vessels and stagnation of blood flow, or internal accumulation of fat and greasy substance, involving the meridians and collaterals and blocking flow of qi and blood, would damage five solid organs, presenting various diseases like chest impediment, dizziness, etc.

肥胖症的体制特点为本虚标实，即以脾肾脏腑虚弱，津液失常为本；痰湿、脂膏积于体内为标。重度肥胖者湿邪日久入络，阻滞血脉，血行滞涩，或膏脂内聚，浸淫脉络，阻滞气血，损伤五脏则百变丛生，可出现胸痹、眩晕诸症。

2 Key to diagnosis

(1) Body weight 10%～19% more than the mean value of reference population in same sex and same height is diagnosed as overweight, and body weight over 20% could be diagnosed as obesity. Among them, 20%～29% of the patients are diagnosed as mild obesity, 30%～49% as medium obesity, and over 50% as severe obesity.

(2) Body mass index (BMI) is the ratio of body weight and the square of body height (kg/m^2) and is another index to evaluate obesity. When BMI is larger than the 95th percentiles, it could be diagnosed as obesity, larger than the 85～95th percentile, as overweight, with a risk of obesity. BMI in the infants varies with age and sex.

2 诊断要点

（1）体重超过同性别、同身高参照人数均值的10%～19%者为超重；超过20%者可诊断为肥胖症，其中20%～29%者为轻度肥胖；30%～49%者为中度肥胖；超过50%者为重度肥胖。

（2）体质指数（BMI）是指体重和身高平方的比值，是评价肥胖的另一种指标。当BMI＞同年龄、同性别的第95百分位数可诊断肥胖；第85～95百分位数为超重，并具有肥胖风险。小儿BMI随年龄、性别而有差异。

3 Pattern identification and treatment

The pathogenesis of obesity lies in deficiency in the constitution and excess in the symptoms: the spleen deficiency and deficiency in the both spleen and kidney are in predominance; excess in the symptoms are phlegm, dampness, blood stasis. Pattern identification is supposed to differentiate between deficiency and excess, but mostly deficiency and excess are mixed. The severity of the disease is different.

The treatment is mainly to fortify the spleen and supplement the kidney, clear away phlegm and eliminate dampness. Together with the medications, it is important to follow the treatment progressively, and it is important to follow consistantly the assisting means like diet control, physical exercises, acumoxatherapy and tuina.

(1) Pattern of spleen deficiency and dampness

Manifestations: Bloated and fat body, heavy sensation in the limbs, puffy swelling of lower limbs, somnolence, profuse sweating, lack of strength and movement, full sensation in the abdomen, poor appetite, little urine, sloppy stool, pale and fat tongue, thin white or slimy white tongue coating, slippery and deep pulse.

Therapeutic method: To fortify the spleen and dissolve phlegm, warm up the Middle Energizer and dry up dampness.

Main Formula: *Sclerotium Poria, Cinnamomi, Atractylodis Macrocephalae, Glycyrrhizae Decoction* (Ling Gui Zhu Gan Tang) with supplementaries.

Commonly used herbs: *Poria* (Fu Ling), *Cinnamomi Ramulus* (Gui Zhi), *Atractylodis Macrocephalae*

3 辨证论治

肥胖症的病机为正虚邪实，以脾虚、脾肾两虚为本，痰、湿、瘀为标，辨证有虚实之分，但多虚实夹杂，病情有轻重之别。

治疗以健脾补肾，涤痰除湿为主。关键重在循序渐进，在药物治疗的同时辅以饮食控制、体育锻炼、针灸推拿，重在持之以恒。

(1) 脾虚夹湿

证候：形体臃肿肥胖，肢体困重，可有下肢浮肿，嗜睡多汗，乏力少动，腹满纳差，尿少便溏，舌淡胖，苔薄白或白腻，脉沉滑。

治法：健脾化痰，温中燥湿。

主方：苓桂术甘汤加味。

常用药：茯苓、桂枝、白术、甘草。

Rhizoma (Bai Zhu), *Glycyrrhizae Radix Et Rhizoma*(Gan Cao).

Modification: For qi deficiency and lack of strength, add *Astragali Radix* (Huang Qi), *Codonopsis Radix*(Dang Shen), *Atractylodis Macrocephalae Rhizoma* (Bai Zhu), and *Crataegi Fructus* (Shan Zha); for cumbersome limbs, slimy tongue coating with heavy dampness, add *Atractylodis Rhizoma* (Cang Zhu), and *Magnoliae Officinalis Cortex* (Hou Pu); for abdomen distention, add *Aucklandiae Radix* (Mu Xiang), and *Arecae Pericarpium*(Da Fu Pi); for profuse sweating, add *Ostreae Concha* (Mu Li), and *Persicae Abnormalis Fructus* (Bie Tao Gan); for sloppy stool, add *Zingiberis Rhizoma Tostum* (Sheng Jiang) and *Alpiniae Oxyphyllae Fructus* (Yi Zhi).

加减:气虚乏力者,加黄芪、党参、白术、山楂;肢困、苔腻湿重者,加苍术、厚朴;腹胀者,加木香、大腹皮;汗多者,加牡蛎、瘪桃干;大便溏者,加煨姜、益智。

(2) Pattern of stomach heat and damp obstruction

(2) 胃热湿阻

Manifestations: Fat physique, fatigue and no desire for activity, head distention, dizziness, quick digestion and easy hunger, foul breath, thirst with preference for drinking, red tongue, slimy or slight yellow tongue coating, slippery pulse.

证候:形体肥胖,倦怠懒动,头胀眩晕,消谷善饥,口臭,口渴喜饮,舌质红,苔腻或微黄,脉滑。

Therapeutic method: To clarify the stomach and drain heat, eliminate dampness and disperse swelling.

治法:清胃泻热,除湿消肿。

Main formula: *Yellow-Draining Powder* (Xie Huang San)

主方:泻黄散加减。

Commonly used herbs: *Folium Agastaches* (Huo Xiang Ye), *Gardeniae fructus* (Zhi Zi Ren), *Gypsum Fibrosum* (Shi Gao), *Radix Glycyrrhizae* (Gan Cao), *Ledebouriellae Radix* (Fang Feng)

常用药:藿香叶、栀子、石膏、甘草、防风。

Modification: For fatigue and cumbersome limbs, add *Alismatis Rhizoma* (Ze Xie), *Coicis Semen* (Yi

加减:倦怠肢困者,加泽泻、薏苡仁、厚朴、苍术;口渴

Yi Ren), *Magnoliae Officinalis Cortex* (Hou Pu), and *Atractylodis Rhizoma* (Cang Zhu); for thirst and foul breath, add *Coptidis Rhizoma* (Huang Lian), and *Trichosanthis Radix* (Tian Hua Fen).

口臭者,加黄连、天花粉。

(3) Pattern of liver heat with dampness

(3) 肝热夹湿

Manifestations: Fat physique, flushed complexion, dizziness and headache, vexation and crying, restless sleep, palpitation, short of breath, bitter taste in the mouth and dry throat, scanty and brown urine, red tongue, yellow or slimy tongue coating, rapid and string-taut pulse, or manifestations of insufficiency of yin deficiency and internal heat due to yang hyperactivity such as feverish sensation in the chest, palms and soles, low-grade fever, night sweating, red tongue tip, rapid, thready and fine pulse.

证候:形体肥胖,面赤,头晕头痛,烦恼多啼,睡卧不宁,心悸气短,口苦咽干,小便黄少,舌质红,苔黄或腻,脉弦数。或见五心烦热,低热盗汗,舌尖红,脉细数等肝阴不足,阳亢内热之象。

Therapeutic method: To tranquilize the liver and clear away heat, regulate qi and dissovle dampness.

治法:平肝清热,理气化湿。

Main formula: *Liver-Normalizing Decoction* (Hua Gan Jian) with modification.

主方:化肝煎加减。

Commonly used herbs: *Citri Reticulatae Pericarpium Viride* (Qing Pi), *Citri Reticulatae Pericarpium* (Chen Pi), *Radix Paeoniae* (Shao Yao), *Moutan Cortex Radicis* (Mu Dan Pi), *Gardeniae Fructus* (Zhi Zi), *Alismatis Rhizoma* (Ze Xie), *Bolbostemmatis Rhizoma* (Tu Bei Mu).

常用药:青皮、陈皮、芍药、牡丹皮、栀子、泽泻、土贝母。

Modification: For dried stool and constipation, add *Cassiae Semen* (Jue Ming Zi), and *Plygoni Multiflori Radix* (He Shou Wu); for bitter taste in the mouth and dry throat, add *Scutellariae Radix* (Huang Qin), *Prunellae Spica* (Xia Ku Cao); for hypochondriac distension and vomiting, add *Aurantii Fructus* (Zhi Qiao), and *Pinelliae Rhizoma*

加减:大便秘结者,加决明子、生何首乌;口苦咽干者,加黄芩、夏枯草;胁胀呕吐者,加枳壳、姜半夏;烦恼不宁者,加灯心草、竹叶;舌质紫黯,有瘀点者,加丹参、郁金、红花、桃仁。

Preparata (Jiang Ban Xia); for vexation and restlessness, add *Junci Medulla* (Deng Xin Cao), and *Folium Phyllostachys* (Zhu Ye); for dark purple tongue with stasis spots, add *Salviae Miltiorrhizae Radix Et Rhizoma* (Dan Shen), *Curcumae Radix* (Yu Jin), *Carthami Flos* (Hong Hua), and *Persicae Semen* (Tao Ren).

(4) Pattern of obstruction of blood stasis in the meridians and collaterals

（4）瘀阻经络

Manifestations: Fat physique, fat end of extremities that turn dark purple with cold, soot-black facial complexion, distending and painful chest and ribs, vexation and irascibility, excessive appetite, dark purple tongue with stasis spots, stringe-taut pulse or thready and hesitant pulse.

证候：形体肥胖，肢端肥胖，遇冷紫黯，面色黧黑，胸胁胀痛，烦躁易怒，食欲亢进，舌质紫黯有瘀点，脉弦或细涩。

Therapeutic method: To warm up the meridians and disperse cold, nourish blood and dredge the meridians.

治法：温经散寒，养血通脉。

Main formula: *Chinese Angelica Counterflow Cold Powder* (Dang Gui Si Ni San) with modifications

主方：当归四逆散加减。

Commonly used herbs: *Angelicae Sinensis Radix* (Dang Gui), *Cinnamomi Ramulus* (Gui Zhi), *Paeoniae Radix* (Shao Yao), *Asari Radix Et Rhizoma* (Xi Xin), *Tetrapanacis Medulla* (Tong Cao), *Jujubae Fructus* (Da Zao), *Glycyrrhizae Radix Et Rhizoma Preparata* (Zhi Gan Cao).

常用药：当归、桂枝、芍药、细辛、通草、大枣、炙甘草。

Modifications: For hypochondriac distension and susceptibility to pain, add *Aurantii Fructus Immaturus* (Zhi Shi), *Uncariae ramulus Cum uncis* (Gou Teng), *Curcumae Radix* (Yu Jin), and *Persicae Semen* (Tao Ren); for sloppy stool, add *Zingiberis Rhizoma Preparata* (Pao Jiang), and *Crataegi Fructus* (Shan Zha); for obvious cold limbs, add

加减：胁胀易痛者，加枳实、钩藤、郁金、桃仁；便溏者，加炮姜、山楂；肢冷明显者，加附子、姜黄；瘀血重者，加乳香、没药。

Aconiti Lateralis Radix Praeparata (Fu Zi), *Rhizoma Curcumae Longae* (Jiang Huang); for severe blood stasis, add *Olibanum* (Ru Xiang), and *Myrrha* (Mo Yao).

(5) Pattern of yang deficiency in the spleen and kidney

（5）脾肾阳虚

Manifestations: Fat and and puffy body, aching soreness and softness in the lumbus and legs, cold sensation in the body and cold limbs, fatigue and lack of strength, slight red tongue, white tongue coating, slow and deep pulse.

证候：肥胖浮肿，腰酸腿软，形寒肢冷，疲乏无力，舌淡红，苔白，脉沉缓。

Therapeutic method: To supplement the spleen and secure the kidney, warm up yang and dissolve dampness.

治法：补脾固肾，温阳化湿。

Main formula: *True Warrior Decoction* (Zhen Wu Tang) with modification.

主方：真武汤加减。

Commonly used herbs: *Poria* (Fu Ling), *Paeoniae Radix* (Shao Yao), *Atractylodis Macrocephalae Rhizoma* (Bai Zhu), *Zingiberis Rhizoma Recens* (Sheng Jiang), and *Aconiti Lateralis Radix Praeparata* (Fu Zi).

常用药：茯苓、芍药、白术、生姜、附子。

Modification: For aching soreness and softness in the lumbus and legs, add *Eucommiae Cortex* (Du Zhong), *Achyranthis Bidentatae Radix* (Niu Xi), *Ligustri Lucidi Fructus* (Nu Zhen Zi); for fat and bloated body and qi deficiency, add *Astragali Radix* (Huang Qi); for aversion to cold and cold limbs, add *Cinnamomi Ramulus* (Gui Zhi); for obvious puffy swelling, add *Plantaginis Semen* (Che Qian Zi), and *Alismatis Rhizoma* (Ze Xie); for sloppy stool and abdominal distention, add *Amomi Fructus* (Sha Ren), and *Crataegi Fructus Ustus* (Jiao Shan Zha).

加减：腰腿酸软者，加杜仲、牛膝、女贞子；肥胖浮肿而气虚者，加黄芪；畏寒肢冷者，加桂枝；浮肿明显者，加车前子、泽泻；便溏腹胀者，加砂仁、焦山楂。

4　Other therapies

4.1　Patent Chinese medicine

Saposhnikovia Sage-Inspired Pill (Fang Feng Tong Shen Wan) is used for obesity in pattern of stomach heat and obstruction of dampness.

4.2　Acumoxatherapy

Acupuncture can be used to promote fat metabo lism in the body and increase heat production, so as to consume the retained fat. For and phlegm and dampness due to the spleen deficiency, select Neiguan (PC 6), Shuifen (CV 9), Tianshu (ST 25), Guanyuan (CV 4), Fenglong (ST 40), Sanyinjiao (SP 6), and Lieque (LU 7). For stomach heat and obstruction of dampness, select Quchi (LI 11), Zhigou (TE 6), Siman (KI 14), and Neiting (ST 44). For deficiency in the spleen and kidney, select Neiguan (PC 6) and Zusanli (ST 36).

4　其他疗法

4.1　中成药

防风通圣丸:适用于肥胖症胃热湿阻证。

4.2　针灸疗法

针刺治疗能促进机体脂肪代谢,使产热增加,从而消耗存积的脂肪。脾虚痰湿:取内关、水分、天枢、关元、丰隆、三阴交、列缺等;胃热湿阻:取曲池、支沟、四满、三阴交、内庭等;脾肾两虚:取内关、足三里、天枢、曲池、丰隆、梁丘、支沟等。

Chapter 4 Diseases of Heart and Hematopoietic System

第4章 心脏及造血系统疾病

Section 1 Viral Myocarditis

第1节 病毒性心肌炎

Viral myocarditis is a disease caused by invasion of virus into the heart, leading to pathological changes of localized or diffuse myocarditis, involving pericardium or endocardium in some cases, and clinically characterized by the symptoms, such as palpitation, oppression in the chest, lack of strength, short of breath, pale facial complexion, cold limbs, profuse sweating, etc. In recent years, with increasing virus infection, viral myocarditis tends to increase in the incidence rate accordingly, and becomes a common infantile cardiac disease.

病毒性心肌炎是由病毒侵犯心脏,引起局限性或弥漫性心肌炎性病变为主的疾病,有的可累及心包或心内膜。临床可见心悸、胸闷、乏力、气短、面色苍白、肢冷、多汗等症。近年来,病毒性心肌炎的发病率有逐渐升高的趋势,成为小儿常见的心脏疾病。

It is mostly seen in children from 3 to 10 years old and can occur throughout the four seasons. It is often secondary to viral diseases, such as common cold, measles, mumps, diarrhea, etc. It belongs to the scope of "palpitation", "anxiety" or "chest impediment pattern" in traditional Chinese medicine.

多见于3～10岁的儿童,四季均可发病。常继发于感冒、麻疹、流行性腮腺炎、腹泻等病毒感染性疾病之后。本病属中医学"心悸""怔忡""胸痹"范畴。

1 Etiology and pathogenesis

1 病因病机

The depletion of the vital energy is an internal cause of the illness, and the invasion of pathogenic

正气亏虚是发病之内因,风温、湿热邪毒侵袭是发

wind and warmth, pathogenic dampness and heat is an external cause.

The main pathological changes are obstruction of the heart meridian and consumption and injury of qi and yin. The static blood and phlegm turbidity are the pathological products. In the course of illness, either deficiency in the constitution and excess in the symptoms would exist, or deficiency in predominance, or deficiency mixed with excess. Because the pathogenesis changes unpredictably, it is important to identify varying patterns. In the clinical treatment, it is necessary to be aware of the transmuted pattern of sudden collapase of yang desertion.

病之外因。

以心脉痹阻，气阴耗伤为主要病理变化，瘀血、痰浊为病理产物。病程中或邪实正虚，或以虚为主，或虚中夹实，病机演变多端，需随证辨识，临证时要警惕发生心阳暴脱的变证。

2 Key to diagnosis

2.1 Diagnostic basis

(1) There is a history of common cold, diarrhea, or urticaria before onset.

(2) There is cardiac insufficiency, cardiac shock or cardiocerebral syndrome, manifested by obvious palpitation, chest oppression, lack of strength, short of breath, cold limbs, profuse sweating, intermittent irregular pulse, etc.

(3) By cardiac auscultation, there could be low and blunt cardiac sound, increased heart rate, arrhythmia, gallop rhythm, etc.

(4) X-ray or ultrasound cardiogram shows cardiac dilatation. Electrocardiogram shows changes in 2 or more than 2 ST-T sections for more than 4 days in I, II aVF, V5 leads, and other severe arrhythmia. Serum creatine kinase (CK-MB) increases, and cardiac troponin (cTnI or cTnT)is positive.

2 诊断要点

2.1 临床诊断依据

（1）发病前有感冒、泄泻、风疹等病史。

（2）心功能不全、心源性休克或心脑综合征。有明显心悸、胸闷、乏力、气短、面色苍白、肢冷、多汗、脉结代等表现。

（3）心脏听诊可有心音低钝，心率加快，心律不齐，奔马律等。

（4）X 线或超声心动图检查示心脏扩大；心电图示Ⅰ、Ⅱ、aVF、V_5导联中 2 个或 2 个以上 ST-T 改变持续 4 天以上，以及其他严重心律失常；血清肌酸激酶同工酶升高，心肌肌钙蛋白阳性。

2.2 Phases of Disease

(1) Acute phase: New onset, obvious and varying symptoms and positive findings from examinations, with duration within half a year.

(2) Prolonged phase: Repeated occurrence of clinical symptoms, lingering indexes of objective examinations, with duration over half a year.

(3) Chronic phase: Progressive heart enlargement, repeated heart failure or arrhythmia, fluctuation in pathologic situation, with duration over a year.

3 Pattern identifications and treatment

Due to different clinical manifestations and mixed syndromes, pattern identification can be complicated. According to clinical manifestations, it is requested to identify deficiency and excess first, and then identify the severity. The short duration, manifested by oppressed and painful sensation in the chest, short of breath and copious phlegm, nausea, vomiting, abdominal pain and diarrhea, red tongue and yellow tongue coating, belongs to excess pattern. The duration over several months, manifested by palpitation, short of breath, pale compelxion, profuse sweating, pale tongue, or red tongue, peeled tongue with little tongue coating, belongs to deficiency pattern. Usually, the acute phase is characterizd by excess pattern, and the prolonged phase and chronic phase are characterized mainly by deficiency pattern or mixed pattern of excess and deficiency. Clear consciousness, comfortable physical expression, rosy and healthy complexion, replete and forceful pulse indicate mild condition. Pale complexion, rapid breathing and panting, extreme

2.2 分期

（1）急性期：新发病，症状及检查阳性发现明显且多变，一般病程在半年以内。

（2）迁延期：临床症状反复出现，客观检查指标迁延不愈，病程多在半年以上。

（3）慢性期：进行性心脏增大，反复心力衰竭或心律失常，病情时轻时重，病程在1年以上。

3 辨证论治

由于临床表现不一，证候错杂，辨证较为复杂。可根据临床表现，首先辨明虚实，其次辨别轻重。凡病程短暂，见胸闷胸痛，气短多痰，或恶心呕吐，腹痛腹泻，舌红苔黄，属实证；病程长达数月，见心悸气短，神疲乏力，面白多汗，舌淡或偏红，舌光少苔，属虚证。一般急性期以实证为主，迁延期、慢性期以虚证为主或虚实夹杂。神志清楚，神态自如，面色红润，脉实有力者，病情轻；若面色苍白，气急喘息，四肢厥冷，口唇青紫，烦躁不安，脉微欲绝或频繁结代者，病情危重。

cold sensation in the limbs, green-blue mouth and lips, vexation and agitation, tiny and disappearing pulse, or frequent intermittent pulse indicate critical condition.

The basic treatment principle is to calm down the heart and dredge the collaterals. It is necessary to dispel evils, nourish the heart and dredge the collaterals in the initial stage; while in the late stage, it is to support the body constitution, enrich the heart and dredge the collaterals predominantly and to dispel evils assistantly. For invasion of pathogens into the heart at initial stage, the treatment is given to clear away heat, resolve toxin, nourish the heart and dredge the collaterals. For invasion of dampness and heat into the heart, the treatment is given to clear away heat, dissolve dampness, calm down the heart and dredge the collaterals. For deficiency and depletion of qi and yin in the late phase, the treatment is given to boost qi and nourish yin, tranquilize the heart and calm down the spirit. For mixture of phlegm and blood stasis, the treatment is given to quicken blood flow and disperse blood stasis, dispel phlegm and dissolve the turbidity. For deficiency and depletion of heart yang, the treatment is given to boost qi, restore yang, and correct counterflow for resuscitation.

以宁心通脉为基本治则。初期以祛邪、养心通脉为要,后期以扶正、养心通脉为主,祛邪为辅。病初邪毒犯心者,治以清热解毒,养心通脉;湿热侵心者,治以清热化湿,宁心通脉;后期气阴亏虚者,治以益气养阴,宁心安神;痰瘀互结者,治以活血化瘀,祛痰化浊。心阳虚衰者,治以益气回阳,救逆固脱。

(1) Invasion of wind and heat into the heart

Manifestations: Aversion to cold, fever, headache, running nose, sore throat, sore muscles, palpitation, short breath, oppression of chest and chest pain, red tongue, thin yellow tongue coating, rapid and floating pulse or abrupt pulse.

Therapeutic method: To expel wind and clear away heat, resolve toxin and safeguard the heart.

(1) 风热犯心

证候:恶寒发热,头痛流涕,咳嗽,咽痛,肌肉酸痛,心悸气短,胸闷胸痛,舌质红,苔薄黄,脉浮数或促。

治法:疏风清热,解毒护心。

Main formula: *Lonicera and Forsythia Powder* (Yin Qiao San) with modification.

主方:银翘散加减。

Commonly used herbs: *Lonicerae Flos Japonicae* (Jin Yin Hua), *Forsythiae Fructus* (Lian Qiao), *Sojae Semen Praeparatum* (Dan Dou Chi), Arctii Fructus(Niu Bang Zi), *Menthae Haploalycis Herba* (Bo He), *Schizonepetae Herba* (Jing Jie), *Platycodonis Radix* (Jie Geng), *Glycyrrhizae Radix Et Rhizoma*(Gan Cao), *Lophatheri Herba* (Dan Zhu Ye), *Phragmitis Rhizoma* (Lu Gen).

常用药:金银花、连翘、淡豆豉、牛蒡子、薄荷、荆芥、桔梗、甘草、淡竹叶、芦根。

Modification: For exuberant evil heat, add *Scutellariae Radix*(Huang Qin), *Gardeniae Fructus* (Zhi Zi), and *Gypsum Fibrosum*(Sheng Shi Gao); for oppression in the chest, add *Aurantii Fructus* (Zhi Qiao) and *Curcumae Radix*(Yu Jin); for chest pain, add *Salviae Miltiorrhizae Radix Et Rhizoma* (Dan Shen) and *Carthami Flos*(Hong Hua); for palpitation and rapid pulse, add *Schisandrae Fructus Chinensis* (Wu Wei Zi), *Platycladi Semen*(Bai Zi Ren), and *Spatholobi Caulis* (Ji Xue Teng); for sore throat, add *Sophorae Tonkinensis Radix Et Rhizoma* (Shan Dou Gen), *Scrophulariae Radix* (Xuan Shen), and *Isatidis Radix* (Ban Lan Gen).

加减:邪热炽盛者,加黄芩、栀子、生石膏;胸闷者,加枳壳、郁金;胸痛者,加丹参、红花;心悸、脉促者,加五味子、柏子仁、鸡血藤;咽痛红肿者,加山豆根、玄参、板蓝根。

(2) Invasion of dampness and heat into the heart

(2) 湿热侵心

Manifestations: Flucturating cold and heat, aching soreness of whole body, nausea, vomiting, abdominal pain, diarrhea, somber facial complexion, fatigue and lack of strength, suppressed chest, palpitation, shortness of breath, frequent sighing, red tongue, yellow slimy tongue coating, rapid and soft pulse or intermittent pulse.

证候:寒热起伏,全身酸痛,恶心呕吐,腹痛腹泻,面色晦暗,倦怠乏力,胸部憋闷,心悸气短,善太息,舌质红,苔黄腻,脉濡数或结代。

Therapeutic method: To clear away heat and dissolve dampness, quiet the heart and dredge the collaterals.

治法:清热化湿,宁心通脉。

Main formula: *Middle Energizer Impediment-Diffusing Decoction* (Zhong Jiao Xuan Bi Tang) with modification.

主方:中焦宣痹汤加减。

Commonly used herbs: *Forsythiae Fructus* (Lian Qiao), *Gardeniae Fructus*(Zhi Zi), *Bombycis Faeces* (Can Sha), *Vignae semen* (Chi Xiao Dou), *Coicis Semen* (Yi Yi Ren), *Armeniacae Semen Amarum* (Ku Xing Ren), *Radix Cocculi* (Mu Fang Ji), *Talcum* (Hua Shi), *Pinelliae Rhizoma* (Ban Xia)

常用药:连翘、栀子、蚕沙、赤小豆、薏苡仁、苦杏仁、木防己、滑石、半夏。

Modification: For stifling oppression in the chest, add *Trichosanthis Pericarpium* (Gua Lou Pi), and *Allii Macrostemonis Bulbus* (Xie Bai); for soreness of limbs and body, add *Angelicae Pubescentis Radix*(Du Huo), *Notopterygii Rhizoma seu Radix* (Qiang Huo), and *Chaenomelis Fructus* (Mu Gua); for palpitation and intermittent pulse, add *Salviae Miltiorrhizae Radix Et Rhizoma* (Dan Shen), *Margaritifera Concha* (Zhen Zhu Mu), and *Os Draconis* (Long Gu).

加减:胸闷气憋者,加瓜蒌皮、薤白;肢体酸痛者,加独活、羌活、木瓜;心悸、脉结代者,加丹参、珍珠母、龙骨。

(3) Deficiency of both qi and yin

(3) 气阴两虚

Manifestations: Palpitation, anxiety, oppression in the chest, shortness of breath, shortage of qi, reluctance to speak, low spirit, dizziness, blurred vision, heat vexation, thirst, spontaneous sweating and night sweating, insomnia, lassitude, red tongue with scanty body fluid, thready and rapid pulse or intermittent pulse.

证候:心悸怔忡,胸闷气短,少气懒言,神疲倦怠,头晕目眩,烦热口渴,自汗盗汗,失眠乏力,舌质红少津,脉细数或结代。

Therapeutic method: To boost qi, nourish yin, quiet the heart and calm down the mind.

治法:益气养阴,宁心安神。

Main formula: *Pulse-engendering Powder* (Sheng Mai San) with modification.

主方:生脉散加减。

Commonly used herbs: *Ginseng Radix* (Ren Shen), *Ophiopogonis Radix*(Mai Dong), *Schisandrae Fructus Chinensis* (Wu Wei Zi), *Pseudostellariae Radix*

常用药:人参、麦冬、五味子、太子参、当归、生地黄、丹参、酸枣仁、炙甘草。

(Tai Zi Shen), *Angelicae Sinensis Radix* (Dang Gui), *Rehmanniae Radix Cruda* (Sheng Di Huang), *Salviae Miltiorrhizae Radix Et Rhizoma* (Dan Shen), *Ziziphi Spinosi Semen* (Suan Zao Ren), *Glycyrrhizae Radix Et RhizomaPraeparata* (Zhi Gan Cao).

Modification: For obvious qi deficiency, add *Astragali Radix* (Huang Qi) and *Radix Panacis Quinquefolii* (Xi Yang Shen); for obvious yin deficiency, add *Rehmanniae Radix Praeparata* (Shu Di Huang) and *Polygonati Odorati Rhizoma*(Yu Zhu); for palpitation, add *Polygoni Multiflori Caulis* (Shou Wu Teng) and *Platycladi Semen* (Bai Zi Ren); for obvious oppression in the chest, add *Curcumae Radix* (Yu Jin) and *Aurantii Fructus* (Zhi Qiao); for spontaneous and night sweating, add *Tritici Levis Fructus* (Fu Xiao Mai), *Ephedrae Radix Et Rhizoma* (Ma Huang Gen); for dry stool, add *Cannabis Fructus*(Huo Ma Ren), *Trichosanthis Semen* (Gua Lou Zi) and *Platycladi Semen*(Bai Zi Ren).

加减:若气虚明显者,加黄芪、西洋参;阴虚明显者,加熟地黄、玉竹;心悸不安者,加首乌藤、柏子仁;胸闷明显者,加郁金、枳壳;自汗盗汗者,加浮小麦、麻黄根;大便偏干者,加火麻仁、瓜蒌子、柏子仁。

(4) Accumulation of phlegm and blood stasis

(4) 痰瘀互结

Manifestations: Palpitation, shortness of breath, oppression in the chest and suffocation, or stabbing pain in the heart, fullness and oppression in the epigastric region, nausea and vomiting, somber facial complexion, green-blue lips and nails, dark purple tongue, stasis speckles on the margin and tip of the tongue, slimy tongue coating, slippery or intermittent pulse.

证候:心悸气短,胸闷憋气或心痛如针刺,脘腹满闷,恶心泛呕,面色晦暗,唇甲青紫,舌质紫黯,舌边尖有瘀点,舌苔腻,脉滑或结代。

Therapeutic method: To quicken blood flow and dissolve blood stasis, dissipate phlegm and open impediment.

治法:活血化瘀,豁痰开痹。

Main formula: *Trichosanthes, Chinese Chive*

主方:瓜蒌薤白半夏汤

and Pinellia Decoction (Gua Lou Xie Bai Ban Xia Tang) and *Sudden Smile Powder* (Shi Xiao San) with modification.

合失笑散加减。

Commonly used herbs: *Trichosanthis Pericarpium* (Gua Lou Pi), *Allii Macrostemonis Bulbus* (Xie Bai), *Pinelliae Rhizoma* (Ban Xia), *Salviae Miltiorrhizae Radix Et Rhizoma* (Dan Shen), *Curcumae Radix* (Yu Jin), *Aurantii Fructus* (Zhi Qiao), *Typhae Pollen* (Pu Huang), *Trogopterorum Faeces* (Wu Ling Zhi).

常用药:瓜蒌皮、薤白、半夏、丹参、郁金、枳壳、蒲黄、五灵脂。

Modification: For obvious heart pain, add *Chuanxiong Rhizoma* (Chuan Xiong), *Carthami Flos* (Hong Hua), and *Dalbergiae Odoriferae Lignum* (Jiang Xiang); for accumulation of phlegm turning into heat, add *Coptidis Rhizoma* (Huang Lian), and *Bambusae Caulis in Taenias* (Zhu Ru); for imsomnia, add *Flos Albiziae* (He Huan Hua), *Polygoni Multiflori Caulis* (Shou Wu Teng), *Ziziphi Spinosi Semen* (Suan Zao Ren).

加减:心痛明显者,加川芎、红花、降香;痰郁化热者,加黄连、竹茹;夜不能寐者,加合欢花、首乌藤、酸枣仁。

(5) Deficient decline of heart yang

(5) 心阳虚衰

Manifestations: Palpitation, anciety, oppression and discomfort of chest, pale facial complexion, cold limbs, dizziness, spontaneous sweating or dripping sweating, extreme cold sensation in the limbs, purple mouth and lips, purple nails, shallow and abrupt breathing, slight dark tongue, thin white tongue coating, thread and rapid pulse or faint pulse.

证候:心悸怔忡,胸闷不舒,面色苍白,四肢不温,头晕自汗,甚则大汗淋漓,四肢厥冷,口唇及指(趾)发紫,呼吸浅促,舌质淡暗,舌苔薄白,脉细数或脉微欲绝。

Therapeutic method: To boost qi and restore yang, correct counterflow for resuscitation.

治法:益气回阳,救逆固脱。

Main formula: *Cinnamon Twig, Licorice, Dragon Bone, and Oyster Shell Decoction* (Gui Zhi Gan Cao Long Gu Mu Li Tang) with modification.

主方:桂枝甘草龙骨牡蛎汤加减。

Commonly used herbs: *Cinnamomi Ramulus*

常用药:桂枝、甘草、龙

(Gui Zhi), *Glycyrrhizae Radix Et Rhizoma* (Gan Cao), *Os Draconis* (Long Gu), *Ostreae Concha* (Mu Li), *Ginseng Radix* (Ren Shen), *Astragali Radix* (Huang Qi), *Chuanxiong Rhizoma* (Chuan Xiong), *Paeoniae Radix Albae* (Bai Shao).

骨、牡蛎、人参、黄芪、川芎、白芍。

Modification: For physical cold sensation and cold limbs, add *Aconiti Lateralis Radix Praeparata* (Fu Zi), and *Zingiberis Rhizoma* (Gan Jiang); for fulminant desertion of yang qi, add *Ophiopogonis Radix* (Mai Dong), *Schisandrae Fructus Chinensis* (Wu Wei Zi), *Aconiti Lateralis Radix Praeparata* (Fu Zi), and *Zingiberis Rhizoma* (Gan Jiang).

加减:形寒肢冷者,加附子、干姜;阳气暴脱者,加麦冬、五味子、附子、干姜。

4 Other therapies

4 其他疗法

4.1 Patent Chinese medicine

4.1 中成药

(1) *Pulse-Engendering Decoction* (Sheng Mai Yin) is used for viral myocarditis in pattern of qi and yin deficiency.

(1) 生脉饮:适用于病毒性心肌炎气阴两虚证。

(2) *Compound Red Sage Pills* (Fu Fang Dan Shen Pian) is used for viral myocarditis in pattern of accumulation of phlegm and blood stasis.

(2) 复方丹参片:适用于病毒性心肌炎痰瘀互结证。

(3) *Red Sage Injection* (Dan Shen Zhu She Ye) is used for viral myocarditis in pattern of accumulation of phlegm and blood stasis.

(3) 丹参注射液:适用于病毒性心肌炎痰瘀互结证。

(4) *Pulse Engendering Injection* (Sheng Mai Zhu She Ye) is used for pattern of qi and yin deficiency.

(4) 生脉注射液:适用于病毒性心肌炎气阴两虚证。

(5) *Ginseng and Aconite Injection* (Shen Fu Zhu She Ye) is used for viral myocarditis in pattern of deficient decline of heart yang.

(5) 参附注射液:适用于病毒性心肌炎心阳虚衰证。

4.2 Acumoxatherapy

4.2 针灸治疗

(1) Body acupuncture: Select Xinshu (BL 15), Juque(CV 14), Jianshi (PC 5), Shenmen (HT 7), Xuehai (SP 10) as the main acupoints, and select

(1) 体针:主穴取心俞、巨阙、间使、神门、血海,配穴取大陵、膏肓、丰隆、内关。

Daling (PC 7), Gaohuang (BL 43), Fenglong (ST 40), and Neiguan (PC6) as the additional acupoints. Puncture with the needling technique for supplementation, and retain the needles after the arrival of the needling sensation.

用补法,得气后留针。

(2) Ear acupuncture: Select the ear points of Pt. Heart, Pt. Sympathetic Nerve, Pt. Ear-Shenmen, and Pt. Subcortex, and embed the ear points with *Semen Vaccariae* (Wang Bu Liu Xing), fix with adhesive plaster, and press every day.

(2) 耳针:取心、交感、神门、皮质下,或用王不留行压穴,用胶布固定,每日按压。

Section 2 Idiopathic Thrombocytopenic Purpura

第 2 节　特发性血小板减少性紫癜

Idiopathic thrombocytopenic purpura, a most common hemorrhagic disease in children, is clinically characterized by the spontaneous bleeding of the skin or mucous membrane, thrombopenia, normal or increased marrow megacaryocyte count, prolonged bleeding time and poor blood clot retraction. It mostly occurs in children aged from 2 to 8 years old, and is clinically manifested by acute and chronic types. The acute type is common in children, accounting for 85%, and the prognosis is relatively good in comparison with the adults.

特发性血小板减少性紫癜是小儿最常见的出血性疾病。其临床特点为皮肤、黏膜自发性出血,血小板减少,骨髓巨核细胞数正常或增多,出血时间延长和血块收缩不良。多见于 2～8 岁的小儿。临床上常分急性型与慢性型,小儿以急性型较多见,约占 85%,其预后相对比成人为好。

It belongs to the scope of "blood pattern", "spontaneous bleeding of the flesh", "purple macules" and "consumptive diseases" in traditional Chinese medicine.

本病属中医学"血证""肌衄""紫斑"和"虚劳"等范畴。

1　Etiology and pathogenesis

1　病因病机

The external causes are related to infection of exogenous pathogenic wind, heat, dryness, and pes-

外因为感受风、热、燥、火、疫毒诸邪,内因为脏腑气

tilential toxin. The internal causes are related to deficiency and debility of qi and blood in the bowels and viscera, causing internal latency of pathogenic heat in Ying-nutrient system and blood, and hence extravasation.

血虚损，使邪热内伏营血，致血液离经外溢。

The acute phase is mostly related to infection of exogenous heat toxin and various pathogens, and invasion of heat toxin, which harass Ying-nutrient system and blood, burn the blood collaterals, force the blood to flow frenetically and spill out of the collaterals, resulting in purpura in the mucous membrane of the skin or other accompanying blood patterns. This mostly belongs to excess pattern. The chronic type is mainly related to qi deficiency and yin deficiency. Spleen deficiency fails to control and contain the blood, leading to blood failing to stay inside the meridians, spilling out of blood vessels and collaterals, and oozeing out over the skin. If fire is hyperactive due to yin deficiency, the deficient fire would burn the blood vessels and collaterals, causing extravasation. After bleeding in this disease, blood would fail to stay inside the meridians and would flow out of blood vessels and collaterals, and the blood out of vessels would often cause internal obstruction of blood stasis, aggravating bleeding or leading to recurrent bleeding, termed as mixed pattern of deficiency and excess.

急性期多因外感热毒诸邪，热毒入侵，内扰营血，灼伤血络，迫血妄行，溢于脉外，出现皮肤黏膜紫癜或伴其他血证，多属实证。慢性者多为气虚、阴虚。脾气虚则不能统摄血液，以致血不循经，溢于脉络之外，渗于皮肤之间；若阴虚火旺则虚火灼伤脉络，血溢脉外。本病出血后，血不归经，血流脉外，离经之血常导致瘀血内阻，使出血加重，或反复出血，则为虚实夹杂之证。

2 Key to diagnosis

2 诊断要点

2.1 Clinical diagnosis

2.1 临床诊断

(1) Clinically, there are bleeding spots over the skin, ecchymosis, and/or mucosal bleeding.

（1）有皮肤出血点、瘀斑和（或）黏膜出血等临床表现。

(2) Platelet count is $<100\times10^9/\mathrm{L}$. The bleeding time is prolonged, with poor blood clots and

（2）血小板计数低于 100×10^9/升。出血时间延

positive beam arm test.

(3) Bone marrow megakaryocyte increases or is normal, with dysmaturity, manily manifested by increased ratio of immature and/or mature megakaryocyte without platelet, and deficient particles and less cytoplasm of megakaryocyte.

(4) No obvious enlargement of the liver, spleen and lymph node.

(5) There is any one of the four items: ① effective treatment by adrenal cortex hormone, ② effective splenectomy, ③ positive platelet-associated antibody (PAIg, PAC_3)or specific anti platelet antibodies, ④ shortened platelet life span.

(6) Exclusion of other diseases that can cause thrombocytopenia, such as aplastic anemia (SS), leukemia, myelodysplastic syndrome (MDS), and other immunological diseases, or drug factors.

2.2 Classification

(1) Acute type: Sudden onset, serious bleeding, and duration in less than 6 months.

(2) Chronic type: Insidious onset, or long disease course usually present with mild bleeding, and duration in over 6 months.

3 Pattern identification and treatment

The pattern identification is based upon the theory of eight principles, and the theory of bowels and viscera. According to the priority of onset and the various clinical manifestations, it is necessary to clearly identify excess pattern, deficiency pattern or

长，血块收缩不良，束臂实验阳性。

（3）骨髓巨核细胞增多或正常，有成熟障碍，主要表现为幼稚型和（或）成熟型无血小板释放的巨核细胞比例增加，巨核细胞颗粒缺乏，胞浆少。

（4）无明显肝、脾、淋巴结肿大。

（5）具有以下四项中任何一项：①肾上腺皮质激素治疗有效；②脾切除有效；③血小板相关抗体（PAIg、PAC_3）或特异性抗血小板抗体阳性；④血小板寿命缩短。

（6）排除其他可引起血小板减少的疾病，如再生障碍性贫血、白血病、骨髓增生异常综合征、其他免疫性疾病及药物性因素等。

2.2 分型

（1）急性型：起病急，出血一般较重，病程<6个月。

（2）慢性型：起病隐匿或病程迁延，出血一般较轻，病程超过6个月。

3 辨证论治

辨证以八纲辨证为主，兼用脏腑辨证。根据起病的缓急和临床不同的证候，分清实证、虚证、虚实夹杂证。

pattern of mixed deficiency and excess.

The acute type mostly belongs to excess pattern, often caused by infection of exogenous pathogenic heat, and is appropriately treated by the methods of clearing away heat, resolving toxin, cooling down blood and stoping bleeding. The chronic type usually belongs to deficiency pattern, mostly caused by deficiency and detriment of bowels and viscera, and is appropriately treated by the methods to boost qi and fortify the spleen, nourish and contain blood. For those with blood stasis, the treatment should be combined with the methods of quickening blood flow and dispersing blood stasis. For those with yin damage due to lingering illness, the treatment should be combined with the methods of enriching yin and clearing away heat.

急性型多属实证，常为外感邪热，治疗宜采用清热解毒、凉血止血之法；慢性型多属虚证，大多因脏腑虚损所致，治疗宜采用益气健脾，养血摄血之法；兼有瘀血者，配合活血化瘀法；久病伤阴者，应用滋阴清热之法。

(1) Injury of collaterals by blood heat

(1) 血热伤络

Manifestations: Sudden onset, stasis macules and stasis speckles on the skin, in bright red color, accompanied by bleeding gums and nosebleed, occasional bloody urine, red face and eyes, vexation and thirst, constipation, scanty urine, red tongue, yellow tongue coating, rapid pulse.

证候：起病急骤，皮肤出现瘀斑瘀点，色红鲜明，伴有齿衄鼻衄，偶有尿血，面红目赤，心烦口渴，便秘尿少，舌红，苔黄，脉数。

Therapeutic method: To clear away heat and resolve toxin, cool down blood and stop bleeding.

治法：清热解毒，凉血止血。

Main formula: *Rhinoceros Horn and Rehmannia Decoction* (Xi Jiao Di Huang Tang) with modification.

主方：犀角地黄汤加减。

Commonly used herbs: *Rhinocerotis Cornu* (Xi Jiao), *Rehmanniae Radix Cruda* (Sheng Di Huang), *Paeoniae Radix* (Shao Yao), *Moutan Cortex Radicis* (Mu Dan Pi).

常用药：犀牛角、生地黄、芍药、牡丹皮。

Modification: For fever, vexation, thirst with preference for drink, add *Cornu Saigae Tataricae*

加减：发热烦渴喜饮者，加羚羊角粉、生石膏、知母清

Pulverata (Ling Yang Jiao Fen), *Gypsum Fibrosum* (Sheng Shi Gao), *Anemarrhenae Rhizoma* (Zhi Mu) to clear away heat and drain fire; for constipation, add *Rhei Radix Et Rhizoma* (Da Huang) to relax the bowels and drain heat; for stasis speckles forming patches, add *Arnebiae Radix* (Zi Cao), *Platycladi cacumen Carbonisatum* (Ce Bai Tan) to cool down blood and resolve toxin; for bloody urine, add *Cirsii Herba* (Xiao Ji), *Imperatae Rhizoma* (Bai Mao Gen), *Agrimoniae Herba* (Xian He Cao) to cool down blood and stop bleeding; for bloody stool, add *Notoginseng Radix Et Rhizoma Pulverata* (San Qi Fen) and *Sanguisorbae Radix* (Di Yu) to astringe and stanch bleeding.

热泻火;便秘者,加大黄通腑泻热;瘀点成片者,加紫草、侧柏炭凉血解毒;尿血者,加小蓟、白茅根、仙鹤草凉血止血;便血者,加三七粉、地榆收敛止血。

(2) Failure of qi in containing blood

(2) 气不摄血

Manifestations: Recurrent stasis macules and speckles over the skin and mucus membrane, in faint green-blue color, accompanied by bleeding gums and nosebleed, fatigued spirit and lack of strength, sallow or somber, pale and lusterless facial complexion, poor appetite, sloppy stool or diarrhea, dizziness, palpitation, slight red tongue, thin tongue coating, thready and weak pulse.

证候:皮肤、黏膜瘀斑瘀点反复发作,色青紫而暗淡,伴鼻衄齿衄,神疲乏力,面色萎黄或苍白无华,食欲不振,大便溏泄,头晕心悸,舌淡红,苔薄,脉细弱。

Therapeutic method: To boost qi and fortify the spleen, contain and nourish blood.

治法:益气健脾,摄血养血。

Main formula: *Spleen-Returning Decoction* (Gui Pi Tang) with modifications.

主方:归脾汤加减。

Commonly used herbs: *Atractylodis Macrocephalae Rhizoma* (Bai Zhu), *Angelicae Sinensis Radix* (Dang Gui), *Poria Alba* (Bai Fu Ling), *Astragali Radix* (Huang Qi), *Longan Arillus* (Long Yan Rou), *Polygalae Radix* (Yuan Zhi), *Ziziphi Spinosi Semen* (Suan Zao Ren), *Aucklandiae Radix* (Mu Xiang), *Glycyrrhizae Radix Et Rhizoma* (Gan

常用药:白术、当归、白茯苓、黄芪、龙眼肉、远志、酸枣仁、木香、甘草。

Cao).

Modification: For continuous bleeding, add *Bletillae Rhizoma* (Bai Ji), *Typhae Pollen Carbonisata* (Pu Huang Tan) to harmonize blood and stanch bleeding; for poor appetite and sloppy stool, remove *Ziziphi Spinosi Semen* (Suan Zao Ren) and *Longan Arillus* (Long Yan Rou), add *Crataegi Fructus Ustus* (Jiao Shan Zha), *Fructus Setariae Germinatus* (Gu Ya) and *Hordei Fructus Germinatus* (Mai Ya), *Citri Reticulatae Pericarpium* (Chen Pi), and *Dioscoreae Rhizoma* (Shan Yao) to fortify the spleen and digest food.

加减:出血不止者,加白及、蒲黄炭和血止血;纳呆便溏者,去酸枣仁、龙眼肉,加焦山楂、谷麦芽、陈皮、山药健脾消食。

(3) Fire hyperactivity due to yin deficiency

(3) 阴虚火旺

Manifestations: Intermittent and scattered stasis mucules and speckles over the skin and mucus membrane, in bright red color, especially in the lower limbs, accompanied by gum bleeding, nosebleed, or bloody urine, low fever, night sweating, feverish sensation in the chest, palms and soles, vexation, flushed cheeks, dry mouth and throat, red tongue with little tongue coating, thready and rapid pulse.

证候:皮肤黏膜散在瘀点瘀斑,下肢尤甚,时发时止,颜色鲜红,伴齿衄、鼻衄或尿血,低热盗汗,手足心热,心烦颧红,口干咽燥,舌红少苔,脉细数。

Therapeutic method: To enrich yin and clear away heat, cool down blood and tranquilize the collaterals.

治法:滋阴清热,凉血宁络。

Main formula: *Major Yin Supplementation Pill* (Da Bu Yin Wan) and *Madder Root Powder* (Qian Gen San) with modification.

主方:大补阴丸合茜根散加减。

Commonly used herbs: *Rehmanniae Radix Praeparata* (Shu Di Huang), *Anemarrhenae Rhizoma* (Zhi Mu), *Phellodendri Cortex Chinensis (Huang Bo)*, *Carapax et Testudinis Carapax Et Plastrum* (Gui Jia), *Rubiae Radix Et Rhizoma* (Qian Gen), *Scutellariae Radix*(Huang Qin), *Gardeniae Fructus*

常用药:熟地黄、知母、黄柏、龟甲、茜根、黄芩、栀子、阿胶。

(Zhi Zi), *Colla Corii Asini* (E Jiao).

Modification: For flaming up of deficiency fire and obvious fever, add *Artemisiae Annuae Herba* (Qing Hao), *Lycii Cortex* (Di Gu Pi), and *Trionycis Carapax Et Rhizoma* (Bie Jia); for obvious night sweating, add *Lycii Cortex* (Di Gu Pi), *Os Draconis Calcinata* (Duan Long Gu), and *Ostreae Concha Calcinata* (Duan Mu Li); for obvious gum bleeding and nosebleed, add *Gardeniae Fructus Ustus* (Jiao Zhi Zi), *Imperatae Rhizoma* (Bai Mao Gen), *Agrimoniae Herba* (Xian He Cao).

加减:虚火内炽、发热明显者,加青蒿、地骨皮、鳖甲;盗汗明显者,加地骨皮、煅龙骨、煅牡蛎;齿衄、鼻衄明显者,加焦栀子、白茅根、仙鹤草。

(4) Qi stagnation and blood stasis

(4) 气滞血瘀

Manifestations: Continuous illness, recurrent bleeding, dark purpra on the skin, somber facial complexion, dark red or purple tongue, or purple patches on the tongue margin, thin white tongue coating, thready and hesitant pulse.

证候:病程缠绵,出血反复不止,皮肤紫癜色暗,面色晦暗,舌暗红或紫或边有紫斑,苔薄白,脉细涩。

Therapeutic method: To quicken blood flow and disperse blood stasis, regulate qi and stanch bleeding.

治法:活血化瘀,理气止血。

Main formula: *Peach Kernel Decoction* (Tao Ren Tang) with modification.

主方:桃仁汤加减。

Commonly used herbs: *Persicae Semen* (Tao Ren), *Rhei Radix Et Rhizoma* (Da Huang), *Natrii Sulfas* (Mang Xiao), *Cinnamomi Cortex Rasus* (Gui Xin), *Angelicae Sinensis Radix* (Dang Gui), *Glycyrrhizae Radix Et Rhizoma* (Gan Cao).

常用药:桃仁、大黄、芒硝、桂心、当归、甘草。

Modification: For qi deficiency, add *Codonopsis Radix* (Dang Shen) and *Astragali Radix* (Huang Qi) to supplement the spleen and boost qi; for bloody urine, add *Imperatae Rhizoma* (Bai Mao Gen) to cool down blood and stanch bleeding; for enduring stasis macules, add *Notoginseng Radix Et Rhizoma Pulverata* (San Qi Fen) to quicken blood

加减:气虚者,加党参、黄芪补脾益气;尿血者,加白茅根凉血止血;瘀斑久不消者,加三七粉活血化瘀。

flow and disperse blood stasis.

4 Other therapies

4.1 Chinese Patent medicine

(1) *Blood-Quieting Syrup* (Nin Xue Tang Jiang) is used for patterns of qi failing to contain blood.

(2) *Yunnan White* (Yun Nan Bai Yao) is used for nosebleed, gum bleeding, and bloody stool.

4.2 External therapy

Fill in powdered *Gardeniae Fructus*(Zhi Zi) at both sides of the nostrils, for purpura accompanied by nosebleed.

4 其他疗法

4.1 中成药

(1) 宁血糖浆:用于气不摄血证

(2) 云南白药:用于鼻衄、齿衄、便血。

4.2 外治疗法

栀子末少许塞两侧鼻孔,用于紫癜伴鼻出血者。

Chapter 5 Diseases of Urinary System

第5章 泌尿系统疾病

Section 1 Acute Glomerulonephritis

第1节 急性肾小球肾炎

Acute glomerulonephritis is abbreviated acute nephritis. It is a common immune response glomerular disease in pediatric clinics, manifested mainly by bloody urine, albuminuria, edema, and hypertension. It mostly occurs after infection, especially after hemolytic streptococcus infection, so it is also called acute post-streptococcal glomerulonephritis.

急性肾小球肾炎简称急性肾炎，是儿科常见的免疫反应性肾小球疾病，以血尿、蛋白尿、水肿和高血压为主要表现。大多发生于感染后，尤其是发生于溶血性链球菌菌珠感染后，故又称为急性链球菌感染后肾小球肾炎。

It often occurs in children of 3 to 8 years old, mostly in the autumn and winter. The infection of the respiratory tract is the most common route, and the skin infection comes the next.

本病好发于3～8岁小儿，以秋冬二季为多。感染途径以呼吸道感染最为常见，其次为皮肤感染。

In traditional Chinese medicine, it belongs to scope of “edema” and “bloody urine”.

本病属中医学“水肿”“尿血”范畴。

1 Etiology and pathogenesis

1 病因病机

It is mainly caused by infection of exogenous pathogenic wind, heat and dampness, and the internal disturbance by exogenous pathogens, leading to functional disorders of the lung, spleen and kidney.

主要因外感风热湿毒，外邪内扰使肺脾肾功能失调所致。

The infection of the external pathogenic wind, dampness, heat and sore toxin would induce the

外感风邪、湿热、疮毒，导致肺脾肾三脏功能失调。

functional disorders of the lung, spleen and kidney. The accumulation of pathogenic wind, heat, toxin and water dampness, dysfunction of regulation in water passage and of transformation and transportation, failure in closing and opening ability, and disorder in water metabolism would lead to edema. The injury of blood collaterals in the Lower Energizer by pathogenic heat would induce bloody urine. Overflow of pathogenic water in severe cases could cause patterns termed as invasion of evils into the heart and liver, invasion of water into the heart and lung, and internal blockage by water toxin.

风、热、毒与水湿互结，通调、运化、开阖失司，水液代谢障碍而为水肿；热伤下焦血络而致血尿。重症水邪泛滥可致邪陷心肝、水凌心肺、水毒内闭之证。

2 Key to diagnosis

2 诊断要点

(1) There is a history of infection in the respiratory tract or skin infection before the disease.

（1）发病前有呼吸道或皮肤感染史。

(2) Edema varies in different degrees. The mild cases could be only manifested by puffy eyelids in the morning. The severe cases would be present with edema in the lower limbs or the whole body, even with hydrothorax and ascites. The edema will not depress when pressed. There is scanty urine or no urine, and bloody urine by naked eyes or under microscope. There can be mild or medium hypertension like dizziness and headache in some cases.

（2）水肿轻重不等。轻者仅有晨起时双睑水肿，重者可有下肢或全身水肿，甚至出现胸水、腹水，水肿大多按之不凹陷。尿少或无尿，肉眼血尿或镜下血尿；部分患儿可出现头晕头痛等轻、中度高血压表现。

The severe cases may present complications and the complications mostly occur within one to two weeks after onset, including mainly severe circulatory congestion, hypertensive encephalopathy, and acute renal insufficiency, etc.

重症病例可以出现合并症，大多在起病1～2周内出现，主要有严重的循环充血、高血压脑病和急性肾功能不全等。

The atypical cases may occur with no symptoms, or only abnormal findings in urine analysis, or with nephrotic syndrome.

非典型病例可无症状或仅有尿检异常，或以肾病综合征的方式起病。

(3) The routine urianlysis could show albumen,

（3）尿常规检查可见蛋

red blood cell, or a little white blood cell, as well as increased erythrocyte sedimentation rate, decreased C_3, and increased anti-"O", etc, in most cases.

白、红细胞或少许白细胞。大多有血沉增快、C_3降低、抗"O"增高等。

3 Pattern identification and treatment

3 辨证论治

It is necessary to identify acute phase or chronic phase for ordinary cases and to identify the bowels and visceras for transmuted patterns. The acute phase of acute nephritis is at a period of exuberance in constitution and excess in pathogens, manifested by rapid onset, quick change, puffiness and obvious bloody urine. The recovery phase is mainly characterized by decrease in puffiness, increase in quantity of urine, no bloody urine by the naked eyes, hematuria and albuminuria under microscope, and lingering retention of dampness and heat. If scanty urine, bloated belly, fullness in the chest, panting and coughing, and palpitation are still present, it could be diagnosed as upward attack of water into the heart and lung. If coma, delirious speech, convulsion, syncope, rapid breathing are still present, it could be diagnosed as penetration of pathogens into the pericardium and internal blockage of Jueyin meridian. If anuresis, nausea, vomiting, foul breath, sloppy stool, and epistaxis are still present, it could be diagnosed as internal accumulation of water and toxin, and failure and exhaustion in the spleen and kidney.

常证辨急性期与慢性期;变证辨脏腑。急性肾炎的急性期为正盛邪实阶段,起病急,变化快,浮肿及血尿多较明显。恢复期共同特点为浮肿已退,尿量增加,肉眼血尿消失,但镜下血尿或蛋白尿未恢复,且多有湿热留恋。若见尿少、腹大、胸满、咳喘、心悸、应考虑水气上凌心肺;若见神昏谵语、抽风痉厥、呼吸急促,应考虑邪陷心包,内闭厥阴;若见尿闭、恶心呕吐、口有秽气、便溏、衄血,为水毒内闭,脾肾败绝。

The disease is mainly excessive in the evils and should be treated accordingly and appropriately by the clarifying, diluting and diffusing method. The common treatment principle is supposed to clear away heat, resolve toxin, diffuse the lung qi and re-

本病以邪实为主,治当因其势而利导之,宜清、宜渗、宜利。常用治则有清热解毒,宣肺利水,疏风利咽,清热利湿。并对变证积极防治。

move water, expel wind and benefit the throat, clear away heat and dissolve dampness. The transmuted patterns should be prevented actively.

3.1 Ordinary patterns

(1) Fighting of wind and water

Manifestations: Puffy eyelids, obvious puffy face, followed by edema in the limbs, and even in the chest and abdomen, shining skin and non-depressed edema, scanty and brown urine, bloody urine in most cases, fever, aversion to wind, cough, sore throat, slight red tongue, thin white tongue coating, and floating pulse.

Therapeutic method: To expel wind and diffuse the lung qi, disinhibit water and disperse swelling.

Main formula: *Ephedra, Forsythia, and Rice Bean Decoction* (Ma Huang Lian Qiao Chi Xiao Dou Tang) with modification.

Commonly used herbs: *Ephedrae Herba* (Ma Huang), *Forsythiae Fructus* (Lian Qiao), *Vignae Semen* (Chi Xiao Dou), *Lonicerae Flos Japonicae* (Jin Yin Hua), *Plantaginis Herba* (Che Qian Cao), *Platycodonis Radix* (Jie Geng), *Imperatae Rhizoma* (Bai Mao Gen), *Glycyrrhizae Radix Et Rhizoma* (Gan Cao).

Modification: For cold exterior, add *Notopterygii Rhizoma seu Radix* (Qiang Huo), and Schizonepetae Herba (Jing Jie); for vexation, thirst and interior heat, add *Gypsum Fibrosum* (Sheng Shi Gao) and *Scutellariae Radix* (Huang Qin); for obvious bloody urine, add *Cirsii Herba* (Xiao Ji) and *Imperatae Rhizoma* (Bai Mao Gen); for sore throat, add *Sophorae Tonkinensis Radix Et Rhizoma* (Shan Dou Gen), and *Rabdosiae Rubescentis Herba* (Dong Ling Cao).

3.1 常证

(1) 风水相搏

证候:眼睑先肿,颜面浮肿明显,继而四肢,甚则胸腹,皮肤光亮,按之不凹陷,小便短黄,多有血尿,或有发热恶风,咳嗽,咽喉肿痛,舌质淡红,苔薄白,脉浮。

治法:疏风宣肺,利水消肿。

主方:麻黄连翘赤小豆汤加减。

常用药:麻黄、连翘、赤小豆、金银花、车前草、桔梗、白茅根、甘草。

加减:若有表寒症状者,加羌活、荆芥;烦躁口渴,有里热者,加生石膏、黄芩;血尿明显者,加小蓟、白茅根;咽喉肿痛者,加山豆根、冬凌草。

(2) Internal invasion of dampness and heat

Manifestations: Edema or no edema, scanty and brown urine, bloody urine in most cases with a history of infection of sores and boils, red tongue, yellow or slimy tongue coating, rapid and slippery pulse.

Therapeutic method: To clear away heat and disinhibit dampness.

Main formula: *Field Thistle Drink* (Xiao Ji Yin Zi) with modification.

Commonly used herbs: *Cirsii Herba* (Xiao Ji), *Typhae Pollen* (Pu Huang), *Angelicae Sinensis Radix* (Dang Gui), *Rehmanniae Radix Cruda* (Sheng Di Huang), *Lophatheri Herba* (Dan Zhu Ye), *Forsythiae Fructus* (Lian Qiao), *Nodus Nelumbinis Rhizomatis* (Ou Jie), *Gardeniae Fructus* (Zhi Zi), *Agrimoniae Herba* (Xian He Cao).

Modification: For severe swelling, add *Plantaginis Herba* (Che Qian Cao) and *Arecae Pericarpium* (Da Fu Pi); for bloody urine, add *Cirsii japonica herba* (Da Ji), *Pyrrosiae Folium* (Shi Wei), and *Moutan Cortex Radicis* (Mu Dan Pi); for skin sores and boils, add *Chrysanthemi Indici Flos* (Ye Ju Hua), *Violae Herba* (Zi Hua Di Ding), *Semiaquilegiae Radix* (Tian Kui Zi), and *Taraxaci Herba* (Pu Gong Ying).

(3) Qi deficiency of the lung and spleen

Manifestations: Fatigue and lack of strength, sallow facial complexion, poor appetite, sloppy stool, spontaneous sweating, susceptibility to common cold, slight red tongue, white tongue coating, slow and weak pulse.

Therapeutic method: To boost qi and secure the defending ability, fortify the spleen and dissolve

(2) 湿热内侵

证候:水肿可有可无,小便短赤,多有血尿,可有皮肤疮毒史,舌质红,苔黄或腻,脉滑数。

治法:清热利湿。

主方:小蓟饮子加减。

常用药:小蓟、蒲黄、当归、生地黄、淡竹叶、连翘、藕节、栀子、仙鹤草。

加减:肿甚者,加车前草、大腹皮;尿血明显者,加大蓟、石韦、牡丹皮;皮肤有疮疡者,加金银花、野菊花、紫花地丁、天葵子、蒲公英。

(3) 肺脾气虚

证候:身倦乏力,面色萎黄,纳少便溏,自汗出,易于感冒,舌淡红,苔白,脉缓弱。

治法:益气固卫,健脾化湿。

dampness.

Main formula: *Ginseng, Poria, and White Atractylodes Powder* (Shen Qin Bai Zhu San) with modification.

主方:参苓白术散加减。

Commonly used herbs: *Codonopsis Radix*(Dang Shen), *Astragali Radix* (Huang Qi), *Poria* (Fu Ling), *Atractylodis Macrocephalae Rhizoma* (Bai Zhu), *Dioscoreae Rhizoma* (Shan Yao), Citri Reticulatae Pericarpium (Chen Pi), *Lablab Semen Album* (Bai Bian Dou), *Coicis Semen* (Yi Yi Ren), *Glycyrrhizae Radix Et Rhizoma*(Gan Cao).

常用药:党参、黄芪、茯苓、白术、山药、陈皮、白扁豆、薏苡仁、甘草。

Modification: For continual bloody urine, add *Notoginseng Radix Et Rhizoma* (San Qi) and *Angelicae Sinensis Radix* (Dang Gui); for copious sweating, add *Os Draconis* (Long Gu), and *Ostreae Concha* (Mu Li); for dark tongue or tongue with stasis speckles, add *Salviae Miltiorrhizae Radix Et Rhizoma* (Dan Shen), *Carthami Flos*(Hong Hua), and *Lycopi Herba*(Ze Lan).

加减:血尿持续不消者,加三七、当归;汗多者,加龙骨、牡蛎;舌质淡暗或有瘀点者,加丹参、红花、泽兰。

3.2 Transmuted patterns

3.2 变证

(1) Water attacking the heart and lung

(1) 水凌心肺

Manifestations: Obvious swelling in the whole body, coughing, short breath, pale facial complexion, palpitation, chest oppression, vexation and agitation, difficult to lie on the back, and even purple lips and nails, dark red tongue, white and slimy tongue coating, thready, rapid and forceless pulse.

证候:全身明显浮肿,咳嗽气急,面色苍白,心悸胸闷,神情烦躁,难以平卧,甚则唇甲青紫,舌质暗红,舌苔白腻,脉细数无力。

Therapeutic method: To drain the lung fire and expel water, warm up yang and support the Vital Energy.

治法:泻肺逐水,温阳扶正。

Main formula: *Stephania, Zanthoxylum, Descurainia, and Rhubarb Pill* (Ji Jiao Li Huang Wan) and *Ginseng and Aconite Decoction* (Shen Fu Tang)

主方:己椒苈黄丸合参附汤加减。

with modifications.

Commonly used herbs: *Stephaniae Tetrandrae Radix* (Fang Ji), *Zanthoxyli Semen* (Jiao Mu), *Descurainiae Lepidii Semen* (Ting Li Zi), *Rhei Radix Et Rhizoma* (Da Huang), *Aconiti Lateralis Radix Praeparata* (Fu Zi), *Ginseng Radix* (Ren Shen), *Mori Cortex* (Sang Bai Pi), *Plantaginis Semen* (Che Qian Zi).

常用药：防己、椒目、葶苈子、大黄、附子、人参、桑白皮、车前子。

Modification: For scanty urine, add *Polyporus* (Zhu Ling), *Alismatis Rhizoma* (Ze Xie). When there is gray and whitish facial complexion, extreme cold limbs, sweating and weak pulse, it is a critical condition of heart yang debilitation, so *Ginseng, Aconite, Dragon Bone, Oyster Shell Counterflow Decoction* (Shen Fu Long Mu Jiu Ni Tang) should be applied immediately.

加减：尿少者，加猪苓、泽泻。若见面色灰白，四肢厥冷，汗出脉微，是心阳虚衰之危象，应急用参附龙牡救逆汤。

(2) Penetration of evils into the heart and liver

(2) 邪陷心肝

Manifestations: Puffiness in the body or face, scanty and brown urine, headache, dizziness, blurred vision, vexation and agitation, vomiting, even convulsion, coma, red tongue, rough and yellow tongue coating, rapid and string-taut pulse.

证候：肢体面部浮肿，小便短赤，头痛，眩晕，视物模糊，烦躁，呕吐，甚或抽搐、昏迷，舌质红，苔黄糙，脉弦数。

Therapeutic method: To calm down the liver, drain fire, clear the heart and disinhibit water.

治法：平肝泻火，清心利水。

Main formula: *Gentian Liver-Draining Decoction* (Long Dan Xie Gan Tang) and *Antelope Horn and Uncaria Decoction* (Ling Jiao Teng Gou Tang) with modification.

主方：龙胆泻肝汤合羚角钩藤汤加减。

Commonly used herbs: *Gentianae Radix Et Rhizoma* (Long Dan), *Chrysanthemi Flos* (Ju Hua), *Scutellariae Radix* (Huang Qin), *Gardeniae Fructus* (Zhi Zi), *Rehmanniae Radix Cruda* (Sheng Di Huang), *Alismatis Rhizoma* (Ze Xie), Plantaginis Semen (Che Qian Zi), *Lophatheri Herba* (Dan

常用药：龙胆、菊花、黄芩、栀子、生地黄、泽泻、车前子、淡竹叶、羚羊角、钩藤、白芍。

Zhu Ye), *Antelopis Tataricae Cornu* (Ling Yang Jiao), *Uncariae ramulus Cum uncis* (Gou Teng), *Paeoniae Radix Albae* (Bai Shao).

Modification: For constipation, add *Rhei Radix Et Rhizoma* (Da Huang), and *Natrii Sulfas* (Mang Xiao); for relatively serious headache and dizziness, add *Prunella Spica* (Xia Ku Cao), and *Haliotidis Concha* (Shi Jue Ming); for nausea and vomiting, add *Pinelliae Rhizoma* (Ban Xia), and *Arisaema Cum Bile* (Dan Nan Xing); for coma and convulsion, add *Bovine Bezoar and Heart-Purifying Pills* (Niu Huang Qing Xin Wan) or *Peaceful Palace Bovine Bezoar Pills* (An Gong Niu Huang Wan).

加减:大便秘结者,加大黄、芒硝;头痛眩晕较重者,加夏枯草、石决明;恶心呕吐者,加半夏、胆南星;昏迷抽搐者,可加服牛黄清心丸或安宫牛黄丸。

(3) Internal blockage of water toxin

(3) 水毒内闭

Manifestations: Puffiness all over the body, scanty urine or anuresis, in tea-like color, dizziness, headache, nausea, vomiting, somnolence or even coma, grimy and slimy tongue coating, rapid and slippery pulse.

证候:全身浮肿,尿少或尿闭,色如浓茶,头晕,头痛,恶心,呕吐,嗜睡甚或昏迷,舌苔垢腻,脉滑数。

Therapeutic method: To open by acrid herbs, descend by bitter herbs, and to repel foulness and resolve toxin.

治法:辛开苦降,辟秽解毒。

Main formula: *Gallbladder-Warming Decoction* (Wen Dan Tang) and *Aconite Heart-Draining Decoction* (Fu Zi Xie Xin Tang) with modification.

主方:温胆汤合附子泻心汤加减。

Commonly used herbs: *Coptidis Rhizoma* (Huang Lian), *Rhei Radix Et Rhizoma* (Da Huang), Scutellariae Radix(Huang Qin), *Pinelliae Rhizoma* (Ban Xia), *Citri Reticulatae Pericarpium* (Chen Pi), *Bambusae Caulis in Taenias* (Zhu Ru), *Aurantii Fructus Immaturus* (Zhi Shi), *Poria* (Fu Ling), *Plantaginis Semen* (Che Qian Zi), *Aconiti Lateralis Radix Praeparata* (Fu Zi), *and Zingiberis Rhizoma Recens* (Sheng Jiang).

常用药:黄连、大黄、黄芩、半夏、陈皮、竹茹、枳实、茯苓、车前子、附子、生姜。

Modification: For obvious nausea and vomiting, add *Jade Pivot Elixir* (Yu Shu Dan); for convulsion, add *Antelopis Tataricae Cornu* (Ling Yang Jiao) and *Purple Snow Elixir* (Zi Xue Dan).

加减:恶心呕吐明显者,加玉枢丹;抽搐者,加羚羊角、紫雪丹。

4 Other therapies

4 其他疗法

4.1 Chinese Patent medicine

4.1 中成药

(1) *Nephritis Recovery Pill* (Shen Yan Kang Fu Pian) is used for nephritis at recovery stage, for those with deficiency in qi and yin.

(1) 肾炎康复片　适用于肾炎恢复期,有气阴不足见症者。

(2) *Anemarrhena, Phellodendron, and Rehmannia Pill* (Zhi Bo Di Huang Wan) is used for the disease at recovery stage, for those with bloody urine due to yin deficiency.

(2) 知柏地黄丸　适用于本病恢复期,阴虚血尿者。

4.2 Acumoxatherapy

4.2 针灸疗法

(1) Body acupuncture: Select Feishu (BL 13), Lieque (LU 7), Hegu (LI 4), Yinlingquan (SF 9), Shuifen (CV 9), Sanjiaoshu (BL 22), puncture by the needling technique for sedation. For sore throat, add Shaoshang (LU 11). For severe puffy face, add Shuigou (GV 26). For hypertension, add Quchi (LI 11) and Taichong (LR 3).

(1) 体针:取肺俞、列缺、合谷、阴陵泉、水分、三焦俞。针刺,均用泻法。咽痛者,配少商;面部肿甚者,配水沟;血压高者,配曲池、太冲。

(2) Ear Acupuncture: Select two to three ear points of Pt. Kidney, Pt. Spleen, Pt. Bladder, Pt. Sympathetic Nerve, and Pt. Endocrine, etc., and puncture by light stimulation, and embed the ear acupoint with the needles after acupuncture for 24 hours. Acupuncture is given once every day, for 10 sessions as one course.

(2) 耳针:从肾、脾、膀胱、交感、肾上腺、内分泌等耳穴中每次选 2～3 穴,轻刺激,刺后可埋针 24 小时,每日 1 次,10 次为 1 个疗程。

4.3 Tuina therapy

4.3 推拿疗法

(1) Acute stage: Tranquilize Pt. Ganjing, clarify Pt. Feijing, Pt. Weijing, Pt. Pijing, Pt. Xiaochangjing, and knead Pt. Liufu.

(1) 急性期:平肝经,清肺经、胃经、脾经、小肠经、退六腑。

(2) Recovery Stage: Tranquilize Pt. Ganjing, clari-

(2) 恢复期:平肝经,清补

fy and supplement Pt. Shenjing, rub Pt. Erma, and clarify Pt. Xiaochang.

肾经、脾经,揉二马,清小肠。

4.4 External therapy

(1) Swelling-Diminishing Formula: Pound *Luffae Pericarpium Pericarpium* (Si Gua Pi), *Benincasae Exocarpium* (Dong Gua Pi), *Maydis Stigma* (Yu Mi Xu), 30g each, and apply to the umbilicus, for acute swelling.

(2) Bathing method: Decoct 20g of each of the followings with water: *Notopterygii Rhizoma seu Radix* (Qiang Huo), *Ephedrae Herba* (Ma Huang), *Atractylodis Rhizoma* (Cang Zhu), *Bupleuri Radix* (Chai Hu), *Perillae Caulis* (Zi Su Geng), *Ledebouriellae Radix* (Fang Feng), Schizonepetae Herba (Jing Jie), Arctii Fructus (Niu Bang Zi), *Caulis Lonicerae* (Ren Dong Teng), *Bulbus Allii Fistulosi* (Cong Bai). After decoction cools down to 40℃, take a bath with it till sweating, once every day.

4.4 外治疗法

（1）消肿方:丝瓜皮、冬瓜皮、玉米须各 30 克,共捣烂,外敷于脐部,适用于急性期水肿。

（2）沐浴法:羌活、麻黄、苍术、柴胡、紫苏梗、防风、荆芥、牛蒡子、忍冬藤、葱白各 20 克。加水煮上药,冷至 40 ℃沐浴。汗出即可。每日 1 次。

4.5 Medicated diet of Chinese medicine

(1) *Saposhnikovia Porridge* (Fang Feng Zhou): *Ledebouriellae Radix* (Fang Feng) 15g, *Bulbus Allii Fistulosi* (Cong Bai) (2 pieces with root hair), non-glutinous rice 100g. First decoct *Ledebouriellae Radix* (Fang Feng) and *Bulbus Allii Fistulosi* (Cong Bai) to take decoction and remove dregs. Cook porridge with non-glutinous rice in the usual way. When it is almost cooked, add the decoction. Drink the cooked porridge. It is applied to the initial stage of wind and water, accompanied by exterior syndrome of wind and cold.

(2) *Wax Gourd Rind and Coix Seed Soup* (Dong Gua Pi Yi Ren Tang): Cook *Benincasae Exocarpium* (Dong Gua Pi) 50g, *Coicis Semen* (Yi Yi Ren) 50g, *Vignae semen* (Chi Xiao Dou) 100g, *Maydis Stigma*

4.5 中药膳食

（1）防风粥:防风 15 克,葱白(连须)2 根,粳米 100 克,先煎防风、葱白取汁去渣,粳米按常法煮粥,粥将熟时,加入药汁,熬成稀粥服食。适用于风水初起,兼风寒表证。

（2）冬瓜皮薏仁汤:冬瓜皮 50 克,薏苡仁 50 克,赤小豆 100 克,玉米须(布包)25 克。加水适量,同煮至赤小

(Yu Mi Xu)(wrapped in cloth) 25g, with adequate amount of water, till *Vignae semen* (Chi Xiao Dou) is fully cooked. Eat beans and drink soup. It is used for obvious swelling at the acute stage, or accompanied by hypertension.

豆熟透，食豆饮汤。适用于急性期水肿明显，或伴有高血压者。

Section 2 Nephrotic Syndrome

第 2 节 肾病综合征

Nephrotic syndrome, simplified as nephropathy, is a clinical syndrome caused by the increased permeability of the glomerular filtration membrane due to a variety of causes, leading to loss of considerable number of plasma proteins from urine, and clinically characterized by loads of proteinuria, hypoproteinemia, hyperlipemia, and edema in varying degrees. It often occurs in children from 2 to 8 years old. The peak incidence is in those from 2 to 5 years old.

肾病综合征简称肾病，是一组由多种原因引起的肾小球滤过膜通透性增加，导致大量血浆蛋白从尿中丢失的临床症候群。临床以大量蛋白尿、低蛋白血症、高脂血症和不同程度的水肿为特征。多发于 2～8 岁小儿，其中以 2～5 岁为发病高峰。

In traditional Chinese medicine, it belongs to the scope of "edema" and "consumptive diseases".

本病属中医学"水肿""虚劳"范畴。

1　Etiology and pathogenesis

The main internal cause is related to insufficiency of the natural endowment and weak body constitution after prolonged illness in the infants, resulting in depletion of the lung, spleen and kidney. The common inducing cause is related to infection of exogenous pathogenic factor. The main pathogenesis is related to the dysfunction of the lung, spleen and kidney, inducing the breakdown of qi dynamics, transportation and transformation, failure in storing ability, outward discharge of the es-

1　病因病机

小儿禀赋不足，久病体虚，致肺脾肾三脏亏虚是主要内因；感受外邪是常见诱因。肺脾肾三脏功能虚弱，气化、运化功能失常，封藏失职，精微外泄，水液停聚则是主要的发病机理。

sential substance, and retention of water and fluid.

The nephrotic syndrome belongs to the scope of "edema and yin water". The pathological location of the disease lies in deficiency of the lung, spleen and kidney. In the course of illness, it is often accompanied by existence of exogenous evils, such as exogenous evils, water, dampness, turbidity, and blood stasis, etc., showing a phenomenon of deficiency in the Vital Energy and excess in the symptoms, and of deficiency and excess complex.

肾病综合征属"水肿阴水"范畴,病位重点在肺脾肾不足,病程中常兼见外邪、水湿、湿浊、瘀血等邪气,呈本虚标实,虚实夹杂之象。

2 Key to diagnosis

(1) Simple nephropathy It complies with the following four features: ① loads of proteinuria (UPRO is often above + + +, 24 h UPRO is > 0.05g/kg); ② hypoproteinemia: plasma albumin< 30g/L; ③ hyperlipemia: blood cholesterol > 5.7mmol/L; ④ obvious edema. Of the 4 items, loads of proteinuria and hypoproteinemia are requisites.

(2) Nephritis nephropathy Besides the four features in simple nephritis, there are one or more features of the following items: ① obvious bloody urine, red blood cell >10/HP (distributed in the three smaples of centrifugal urine in two weeks); ② continuous or recurrent hypertension (blood pressure of school children >130/90 mmHg, blood pressure of preschool children>120/80mmHg, by exclusion of the condition not caused by hormone; ③ continuous azotemia (Blood urea nitrogen > 10.7mmol/L), by exclusion of the condition not

2 诊断要点

(1) 单纯性肾病 符合以下四大特征:①大量蛋白尿(尿蛋白定性常在+++以上,24小时尿蛋白定量>0.05克/千克);②低白蛋白血症:血浆白蛋白<30克/升;③高脂血症:血胆固醇>5.7毫摩尔/升;④明显水肿。以上4项中以大量蛋白尿和低蛋白血症为必备条件。

(2) 肾炎性肾病 除单纯型肾病四大特征外,还具有以下四项之一或多项。①明显血尿:尿中红细胞>10个/高倍视野(分布于2周内3次离心尿标本);②高血压持续或反复出现(学龄儿童血压>130/90毫米汞柱,学龄前儿童血压>120/80毫米汞柱,并排除激素所致者;③持续性氮质血症(血尿素

caused by hypovolemia, and ④ repeated decrease of total complement (CH_{50}) or hemalexin C_3.

氮>10.7 毫摩尔/升，并排除血容量不足所致者；④血总补体量（CH_{50}）或血补体 C_3 反复降低。

3　Pattern identification and treatment

3　辨证论治

It is mainly necessary to identify between bowels and viscera: relatively severe puffiness in the eyelids and face, accompanied by symptoms of the lung system, mostly belongs to wind and is related to the lung pathologically. Severe edema under the waist, accompanied by symptoms of spleen dampness, belongs to the spleen. Extremely severe edema under the waist and abdomen, accompanied by aversion to cold, lack of warmth in the four limbs, poor appetite and sloppy stool, shows involvement of the spleen and kidney.

主要辨脏腑：眼睑及颜面浮肿较甚，兼有肺系症状者，多属风，病在肺；腰以下肿甚，兼有脾湿症状者，病在脾；腰腹以下剧肿，兼有畏寒怕冷，四肢不温，纳差便溏者，病在脾肾。

The basic therapeutic principle is to support the Vital Energy and build up the constitutional foundation, by boosting qi, fortifying the spleen, supplementing the kidney, and regulating yin and yang in predominance; meanwhile in order to treat the clinical symptoms, there can be a combination of the methods to promote the lung, disinhibit water, clear away heat, disperse blood stasis and dampness, and downbear the turbidity.

以扶正培本为基本治则，重在益气健脾补肾、调理阴阳，同时注意配合宣肺、利水、清热、化瘀、化湿、降浊等祛邪之法以治其标。

(1) Accumulation of dampness due to spleen deficiency

（1）脾虚湿困

Manifestations: Puffiness in the limbs and body, in depression by pressure, sallow facial complexion, fatigued spirit and lack of strength, oppression in the chest, abdominal distention, reduced food intake, sloppy stool, scanty urine, lack of warmth in the limbs, pale tongue, white glossy

证候：肢体浮肿，按之深陷，面色萎黄，神疲乏力，胸闷腹胀，纳少便溏，小便短少，四肢欠温，舌质淡，苔白滑，脉缓或细弱。

tongue coating, slow or thready and weak pulse.

Therapeutic method: To warm up the Middle Energizer and promote transportation, circulate qi and disinhibit water.

治法:温运中阳,行气利水。

Main formula: *Spleen-Strengthening Decoction* (Shi Pi Yin) with modification.

主方:实脾饮加减。

Commonly used herbs: *Aconiti Lateralis Radix Praeparata* (Fu Zi), *Zingiberis Rhizoma* (Gan Jiang), *Astragali Radix* (Huang Qi), *Poria* (Fu Ling), *Atractylodis Macrocephalae Rhizoma* (Bai Zhu), *Chaenomelis Fructus* (Mu Gua), *Magnoliae Officinalis Cortex* (Hou Pu), *Arecae semen* (Bing Lang), *Fructus Tsaoko* (Cao Guo), *Glycyrrhizae Radix Et Rhizoma* (Gan Cao).

常用药:附子、干姜、黄芪、茯苓、白术、木瓜、厚朴、槟榔、草果、甘草。

Modification: For obvious puffiness, add *Five-Peel Decoction* (Wu Pi Yin); for spontaneous sweating and susceptible to getting cold, use *Astragali Radix* (Huang Qi) in high dose, and add *Ledebouriellae Radix* (Fang Feng), and *Ostreae Concha* (Mu Li); for accompanied aching pain in the lumbar spine, add *Schisandrae Fructus Chinensis* (Wu Wei Zi), *Cuscutae Semen* (Tu Si Zi), *Cistanchis Herba* (Rou Cong Rong), etc.

加减:浮肿明显者,加五皮饮;自汗易感冒者,重用黄芪,加防风、牡蛎;伴腰脊酸痛者,加用五味子、菟丝子、肉苁蓉等。

(2) Yang deficiency of spleen and kidney

(2) 脾肾阳虚

Manifestations: Severe puffiness, in depression by finger pressure, puffy eyelids, hydrothorax, acites, worse in the abdomen and the lower limbs, bright pale facial complexion, fatigued spirit and lack of strength, fear of cold, lack of warmth in the limbs, poor appetite, sloppy stool, and even cough and gasping, fullness in the chest and rapid panting, difficult to lie down, pale tongue, white tongue coating, thready and weak pulse.

证候:高度浮肿,按之没指,目胞浮肿,胸水腹水,腰腹下肢为甚,面色晄白,神疲乏力,畏寒怕冷,四肢不温,纳差便溏,甚则咳逆上气,胸满喘急,难以平卧,舌质淡,苔白,脉细无力。

Therapeutic method: To warm up the kidney

治法:温肾健脾,化气

and fortify the spleen, transform qi and circulate water.

行水。

Main formula: *True Warrior Decoction* (Zhen Wu Tang) and *Five-Peel Decoction* (Wu Pi Yin) with modification.

主方: 真武汤合五皮饮加减。

Commonly used herbs: *Aconiti Lateralis Radix Praeparata* (Fu Zi), *Astragali Radix* (Huang Qi), *Poria* (Fu Ling), *Atractylodis Macrocephalae Rhizoma* (Bai Zhu), *Paeoniae Radix Albae* (Bai Shao), *Arecae Pericarpium* (Da Fu Pi), *Citri Reticulatae Pericarpium* (Chen Pi), *Zingiberis Rhizoma Recens* (Sheng Jiang), *Glycyrrhizae Radix Et Rhizoma* (Gan Cao).

常用药: 附子、黄芪、茯苓、白术、白芍、大腹皮、陈皮、生姜、甘草。

Modification: For severe kidney yang deficiency, add *Trigonellae Semen* (Hu Lu Ba), *Cinnamomi Cortex* (Rou Gui), and *Epimedii Folium* (Yin Yang Huo); for severe water and dampness, add *Cinnamomi Ramulus* (Gui Zhi), *Polyporus* (Zhu Ling), and *Alismatis Rhizoma* (Ze Xie); for scanty urine and difficult urination, add *Zanthoxyli Semen* (Jiao Mu); for diarrhea, add *Baked Zingiberis Rhizoma Recens* (Pao Jiang), and *Psoraleae Fructus* (Bu Gu Zhi).

加减: 肾阳虚重者,加胡芦巴、肉桂、淫羊藿;水湿重者,加桂枝、猪苓、泽泻;尿少不利者,加椒目;腹泻者,加炮姜、补骨脂。

(3) Yin deficiency of liver and kidney

(3) 肝肾阴虚

Manifestations: Mild edema or no edema, tidal reddening of the face, vexing heat in the five hearts, night sweating, headache, dizziness, profuse dreaming and susceptible to fright, limp aching of lumbus and knees, dry stool, red tongue, little tongue coating, thread, rapid and string-taut pulse.

证候: 水肿不重或无水肿,面色潮红,五心烦热,盗汗,头痛眩晕,多梦易惊,腰膝酸软,便干,舌质红,苔少,脉弦细数。

Therapeutic method: To enrich the liver and kidney, foster yin and subdue yang.

治法: 滋补肝肾,育阴潜阳。

Main formula: *Anemarrhena, Phellodendron, and Rehmannia Pill* (Zhi Bo Di Huang Wan) with

主方: 知柏地黄丸加减。

modification.

Commonly used herbs: *Rehmanniae Radix Cruda* (Sheng Di Huang), *Anemarrhenae Rhizoma* (Zhi Mu), *Corni Fructus* (Shan Zhu Yu), *Phellodendri Cortex Chinensis*(Huang Bo), Moutan Cortex *Radicis* (Mu Dan Pi), *Poria* (Fu Ling), *Alismatis Rhizoma* (Ze Xie), *Ecliptae Herba* (Mo Han Lian), and *Glycyrrhizae Radix Et Rhizoma*(Gan Cao).

常用药:生地黄、知母、山茱萸、黄柏、牡丹皮、茯苓、泽泻、墨旱莲、甘草。

Modification: For fire hyperactivity due to yin deficiency, use *Rehmanniae Radix Cruda* (Sheng Di Huang), *Anemarrhenae Rhizoma* (Zhi Mu), and *Phellodendri Cortex Chinensis*(Huang Bo) in large dose. For yin deficiency and heat toxin, add *Lonicerae Flos Japonicae* (Jin Yin Hua), *Hedyotis Diffusae Herba* (Bai Hua She She Cao), and *Isatidis Radix* (Ban Lan Gen); for edema, add *Plantaginis Semen*(Che Qian Zi).

加减:阴虚火旺者,重用生地黄、知母、黄柏;阴虚热毒者,加金银花、白花蛇舌草、板蓝根;有水肿者,加车前子。

(4) Qi stagnation and blood stasis

(4) 气滞血瘀

Manifestations: Somber or soot-black facial complexion, squamous and dry skin, lingering edema, accompanied by lumbus pain or bloody urine, dark and purple tongue, rough or string-taut pulse.

证候:面色晦暗或黧黑,肌肤甲错,水肿难消,常伴腰痛或血尿,舌质紫暗,或有瘀点,脉涩或弦。

Therapeutic method: To quicken blood flow and disperse blood stasis.

治法:活血化瘀。

Main formula: *Peach Kernel and Safflower Four Agents Decoction* (Tao Hong Si Wu Tang) with modification.

主方:桃红四物汤加减。

Commonly used herbs: *Angelicae Sinensis Radix* (Dang Gui), *Chuanxiong Rhizoma* (Chuan Xiong), *Persicae Semen* (Tao Ren), *Carthami Flos* (Hong Hua), Paeoniae Radix *Albae* (Bai Shao), and *Rehmanniae Radix Praeparata* (Shu Di Huang).

常用药:当归、川芎、桃仁、红花、白芍、熟地黄。

Modification: For severe blood stasis, add *Rubiae Radix Et Rhizoma* (Qian Cao), *Sparganii*

加减:若瘀血重者,加茜草、三棱、泽兰;血尿不止者,

Rhizoma (San Leng), and *Lycopi Herba* (Ze Lan); for incessant bloody urine, add *Typhae Pollen Carbonisatae* (Pu Huang Tan), *Cirsii Herba* (Xiao Ji), and *Angelicae Sinensis Radix Carbonisatae* (Dang Gui Tan); for accompanying qi deficiency, add *Astragali Radix* (Huang Qi), and *Codonopsis Radix* (Dang Shen).

加蒲黄炭、小蓟、当归炭；兼气虚者，加黄芪、党参。

4 Other therapies

4 其他疗法

4.1 Chinese Patent medicine

4.1 中成药

(1) *Glucosidorum Tripterygll Totorum Tablets* (Lei Gong Teng Duo Dai Pian) is used for various patterns of renal diseases.

（1）雷公藤多甙片：适用于肾病各个证型。

(2) *Chronic Nephritis Tablets* (Shen Kang Ning Pian) is used for pattern of accumulation of blood stasis and water due to deficiency of kidney yang.

（2）肾康宁片：适用于肾病肾阳虚弱、瘀水互结证。

(3) *Six-Ingredient Rehmannia Pill* (Liu Wei Di Huang Wan) is used for pattern of yin deficiency in the liver and kidney.

（3）六味地黄丸：适用于肾病肝肾阴虚证。

4.2 Acumoxatherapy

4.2 针灸疗法

(1) Body acupuncture: Select Shenshu (BL 23), Pishu (BL 20), Taixi (KI 3), Zusanli (ST 36), Sanyinjiao (SP 6), Qihai (CV 4), Shuifen (CV 9), and puncture by the needling technique for tonification. Apply 3 moxa cones for moxibustion on each acupoint.

（1）体针：取肾俞、脾俞、太溪、足三里、三阴交、气海、水分。针刺，均用补法。灸法各3壮。

(2) Ear acupuncture: Select the ear points of Pt. Spleen, Pt. Kidney, Pt. Subcortex, and Pt. Bladder, two to three ear points each time bilaterally, and puncture by the medium stimulation, and retain the needles for 30 minutes, or embed the intradermal needles for 24 hours, once every day, for 10 sessions as one course.

（2）耳针：取脾、肾、皮质下、肾上腺、膀胱。每次取2～3穴，双侧，用中等刺激，留针30分钟，或埋皮内针24小时，隔日1次，10次为1个疗程。

4.3 Tuina therapy

(1) For yang deficiency in the spleen and kidney, supplement the kidney for 3 minutes, rub Pt. Erma for 2 minutes, rub Pt. Dantian for 2 minutes, rub Shenque (CV 8) for 2 minutes, and push Pt. Sanguan for 2 minutes.

(2) For yin deficiency of the liver and kidney, balance the liver for 2 minutes, supplement the kidney for 2 minutes, rub Pt. Erma for 2 minutes, rub Sanyinjiao (SP 6) for 2 minutes.

4.3 推拿疗法

(1) 脾肾阳虚者,补肾 3 分钟,揉二马 2 分钟,揉丹田 2 分钟,揉神阙 2 分钟,推三关 2 分钟。

(2) 肝肾阴虚者,平肝 2 分钟,补肾 2 分钟,揉二马 2 分钟,揉三阴交 2 分钟。

4.4 Dietetic therapy

(1) Recommendation and restriction: ① In edema and hypertension, give a diet of low salt or no salt temporarily. ② Restrict water intake in scanty urine. ③ Supplement Vitamin D and calcium in defined amount. ④ Supply protein and energy in normal needs for children at the same age. For children with large volume of protein urine, injection of protein should be restricted properly.

(2) Chinese medicated diet: ① Cook one carp with 50g of *Vignae semen* (Chi Xiao Dou) and eat after it is fully cooked. ② Cook a soup with 50g of *Astragali Radix* (Huang Qi) and soft-shelled turtle or chicken.

4.4 饮食疗法

(1) 饮食宜忌:①有水肿和高血压时,给予低盐或短暂无盐饮食。②尿少病例应限制入水量。③适量补充维生素 D 和钙剂。④蛋白质和热量需要按同龄儿童正常需要供应,大量蛋白尿的患儿要适当限制蛋白质的摄入量。

(2) 中药药膳:①鲤鱼 1 条,赤小豆 50 克,煮熟后食用;②黄芪 50 克,煎汤煮甲鱼或炖鸡肉。

Section 3 Urinary Infection

The urinary infection of the urinary system, also known as urinary tract infection, simplified as urinary infection, refers to an inflammation caused by invasion of pathogen into the urinary tract directly. According to the invaded and attacked locations by pathogen, it is generally divided into ne-

第3节 泌尿系感染

泌尿系感染又称尿路感染,简称尿感,是指病原体直接侵入尿路而引起的炎症。按病原体侵袭的部位不同,一般分为肾盂肾炎、膀胱炎、尿道炎。肾盂肾炎又称上尿

phropyelitis, cystitis and urethritis. Nephropyelitis is also called upper urinary tract infection, and cystitis and urethritis are jointly called lower urinary tract infection. Because infection of urinary tract is seldom to be limited in a certain location in the infanthood, clinically it is difficult to determine the location. Therefore, it is known collectively as urinary tract infection.

路感染，膀胱炎和尿道炎合称为下尿路感染。由于小儿时期感染局限在尿路某一部位者少见，临床定位困难，故统称为尿路感染。

This disease can occur at any age during infanthood, mostly common in the infants under 2 years old. It belongs to the scope of "frequent urination", "strangury patterns" in traditional Chinese medicine.

小儿时期任何年龄均可发病，2 岁以下幼儿多见。本病属中医学"尿频""淋证"等范畴。

1　Etiology and pathogenesis

1　病因病机

Mainly, it is caused by accumulation of dampness and heat in the bladder, or breakdown of qi dynamics in the bladder, due to constitutional insufficiency of the spleen and kidney.

主要由湿热蕴结膀胱，或素体脾肾不足，膀胱气化失司所致。

Because of short urinary tract and exposed urethral orifice, the girls are susceptible to impact from external evils and heat toxin. Because of dirty scales in phimosis or constipation, urine holding, overfilling bladder, the boys are susceptible to infection of the pathogenic dampness and heat. Over ingestion of sweet, fatty and greasy food, internal injury of milk feeding, and production of heat by accumulated dampnesss, leading to internal retention of dampness and heat in the bladder, and hence dysfunction of qi dynamics, would also cause frequent urination. If the spleen qi is deficient and fails to perform its transportation and transformation and fails to ascend the clear, water and body fluids cannot be distributed. When the kidney is deficient and

女孩尿道短，外口显露，易受外邪热毒影响；男孩包茎积垢或因便秘、憋尿、膀胱过度充盈，易为湿热邪毒所染；恣食肥甘厚味，内伤乳食，酿湿生热，湿热内伏，蕴郁膀胱，气化失司，引起尿频。脾气虚弱，运化无力，升清无能，水津不布；肾虚则不能温煦，气化失常，均可致尿频。若病程迁延日久，脾肾气虚损及脾肾之阳，则可伴浮肿、神疲乏力、面黄肢冷。

unable to perform the warming ability, causing dysfunction of qi dynamics, there will be frequent urination. If the duration lingers for a long time, qi deficiency in the spleen and kidney would involve the spleen yang and kidney yang, leading to puffiness, fatigued spirit and lack of strength, sallow face, cold limbs.

The diseased location lies in the kidney and bladder. The pathogenic cause is mainly related to dampness and heat. Excess pattern is mainly characterized by retention of pathogenic dampness and heat in the bladder. Deficiency pattern is predominantly induced by dysfunction of qi dynamics in the bladder, due to constitutional insufficiency in the spleen and kidney.

病位在肾与膀胱，病因多为湿热。湿热之邪蕴结膀胱者，实证为主；若因素体脾肾不足，膀胱气化失司所致者，则以虚证为主。

2 Key to diagnosis

(1) Urinary tract infection: Frequent urination, urinary urgency, painful urination, possibly accompanied by symptoms like fever, vomiting, etc, plus white blood cells in routine urine test, and bacteria growth in bacterial culture of urine.

(2) Daytime frequency syndrome: It often occurs in the infanthood, manifested by frequent urinary desire in the daytime. Urinary desire disappears after sleep at night, and it is negative in routine urine test and bacterial culture of urine. It can disappear on its own.

2 诊断要点

(1) 尿路感染：尿频、尿急、尿痛，可伴有发热、呕吐等症。尿常规可见白细胞，尿细菌培养可见细菌生长。

(2) 白天尿频综合征：多发生在婴幼儿时期。患儿白天尿意频繁，但夜间入睡后消失，尿常规、尿细菌培养均阴性，可自行消失。

3 Pattern identification and treatment

It is necessary to identify excess and deficiency: the excess pattern is manifested by sudden onset, short duration, frequency of urination, scanty and brown urine, burning pain in the urinary tract, turbid or bloody urine, and aversion to cold, fever and

3 辨证论治

本证重在辨别虚实：属实证者起病急，病程短，小便频数短赤，尿道灼热疼痛，尿浊或血尿，可见恶寒发热、呕吐等症；虚中夹实证病势缓，

vomiting. The pattern of deficiency mixed with excess is characterized by slow development of illness, long duration, and manifested by frequent urination, dribbling urination, clear urine without pain, fatigued spirit, aching lumbus and lack of strength.

病程较长,以小便频数,淋漓不畅,尿清无痛,精神倦怠,腰酸乏力为特征。

The therapeutic principle is mainly supposed to clear away heat and remove dampness for the excess pattern and to supplement the spleen and kidney by the warm herbs for deficiency pattern. Additionaly, the treatment should be stressed particularly in certain aspect according to different patterns. It is appropriate to dredge the bowels and discharge heat for accumulation of heat in the spleen and stomach, and to clarify and promote the liver and gallbladder, discharge fire and resolve toxin for accumulated heat in the liver and gallbladder. The prolonged duration and repeated seizure are mostly attributed to pattern of deficiency in the Vital Energy and tip excess in the symptoms, and of mixture of deficiency and excess. Therefore, the treatment should be given to deal with the constitutional energy and symptoms, by both the attacking and reinforcing techniques.

属实证者,以清热利湿为主要治则,虚证宜温补脾肾。又根据不同证型有所侧重,有脾胃积热者,宜通腑泻热;有肝胆郁热者,宜清利肝胆,泻火解毒;病程日久或反复发作者,多为本虚标实、虚实夹杂之候,治疗要标本兼顾,攻补兼施。

(1) Downward infusion of dampness and heat

Manifestations: Quick onset, frequent urination, scanty, brown and turbid urine, scorching pain in the urethera, aching lumbus, intermittent crying in the infants, often accompanied by fever, vexation, thirst, headache, body pain, nausea, vomiting, bitter and sticky taste in the mouth, red tongue, slimy and yellow tongue coating, rapid and slippery pulse, purple fingerprints.

(1) 湿热下注

证候:起病较急,小便频数、短赤,尿液混浊,尿道灼痛,腰部酸痛,婴儿则时作啼哭。常伴发热,烦躁口渴,头痛身痛,恶心呕吐,口苦口黏,舌质红,苔黄腻,脉滑数,指纹紫。

Therapeutic method: To clear away heat and remove dampness.

治法:清热利湿。

Main formula: *Eight Corrections Powder* (Ba Zheng San) with modification.

主方:八正散加减。

Commonly used herbs: *Polygoni Avicularis Herba* (Bian Xu), *Dianthi Herba* (Qu Mai), *Tetrapanacis Medulla* (Tong Cao), *Talcum* (Hua Shi), *Gardeniae Fructus* (Zhi Zi), *Alismatis Rhizoma* (Ze Xie), *Rhei Radix Et Rhizoma* (Da Huang), *Glycyrrhizae Radix Et Rhizoma* (Gan Cao).

常用药:萹蓄、瞿麦、通草、滑石、栀子、泽泻、大黄、甘草。

Modification: For fever and aversion to cold, add *Bupleuri Radix* (Chai Hu), and *Scutellariae Radix* (Huang Qin); for nausea and vomiting, add *Bambusae Caulis in Taenias* (Zhu Ru), *Pogostmonis Herba* (Huo Xiang), and *Pinelliae Rhizoma* (Ban Xia); for distention in the lower abdomen and difficult urination, add *Bupleuri Radix* (Chai Hu), *Toosendan Fructus* (Chuan Lian Zi), and *Corydalis Rhizoma* (Yan Hu Suo); for abdominal fullness and sloppy stool, get rid of *Rhei Radix Et Rhizoma* (Da Huang), and add *Arecae Pericarpium* (Da Fu Pi), and *Amomi Fructus Rotundus* (Bai Dou Kou); for bloody urine, scorching pain in the urethera, and interrupted urination, add *Lysimachiae Herba* (Jin Qian Cao), *Lygodii Spora* (Hai Jin Sha), and *Galli Endothelium Corneum Gigerii* (Ji Nei Jin).

加减:发热恶寒者,加柴胡、黄芩;恶心呕吐者,加竹茹、藿香、半夏;少腹作胀,排尿不利者,加柴胡、川楝子、延胡索;腹满便溏者,去大黄,加大腹皮、肉豆蔻;小便带血,尿道灼痛,排尿中断者,可加金钱草、海金沙、鸡内金。

(2) Qi deficiency of the spleen and kidney

(2) 脾肾气虚

Manifestations: Prolonged illness, repeated seizure, frequent urination, sallow facial complexion, poor appetite, even aversion to cold, fear of cold, lack of warmth in the hands and feet, aching lumbus and knees, loose stool, swelling eyelids, pale tongue or with teeth marks, slimy and thin tongue coating, thready and weak pulse.

证候:病程日久,反复不愈,小便频数,面色苍黄,食欲不振,甚则畏寒怕冷,手足不温,腰膝酸痛,大便稀薄,眼睑浮肿,舌质淡或有齿痕,苔薄腻,脉细少力。

Therapeutic method: To supplement the spleen and kidney by warm herbs.

治法:温补脾肾。

Main formula: *Stream Reducing Pills* (Suo Quan Wan) with supplements.

主方:缩泉丸加味。

Commonly used herbs: *Alpiniae Oxyphyllae Fructus* (Yi Zhi), *Dioscoreae Rhizoma* (Shan Yao), *Linderae Radix* (Wu Yao), *Poria* (Fu Ling), *Euryales Semen* (Qian Shi), Plantaginis Semen(Che Qian Zi), *Glycyrrhizae Radix Et Rhizoma* (Gan Cao).

常用药:益智、山药、乌药、茯苓、芡实、车前子、甘草。

Modification: For frequency of micturation at night, add *Mantidis Oötheca* (Sang Piao Xiao), and *Os Draconis Cruda* (Sheng Long Gu).

加减:夜尿增多者,加桑螵蛸、生龙骨。

4 Other therapy

4 其他疗法

4.1 Chinese Patent medicine

4.1 中成药

(1) *Golden Three Pills* (San Jin Pian) is used for urinary infection in pattern of downward infusion of dampness and heat.

(1) 三金片:适用于尿路感染湿热下注证。

(2) *Gentian Liver-Draining Pills* (Long Dan Xie Gan Wan) is used for urinary infection in pattern of downward infusion of dampness and heat.

(2) 龙胆泻肝丸:适用于尿路感染湿热下注证。

(3) *Life Saver Kidney Qi Pills* (Ji Sheng Shen Qi Wan) is used for urinary infection in pattern of qi deficiency in the spleen and kidney.

(3) 济生肾气丸:适用于尿路感染脾肾气虚证。

4.2 Acumoxatherapy

4.2 针灸疗法

Body acupoints: Shenshu (BL 23), Sanyinjiao (SP 6). Ear acupoints: Pt. Adrenal Gland, and puncture once every day. Or select Zhongji (CV 3), Guanyuan (CV 4), Sanyinjiao (SP 6), Pangguangshu (BL 28), and puncture with strong stimulation. Or select Lieque (LU 7), insert the filiform needle obliquely for 0.5 inch, with the needle tip slightly upward. Do not twist and rotate the needle in inserting the needle, till a response appears. Then, twist the needle with the thumb forward for several times

体穴肾俞、三阴交,耳穴肾上腺,每日针刺1次。或取中极、关元、三阴交、膀胱俞等穴,强刺激。亦可取列缺穴,用毫针,针尖稍向上斜刺5分,进针时不捻转,待有感应时再行捻转手法,大指向前推捻数次出针。

before taking out the needle.

4.3 Tuina therapy

Rub Pt. Dantian for 200 times, rub abdomen for 20 minutes, rub Guiwei (GV 1) for 30 times. Use the chafing method for elder children, to chafe Shenshu (BL 23), Shangliao (BL 31), Ciliao (BL 32), Zhongliao (BL 33) and Xiaoliao (BL 34) horizontally till a warm sensation appears, for qi deficiency of the spleen and kidney.

4.3 按摩疗法

揉丹田 200 次，摩腹 20 分钟，揉龟尾 30 次，较大儿童可用擦法，横擦肾俞、八髎，以热为度。适用于脾肾气虚者。

4.4 External therapy

(1) Select *Lonicerae Flos Japonicae* (Jin Yin Hua), *Taraxaci Herba* (Pu Gong Ying), *Phellodendri Cortex Chinensis* (Huang Bo), *Kochiae Fructus* (Di Fu Zi), and *Stemonae Radix* (Bai Bu), each 30g. Decoct with water and take bath for once or twice each day, 30 min every time, for pattern of dampness and heat in the bladder, manifested by frequent urination, urgent urination and painful urination.

(2) Select *Sophorae Flavescentis Radix* (Ku Shen), Phellodendri Cortex Chinensis(Huang Bo), each 15g, *Smilacis Glabrae Rhizoma* (Tu Fu Ling), *Cnidii Fructus* (She Chuang Zi), each 10g. Decoct with water and take bath twice per day, 1 dose every day, for accumulation of heat in the liver and bladder, manifested by frequency of urination and urgency of urination.

4.4 外治疗法

(1) 金银花、蒲公英、黄柏、地肤子、百部各 30 克，水煎坐浴，每日 1～2 次，每次 30 分钟。用于膀胱湿热证，症见尿频、尿急、尿痛者。

(2) 苦参、黄柏各 15 克，土茯苓、蛇床子各 10 克，水煎坐浴，每日 1 剂，坐浴 2 次，用于肝胆郁热证，症见尿频、尿急者。

Chapter 6 Diseases of Nervous System

第6章 神经系统疾病

Section 1 Epilepsy

第1节 癫痫

Epilepsy is paroxysmal cerebral dysfunction caused by various reasons, characterized by sudden and transient cerebral dysfunction in relation to repeated and paroxysmal excessive discharge of electricity in the neurons of the brain, and clinically manifested by functional disorders in motion, sense, behavior, perception or consciousness.

In traditional Chinese medicine, it belongs to the scope of "epileptic disease" and "epilepsy".

癫痫是由多种原因引起的发作性脑功能障碍疾病，其特征是脑内神经元群反复发作性过度放电引起的突发性、一过性脑功能失常，临床出现运动、感觉、行为、知觉或意识方面的功能障碍。

本病属中医学“痫病”“癫痫”等范畴。

1 Etiology and pathogenesis

1 病因病机

The pathogenic factors can be prenatal or postnatal. The prenatal factors are mainly related to fright in embryo, and improper care in pregnancy. The postnatal factors are related to internal retention of obstinate phlegm, exposure to sudden fear and fright, frequent infantile convulsion, traumatic injury of the skull and brain, etc.

致病因素有先天与后天之分，先天之因主要为胎中受惊，孕期调护失宜，后天之因有顽痰内伏、暴受惊恐、惊风频发、颅脑外伤等。

Because the infants are often insufficient in the spleen, phlegm and fluids could be produced internally, leading to obstruction of the meridians and collaterals by phlegm, and hence there is upward counterflow to the orifice. When the fetus is inside the mother's body, if the mother is frightened ex-

小儿脾常不足，内生痰饮，痰阻经络，上逆窍道。儿在母腹之中，若母惊于外，则胎感于内。小儿神气怯弱，若乍见异物，卒闻异声，或不慎跌仆，暴受惊恐，可致气机

ternally, the fetus will feel internally. The infants are timid and weak in the spirit and qi. When seeing or hearing something strange, or falling down accidentally, the infants will be frightened, causing chaotic counterflow of qi dynamic. When phlegm flows reversely with qi, it would mist the clear orifices, and obstruct the meridians and collaterals. Epilepsy could occur, when the exogenous pestilent factors and toxins are infected, which transform into heat and fire, and produce wind due to preponderance of fire, and further produce phlegm due to preponderance of wind, causing upward stirring of wind and fire and mixture of phlegm and fire. If epilepsy frequently reoccurs, without complete eradication, the pathogenic wind and retained phlegm would struggle with each other, further obstructing the meridians and collaterals and disturbing the mind and spirit. The operation for difficult labor or traumatic injury of skull and brain may damage blood vessels, inducing extravasation. The retention and accumulation of blood stasis would mist the brain, inducing loss of the bright spirit, confusion in the mind, malnutrition of the tendons and frequent seizure of convulsion. All the above factors and problems related to wind, fright, phlegm, and blood stasis can cause epilepsy.

逆乱，痰随气逆，蒙蔽清窍，阻滞经络。外感瘟疫邪毒，化热化火，火盛生风，风盛生痰，风火相煽，痰火交结，可发痫证。癫痫频作，未得根除，风邪与伏痰相搏，进而闭塞经络，扰乱神明。难产手术或颅脑外伤，血络受损，血溢络外，瘀血停积，脑窍不通，以致精明失主，昏乱不知人，筋脉失养，抽搐顿作。以上种种，风、惊、痰、瘀为患，皆可致痫。

2 Key to diagnosis

(1) General and paroxysmal sudden fainting, rigidity in the nape and back, tremor in the limbs, or staring with the two eyes, no response to any call, dropping head, flaccid and weak limbs.

(2) In partial seizure, manifested in multiple ways by local convulsion of the mouth, eye, or hand

2 诊断要点

(1) 全身性发作时突然昏倒，项背强直，四肢抽搐。或仅两目瞪视，呼之不应，或头部下垂，肢软无力。

(2) 部分性发作时可见多种形式，如口、眼、手等局

but without sudden fainting, or visual hallucination, or vomiting, profuse sweating, or speech disorder, or unconscious movements, etc.

部抽搐而无突然昏倒，或幻视，或呕吐，多汗，或言语障碍，或无意识的动作等。

(3) Sudden onset, normal like ordinary person after waking up, repeated seizure.

(3) 起病急骤，醒后如常人，反复发作。

(4) There is often a family history, induced every time by fear and fright, fatigue, or extreme emotional activity.

(4) 多有家族史，每因惊恐、劳累、情志过极等诱发。

(5) There are often premonitory signs of vertigo and stuffy sensation in the chest before seizure.

(5) 发作前常有眩晕、胸闷等先兆。

(6) Electroencephalography (EEG) is positive. The examinations by CT, nuclear magnetic resonance are needed, if available.

(6) 脑电图检查有阳性表现，有条件做CT、核磁共振检查。

3 Pattern identifications and treatment

3 辨证论治

In pattern identification for this disease, it is necessary to identify the severity first, and then to identify the causes of disease.

本病辨证，应首分轻重，继辨病因。

The mild cases are often characterized by fewer seizures, short duration, long intervals, slight convulsion, short period of loss of consciousness, slight degree of abnormal electroencephalography (EEG), no abnormality seen by MRI. The severe cases are characterized by sudden onset, frequent and severe convulsion, loss of consciousness, long duration, frequent seizure, seriously abnormal EEG, or organic diseases seen by MRI, and difficulty to be controlled by anti-epilepsy drugs. Prior to the epilepsy due to fright, there is a history of being frightened. During seizure, it is often accompanied by mental symptoms, like screaming and fear. Epilepsy due to wind is often induced by infection of exogenous wind and heat, manifested by obvious convulsion during seizure or accompanied by fever.

发作次数少、持续时间短、间隔时间长，抽搐轻微，意识丧失时间短，脑电图异常程度较轻，颅脑影像学检查未见异常者多属轻症。若起病急骤，抽搐频剧，意识丧失，持续时间长，发作频繁，脑电图异常程度重，或颅脑影像学检查有器质性疾病，抗痫药物难以控制者，则属重症。惊痫发病前常有惊吓史，发作时常伴惊叫、恐惧等精神症状；风痫多由外感发热所诱发，发作时抽搐明显，或伴发热等症；痰痫发作以神识异常为主，常有一过性

Epilepsy due to phlegm is mainly manifested by abnormal consciousness, transient absence of mind, tumble, or object falling down from the hand, and possibly accompanied by symptoms of excessive sputum and saliva. Epilepsy due to blood stasis usually has an obvious history of traumatic injury of the skull and brain, and a relatively localized painful position of the head.

失神、摔倒，手中持物坠落，可伴痰涎壅盛等症；瘀血痫通常有明显的颅脑外伤史，头部疼痛位置较为固定。

In the treatment of epilepsy, it is necessary to distinguish between Vital Energy and clinical symptoms, and between deficiency and excess. The clinical symptoms should be mainly treated for frequent seizure, by dissipating phlegm and extinguishing wind, and opening the aperture and stopping epilepsy. The Vital Energy should be mainly treated for lingering illness leading to deficiency, by strengthening the spleen and dissolving phlegm, or benefiting the kidney and replenishing essence. For persistent status of epilepsy, the medications from both Chinese medicine and Western medicine should be combined to save patients.

癫痫的治疗，应分标本虚实，频繁发作者治标为主，着重豁痰息风，开窍定痫；病久致虚者，以治本为重，或健脾化痰，或益肾填精。癫痫持续状态须中西药配合抢救。

(1) Epilepsy due to fright

(1) 惊痫

Manifestations: Screaming by fright at seizure, urgent crying, fright and fear, abstraction of the spirit and mind, intermittent red or pale facial complexion, convulsion in the four limbs, mental confusion, constitutional timidity and easy frightenedness, spiritual fearfulness, or vexation and irascibility, restless sleep, slight red tongue, white tongue coating, slippery and string-taut pulse, green-blue fingerprint.

证候：发作时惊叫，急啼，惊惕不安，神志恍惚，面色时红时白，四肢抽搐，神昏，平素胆小易惊，精神恐惧或烦躁易怒，夜寐不安，舌淡红，苔白，脉弦滑，指纹青。

Therapeutic method: To settle the fright and calm down the spirit.

治法：镇惊安神。

Main formula: *Fright Settling Pills* (Zhen Jing

主方：镇惊丸加减。

Wan) with modification.

Commonly used herbs: *Poria Cum Ligno Hospite* (Fu Shen), *Ziziphi Spinosi Semen* (Suan Zao Ren), *Acori Rhizoma Tatarinowii* (Shi Chang Pu), *Polygalae Radix* (Yuan Zhi), *Uncariae Ramulus Cum Uncis* (Gou Teng), *Gastrodiae Rhizoma* (Tian Ma), *Arisaema Cum Bile* (Dan Nan Xing), *Pinelliae Rhizoma* (Ban Xia), *Coptidis Rhizoma* (Huang Lian), *Aquilariae Lignum Resinatum* (Chen Xiang).

常用药:茯神、酸枣仁、石菖蒲、远志、钩藤、天麻、胆南星、半夏、黄连、沉香。

Modification: For frequent convulsion, add *Scolopendra* (Wu Gong), *Scorpio* (Quan Xie), and *Bombyx Batryticatus* (Jiang Can); for night crying and fright, add *Magnetitum* (Ci Shi), *Ferric Oxide* (Tie Luo Hua), *Succini Pulvis* (Hu Po Fen) (Take after infused with water); for headache, add *Chrysanthemi Flos* (Ju Hua), and *Haliotidis Concha* (Shi Jue Ming).

加减:抽搐发作频繁者,加蜈蚣、全蝎、僵蚕;夜惊哭闹者,加磁石、铁落花、琥珀粉(冲服);头痛者,加菊花、石决明。

(2) Epilepsy due to phlegm

(2) 痰痫

Manifestations: Sudden tumble and prostration in seizure, staring straight forward, phlegm rale in the throat, convulsion of limbs or partial convulsion, or unobvious convulsion, loss of consciousness or abstraction of spirit, spiritlessness, or headache, abdominal pain, body pain, sticky mouth with profuse sputum, oppression in the chest, vomiting, nausea, possible low intelligence, white and slimy tongue coating, slippery pulse.

证候:发作时突然跌仆,瞪目直视,喉中痰鸣,四肢抽搐,或局部抽动,或抽搐不明显,意识丧失,或神志恍惚,失神,或头痛,腹痛,肢体疼痛,口黏多痰,胸闷呕恶,可伴有智力低下,舌苔白腻,脉滑。

Therapeutic method: To dissipate phlegm and open the orifice.

治法:豁痰开窍。

Main formula: *Phlegm-Flushing Decoction* (Di Tan Tang) with modification.

主方:涤痰汤加减。

Commonly used herbs: *Acori Rhizoma Tatarinowii* (Shi Chang Pu), *Arisaema Cum Bile*

常用药:石菖蒲、胆南星、陈皮、清半夏、枳壳、沉

(Dan Nan Xing), *Citri Reticulatae Pericarpium* (Chen Pi), *Pinelliae Rhizoma Praeparata* (Qing Ban Xia), *Aurantii Fructus* (Zhi Qiao), *Aquilariae Lignum Resinatum* (Chen Xiang), *Chuanxiong Rhizoma* (Chuan Xiong), *Massa Medicata Fermentata* (Liu Shen Qu), *Gastrodiae Rhizoma* (Tian Ma), *Canarii Fructus* (Qing Guo), *Chloriti Lapis* (Qing Meng Shi)(decoct first).

香、川芎、六神曲、天麻、青果、青礞石(先煎)。

Modification: For winking, nodding, and frequent seizure, add *Bambusae Concretio Silicea* (Tian Zhu Huang), *Succini Pulvis* (Hu Po Fen) (take after infused with water), and *Nelumbinis Plumula* (Lian Zi Xin); for headache, add *Chrysanthemi Flos* (Ju Hua); for abdominal pain, add *Corydalis Rhizoma* (Yan Hu Suo), *Toosendan Fructus* (Chuan Lian Zi), *Paeoniae Radix Albae* (Bai Shao), *Glycyrrhizae Radix Et Rhizoma* (Gan Cao); for vomiting, add *Haematitum* (Zhe Shi), and *Bambusae Caulis in Taenias* (Zhu Ru); for body pain, add *Clematidis Radix Et Rtrhizoma* (Wei Ling Xian) and *Spatholobi Caulis* (Ji Xue Teng).

加减:眨眼、点头、发作较频者,加天竺黄、琥珀粉(冲服)、莲子心;头痛者,加菊花;腹痛者,加延胡索、川楝子、白芍、甘草;呕吐者,加赭石、竹茹;肢体疼痛者,加威灵仙、鸡血藤。

(3) Epilepsy due to wind

(3) 风痫

Manifestations: Sudden prostration in seizure, staring upward or sideward, clenched jaw, foaming at the mouth, green-blue mouth, lips and facial complexion, rigidity of neck and back, frequent convulsion, coma, slight red tongue, white tongue coating, slippery and string-like pulse.

证候:发作时突然仆倒,两目上视或斜视,牙关紧闭,口吐白沫,口唇及面部色青,颈项强直,频繁抽搐,神志昏迷,舌质淡红,苔白,脉弦滑。

Therapeutic method: To extinguish wind and check tetany.

治法:息风止痉。

Main formula: *Fit-Settling Pills* (Ding Xian Wan) with modification.

主方:定痫丸加减。

Commonly used herbs: *Gastrodiae Rhizoma* (Tian Ma), *Scorpio* (Quan Xie), *Scolopendra* (Wu

常用药:天麻、全蝎、蜈蚣、石菖蒲、远志、胆南星、半

Gong), *Acori Rhizoma Tatarinowii* (Shi Chang Pu), *Polygalae Radix* (Yuan Zhi), *Arisaema Cum Bile* (Dan Nan Xing), *Pinelliae Rhizoma* (Ban Xia), *Chloriti Lapis* (Qing Meng Shi), *Citri Reticulatae Pericarpium* (Chen Pi), *Poria* (Fu Ling), *Succinum* (Hu Po) (Take after infused with water), *Chuanxiong Rhizoma* (Chuan Xiong), *Aurantii Fructus* (Zhi Qiao), *Uncariae ramulus Cum uncis* (Gou Teng).

夏、青礞石、陈皮、茯苓、琥珀（冲服）、川芎、枳壳、钩藤。

Modification: For high fever, add *Gypsum Fibrosum* (Sheng Shi Gao), Forsythiae Fructus (Lian Qiao), *Antelopis Tataricae Cornu* (Ling Yang Jiao) (grind and take after infused with water); for constipation, add *Rhei Radix Et Rhizoma* (Da Huang), *Natrii Sulfas Exsiccatus* (Xuan Ming Fen) (take after infused with water), and *Aloe* (Lu Hui); for vexation and agitation, add *Coptidis Rhizoma* (Huang Lian), *Gardeniae Fructus* (Zhi Zi), and *Lophatheri Herba* (Dan Zhu Ye); for lingering condition manifested by yin deficiency of the liver and kidney and internal stirring of deficient wind, add *Paeoniae Radix Albae* (Bai Shao), *Carapax et Testudinis Carapax Et Plastrum* (Gui Jia), *Angelicae Sinensis Radix* (Dang Gui), and *Rehmanniae Radix Cruda* (Sheng Di Huang).

加减：高热者，加生石膏、连翘、羚羊角（研末冲服）；大便秘结者，加大黄、玄明粉（冲服）、芦荟；烦躁不安者，加黄连、栀子、淡竹叶；久治不愈，出现肝肾阴虚、虚风内动之象者，可加用白芍、龟甲、当归、生地黄。

(4) Epilepsy due to blood stasis

(4) 瘀血痫

Manifestations: Repeated and lingering convulsion, fixed position of headache. seizures related to menstrual period in the elder girls, seizure before menstrual cycle, distention and fullness in the breasts, hypochondriac region and lower abdomen at the ordinary times, dark purple tongue or with stasis speckles, scanty tongue coating, hesitant pulse, deep and stagnant fingerprints.

证候：反复抽搐，经久不愈，头痛有定处，年长女孩的发作往往与月经周期有关，行经前易发作，平素易胸胁少腹胀满，舌质紫暗或有瘀点，苔少，脉涩，指纹沉滞。

Therapeutic method: To activate blood and extinguish wind.

治法：活血息风。

Main formula: *Orifices Opening and Blood Activating Decoction* (Tong Qiao Huo Xue Tang) with modification.

主方：通窍活血汤加减。

Commonly used herbs: *Persicae Semen* (Tao Ren), *Carthami Flos* (Hong Hua), *Chuanxiong Rhizoma* (Chuan Xiong), *Paeoniae Radix Rubra* (Chi Shao), *Alliium Fistulosum Vetum* (Lao Cong), *Acori Rhizoma Tatarinowii* (Shi Chang Pu), *Gastrodiae Rhizoma* (Tian Ma), *Notopterygii Rhizoma seu Radix* (Qiang Huo).

常用药：桃仁、红花、川芎、赤芍、老葱、石菖蒲、天麻、羌活。

Modification: For recurrent convulsion, add *Scorpio* (Quan Xie), and *Zaocys* (Wu Shao She); for severe headache, add *Salviae Miltiorrhizae Radix Et Rhizoma* (Dan Shen), and *Trogopterorum Faeces* (Wu Ling Zhi); for constipation, add *Aloe* (Lu Hui), and *Cannabis Fructus*(Huo Ma Ren).

加减：抽搐频繁者，加全蝎、乌梢蛇；头痛剧烈者，加丹参、五灵脂；大便秘结者，加芦荟、火麻仁。

(5) Abundance of phlegm due to spleen deficiency

（5）脾虚痰盛

Manifestations: Repeated seizure, forceless convulsion, lusterless facial complexion, occasional dizziness, fatigued spirit, lack of strength, stuffy sensation in the chest and epigastric region, poor appetite, sloppy stool, slight red tongue, white and slimy tongue coating, thready and weak pulse, slight red fingerprint.

证候：反复发作，抽搐无力，面色无华，时作头晕，神疲乏力，胸脘痞闷，纳呆便溏，舌质淡红，苔白腻，脉细软，指纹淡红。

Therapeutic method: To strengthen the spleen and dissolve phlegm.

治法：健脾化痰。

Main formula: *Six Gentlemen Decoction* (Liu Jun Zi Tang) with modification.

主方：六君子汤加减。

Commonly used herbs: *Ginseng Radix* (Ren Shen), *Atractylodis Macrocephalae Rhizoma* (Bai Zhu), *Poria* (Fu Ling), *Glycyrrhizae Radix Et*

常用药：人参、白术、茯苓、甘草、陈皮、半夏、天麻、钩藤、乌梢蛇。

Rhizoma (Gan Cao), *Citri Reticulatae Pericarpium* (Chen Pi), *Pinelliae Rhizoma* (Ban Xia), *Gastrodiae Rhizoma* (Tian Ma), *Uncariae Ramulus Cum Uncis* (Gou Teng), *Zaocys* (Wu Shao She).

Modification: For loose stool, add *Dioscoreae Rhizoma* (Shan Yao), *Lablab Semen Album* (Bai Bian Dou), and *Pogostmonis Herba* (Huo Xiang); for poor appetite, add *Crataegi Fructus Ustus* (Jiao Shan Zha), *Massa Medicata Fermentata* (Liu Shen Qu), and *Amomi Fructus* (Sha Ren).

加减:大便稀薄者,加山药、白扁豆、藿香;纳呆食少者,加焦山楂、六神曲、砂仁。

(6) Depletion of kidney essence

(6) 肾精亏虚

Manifestations: Prolonged illness, recurrent seizure, chronic convulsion, intermittent dizziness, aching soreness in the lumbus and knees, fatigued spirit and lack of strength, deficiency of qi and reluctance in speaking, lack of warmth in the limbs, possible accompanied by retarded mental development, poor memory, pale tongue, white tongue coating, thready, deep and forceless pulse, slight red fingerprints.

证候:发病日久,屡发不止,瘛疭抖动,时有头晕,腰膝酸软,神疲乏力,少气懒言,四肢不温,可伴智力发育迟滞,记忆力差,舌质淡,苔白,脉沉细无力,指纹淡红。

Therapeutic method: To benefit the kidney and replenish essence.

治法:益肾填精。

Main formula: *Human Placenta and Eight-Ingredient Pill* (He Che Ba Wei Wan) with modification.

主方:河车八味丸加减。

Commonly used herbs: *Hominis Placenta* (Zi He Che) (grind and take after infused with water), *Rehmanniae Radix Cruda* (Sheng Di Huang), *Poria* (Fu Ling), *Dioscoreae Rhizoma* (Shan Yao), *Alismatis Rhizoma* (Ze Xie), *Schisandrae Fructus Chinensis* (Wu Wei Zi), *Ophiopogonis Radix* (Mai Dong), *Moutan Cortex Radicis* (Mu Dan Pi), *Cinnamomi Cortex* (Rou Gui), *Aconiti Lateralis Radix Praeparata* (Fu Zi).

常用药:紫河车(研粉冲服)、生地黄、茯苓、山药、泽泻、五味子、麦冬、牡丹皮、肉桂、附子。

Modification: For frequent convulsion, add *Trionycis Carapax Et Rhizoma* (Bie Jia), and *Paeoniae Radix Albae* (Bai Shao); for retarded intelligence, add *Alpiniae Oxyphyllae Fructus* (Yi Zhi Ren), and *Acori Rhizoma Tatarinowii* (Shi Chang Pu); for sloppy stool, add *Lablab Semen Album* (Bai Bian Dou), and *Baked Zingiberis Rhizoma Recens* (Sheng Jiang).

加减:抽搐频繁者,加鳖甲、白芍;智力迟钝者,加益智仁、石菖蒲;大便稀溏者,加白扁豆、炮姜。

4 Other therapies

4 其他疗法

4.1 Chinese Patent medicine

4.1 中成药

(1) *Anti-epilepsy Capsules for Children* (Xiao Er Kang Xian Jiao Nang) is used for epilepsy in pattern of abundance of phlegm due to spleen deficiency.

(1) 小儿抗痫胶囊:适用于癫痫脾虚痰盛证。

(2) *Epilepsy Treatment Pills* (Yi Xian Wan) is used for epilepsy due to wind.

(2) 医痫丸:适用于风痫。

(3) *Amber Dragon-Embracing Pill* (Hu Po Bao Long Wan) is used for epilepsy due to fright.

(3) 琥珀抱龙丸:适用于惊痫。

(4) *Alum and Curcuma Pill* (Bai Jin Wan) is used for epilepsy due to phlegm.

(4) 白金丸:适用于痰痫。

4.2 Simple formula and empirical formula

4.2 单方验方

(1) *White Replacement Powder* (Dai Bai San): Grind *Piperis Fructus Albicatus* (Bai Hu Jiao), *Haematitum* (Zhe Shi), in proportion of 1:2, for further use. Take 1～3g. each time, for 2～3 times per day, with raddish soup or boiled water. The treatment course lasts for 3 to 6 months. It is used for epilepsy due to fright.

(1) 代白散:白胡椒、赭石,配方比例为1∶2,共为细末,备用。每次服1～3克,每日2～3次,白萝卜汤或白开水送服。每个疗程3～6个月。适用于惊痫。

(2) Take one piece of *Hominis Placenta* (Zi He Che), and 10g of *Cinnabaris* (Zhu Sha), and bake *Hominis Placenta* (Zi He Che) dry and grind it together with *Cinnabaris* (Zhu Sha) into fine powder. Take 2～4g each time, for once or twice per

(2) 紫河车1个,朱砂10克。紫河车焙干与朱砂共为细末。每次服2～4克,每日1～2次,白开水送服。适用于各型癫痫伴体虚者。

day. It is used for various types of epilepsy accompanied by deficiency of body constitution.

(3) Grind *Cicadae Periostracum* (Chan Tui), *Bombyx Batryticatus* (Jiang Can), *Scorpio* (Quan Xie), and *Scolopendra* (Wu Gong), in equal proportion, into fine powder and mix them well. Take 2g each time, twice a day, for epilepsy due to wind.

(3) 蝉蜕、僵蚕、全蝎、蜈蚣各等份，共研细末和匀。每次 2 克，每日 2 次，开水送服。适用于风痫。

4.3 Acumoxatherapy

4.3 针灸疗法

(1) Body acupuncture: During seizure, select and puncture Renzhong (GV 26), Hegu (LI 4), Shixuan (EX-UE 11), Neiguan (PC 6), and Yongquan (KI 1), by the needling technique for sedation. During dormant phase, select and puncture Dazhui (GV 14), Shenmen (HT 7), Xinshu (BL 15), Hegu (LI 4), and Fenglong (ST 40), by the moderate needling technique, for once every other day. Choose Baihui (GV 20), Zusanli (ST 36), and Shousanli (LI 10) for moxibustion, 3 moxa cones for each acupoint, once every other day.

（1）体针：发作期取人中、合谷、十宣、内关、涌泉针刺，用泻法；休止期取大椎、神门、心俞、合谷、丰隆针刺，平补平泻法，隔日 1 次。百会、足三里、手三里灸治，每次 3 壮，隔日 1 次。

(2) Ear acupuncture: Select and puncture ear acupoints of Pt. Stomach, Pt. Subcortex, Pt. Ear-Shenmen, Pt. Occiput, and Pt. Heart, 3～5 acupoints each time, and retain the needles for 20 to 30 minutes, and manipulate the needles intermittently, or embed the needles for 3～7 days.

（2）耳针：取胃、皮质下、神门、枕、心。每次选用 3～5 穴，留针 20～30 分钟，间歇捻针。或埋针 3～7 天。

4.4 Catgut-embedding method

4.4 埋线疗法

Commonly used acupoints: Dazhui (GV 14), Yaoqi (EX-B 9), Jiuwei (CV 15); Backup acupoints: Yiming (EX-HN 14), Shenmen (HT 7). Choose 2～3 acupoints each time, and embed catgut, once every 20 days. The commonly used acupoints and backup acupoints are used in alternation.

常用穴：大椎、腰奇、鸠尾。备用穴：翳明、神明。每次选用 2～3 穴，埋入医用羊肠线，隔 20 日 1 次，常用穴和备用穴轮换使用。

Section 2 Cerebral Palsy

Cerebral palsy refers to a syndrome caused by non-progressive brain damage and developmental defect starting from fertilization to infanthood, mainly manifestated by motor disorders and abnormal posture, and often accompanied by mental retardation, convulsive attack, abnormal behavior, hearing disorders, or visual disorders, etc.

It belongs to the scope of "five types of retardation", "five types of flaccidity" and "five types of stiffness", etc. in traditional Chinese medicine.

1 Etiology and pathogenesis

The main cause is related to insufficiency of the natural endowment of the sick child. "Brain is the sea of bone marrow". Only when brain marrow is rich, can it govern the spirit and mind. If the pregnant mother is not appropriately cared or nourished, the fetus will be affected, resulting in the insufficiency of prenatal kidney essence, and malnutrition of the brain marrow. Or if the collaterals of the brains are obstructed by blood stasis and turbid phlegm resulted during or after birth, the dysfrunciton of brain marrow could also be induced. "The kidney stores essence, governs the bones and engenders marrow". "The liver stores blood and governs the tendons". "The spleen is a postnal foundation and governs the muscles and four limbs". Therefore, the morbidity of cerebral palsy is closely related to the liver, spleen and kidney. The dysfunction of the three organs will impair brain marrow, resulting in this disease. Therefore, this disease mostly belongs to deficiency pattern. If the brain is blocked by re-

第2节 脑性瘫痪

脑性瘫痪是指受孕开始至婴儿期非进行性脑损伤和发育缺陷所致的综合征，主要表现为运动障碍及姿势异常，可伴有智力低下、惊厥发作、行为异常、听力障碍、视力障碍等。

本病属于中医学“五迟”“五软”“五硬”等范畴。

1 病因病机

主要原因为患儿先天禀赋不足，“脑为髓之海”，脑髓充实，方能职司神明。产前孕母将养失宜，损及胎儿，导致小儿先天肾精不充，脑髓失养；或产时及产后因素导致瘀血、痰浊阻于脑络，而致脑髓失其所用。

“肾藏精，主骨生髓”，“肝藏血，主筋”，“脾为后天之本，主肌肉四肢”，因此，脑瘫的发病与肝、脾、肾关系密切，三脏功能失调则能损伤脑髓，导致本病发生。故本病大多属虚证，若血瘀痰阻，脑窍闭塞，亦可见实证。

tention of blood stasis and phlegm, excess patterns can also be seen.

2 Key to diagnosis

(1) Cerebral palsy caused by non-progressive brain injury (shortened as brain palsy).

(2) Symptoms appear during infanthood.

(3) The pathological location causing motor disorders lies in the brain.

(4) Sometimes, it can be complicated with mental retardation, epilepsy, sensory disorder, perceptual disorder and other abnormality.

(5) Exclusion of the central motor disorders caused by progressive diseases and temporary retardation in the motor development of the normal children.

3 Pattern identification and treatment

It is necessary to identify the bowels and viscera, and deficiency and excess: if the sick child shows athetosis or dysnoesia, the problem mostly lies in the liver and kidney. If the muscles are flaccid and forceless, and there are flaccid and soft hands, feet and body, it mostly lies in spleen and kidney, as deficiency pattern. If the sick child shows rigidity and hypertonicity of the limbs, emaciation, it mostly lies in the liver and spleen, as mixed pattern of deficiency and excess.

The treatment is mainly given to fortify the spleen, soften the liver, and supplement the kidney. For prolonged illness resulting in exhaustion of qi and blood, it is requested to boost qi and nourish blood additionaly. It is also important to start early rehabilitation treatment, especially in the period within 3 to 9 months after birth, including compre-

2 诊断要点

（1）非进行性的脑损伤引起的脑性瘫痪(简称脑瘫)。

（2）症状在婴儿期出现。

（3）引起运动障碍的病变部位在脑部。

（4）有时合并智力障碍、癫痫、感知觉障碍及其他异常。

（5）除外进行性疾病所致的中枢性运动障碍及正常小儿暂时性的运动发育迟缓。

3 辨证论治

主要辨脏腑及虚实:如患儿主要表现为手足徐动或智力障碍者,多病在肝肾。肌肉软弱无力,手足躯体痿软者,多病在脾肾,为虚证。患儿表现为肢体强直拘挛,肌肉瘦削者,多病在肝脾,为虚实夹杂证。

治疗以健脾、柔肝、补肾为主,病久而有气血虚惫之候者,则佐以益气养血。重视早期康复治疗,特别是出生后3～9个月的阶段内采取中西医综合康复疗法,中医辨证施治,推拿、针灸与西

hensive rehabilitatory therapy of both Chinese medicine and Western medicine, treatment based on pattern identification, Tuina therapy and Acu-moxatherapy of Chinese medicine, and exercise theapy, occupational therapy, language training of Western medicine, in order to correct abnormal posture, promote motor development and seek over-all rehabilitation of the sick child.

医运动疗法、作业疗法、语言训练等相结合,纠正患儿异常姿势,促进运动发育,力求患儿全面的康复。

(1) Depletion of the liver and kidney

(1) 肝肾亏虚

Manifestations: Involuntary movements of limbs, inflexible joints, slight athetosis or tremor of hand and feet, uncoordinated movements, or difficult speech, or loss of hearing or sight, deafness, pale tongue, white and thin tongue coating, thready and weak pulse.

证候:肢体不自主运动,关节活动不灵,手足徐动或震颤,动作不协调。或语言不利,或失听失明,或失聪,舌淡,苔薄白,脉细软。

Therapeutic method: To enrich the liver and kidney, strengthen the tendons and bones.

治法:滋补肝肾,强筋健骨。

Main formula: *Six-Ingredient Rehmannia Pill* (Liu Wei Di Huang Wan) and *Hidden Tiger Pill* (Hu Qian Wan) with modification.

主方:六味地黄丸合虎潜丸加减。

Commonly used herbs: *Rehmanniae Radix Praeparata* (Shu Di Huang), *Corni Fructus* (Shan Zhu Yu), *Dioscoreae Rhizoma* (Shan Yao), *Alismatis Rhizoma* (Ze Xie), *Moutan Cortex*(Dan Pi), Poria (Fu Ling), *Phellodendri Cortex Chinensis* (Huang Bo), *Testudinis Carapax Et Plastrum* (Gui Ban), *Anemarrhenae Rhizoma* (Zhi Mu), *Rehmanniae Radix Cruda* (Sheng Di Huang), *Citri Reticulatae Pericarpium* (Chen Pi), *Paeoniae Radix Albae* (Bai Shao), *Herba Cynomorii* (Suo Yang), *Zingiberis Rhizoma* (Gan Jiang).

常用药:熟地黄、山茱萸、山药、泽泻、丹皮、茯苓、黄柏、龟板、知母、生地黄、陈皮、白芍、锁阳、干姜。

Modification: For loss of sight, add *Mori Fructus* (Sang Shen Zi), and *Astragali Complanati Semen* (Sha Yuan Ji Li) to nourish the liver and

加减:失明者,加桑椹子、沙苑蒺藜养肝明目;失语者,加远志、郁金、石菖蒲化

brighten the eyes; for loss of speech, add *Polygalae Radix*(Yuan Zhi), *Cur Cumae Radix*(Yu Jin), and *Acori Rhizoma Tatarinowii* (Shi Chang Pu) to dispel phlegm and open the orifices.

痰开窍。

(2) Dual depletion of spleen and kidney

(2) 脾肾两亏

Manifestations: Weak and soft neck, unable to uplift, flaccid mouth and lips, difficult to suck or chew, flaccid and weak muscles, pale face, pale tongue, white and thin tongue coating, weak and deep pulse.

证候:头项软弱,不能抬举。口软唇弛,吸吮或咀嚼困难。肌肉松软无力,面白,舌淡,苔薄白,脉沉无力。

Therapeutic method: To fortify the spleen and supplement the kidney, engender flesh and strengthen the bones.

治法:健脾补肾,生肌壮骨。

Main formula: *Center-Supplementing Qi-Boosting Decoction* (Bu Zhong Yi Qi Tang) and *Kidney-Supplementing Rehmannia Pill* (Bu Shen Di Huang Wan) with modification.

主方:补中益气汤合补肾地黄丸加减。

Commonly used herbs: *Astragali Radix* (Huang Qi), *Ginseng Radix* (Ren Shen), *Atractylodis Macrocephalae Rhizoma* (Bai Zhu), *Glycyrrhizae Radix Et Rhizoma* (Gan Cao), *Angelicae Sinensis Radix* (Dang Gui), *Citri Reticulatae Pericarpium* (Chen Pi), *Cimicifugae Rhizoma* (Sheng Ma), *Bupleuri Radix* (Chai Hu), *Zingiberis Rhizoma Recens* (Sheng Jiang), *Jujubae Fructus* (Da Zao), *Dioscoreae Rhizoma* (Shan Yao), *Corni Fructus* (Shan Zhu Yu), *Rehmanniae Radix Praeparata* (Shu Di Huang), *Cyathulae Radix* (Chuan Niu Xi), *Moutan Cortex Radicis* (Mu Dan Pi), *Poria Alba* (Bai Fu Ling), *Alismatis Rhizoma* (Ze Xie).

常用药:黄芪、人参、白术、甘草、当归、陈皮、升麻、柴胡、生姜、大枣、山药、山茱萸、熟地黄、川牛膝、牡丹皮、白茯苓、泽泻。

Modification: For insufficiency of Yuan-original qi and weak crying, add *Ginseng Radix* (Ren Shen) or *Pseudostellariae Radix* (Tai Zi Shen); for dry mouth, add *Dendrobii Herba* (Shi Hu) and

加减:伴元气不足而哭声无力者,加人参或太子参;口干者,加石斛、玉竹滋养胃阴;大便秘结者,加当归、火

Polygonati Odorati Rhizoma (Yu Zhu) to nourish stomach yin; for constipation, add *Angelicae Sinensis Radix* (Dang Gui) and *Cannabis Fructus* (Huo Ma Ren) to moisten the intestines and free the stool.

麻仁润肠通便。

(3) Hyperactivity of the liver and weakness of the spleen

(3) 肝强脾弱

Manifestations: Rigidity and hypertonicity of limbs, disuse due to stiffness, vexation and irascibility, aggravated by external stimulation, poor appetite, emaciation, fatty and big tongue or thin tongue, little or white and slimy tongue coating, deep and weak pulse or thready pulse.

证候:肢体强直拘挛,强硬失用,烦躁易怒,遇到外界刺激后加重,食少纳呆,肌肉瘦削,舌质胖大或瘦薄,舌苔少或白腻,脉沉弱或细。

Therapeutic method: To soften the liver and fortify the spleen, boost qi and nourish blood.

治法:柔肝健脾,益气养血。

Main formula: *Six Gentlemen Decoction* (Liu Jun Zi Tang) and *Sinew-Soothing Decoction* (Shu Jin Tang) with modification.

主方:六君子汤合舒筋汤加减。

Commonly used herbs: *Ginseng Radix* (Ren Shen), *Atractylodis Macrocephalae Rhizoma* (Bai Zhu), *Poria* (Fu Ling), *Glycyrrhizae Radix Et Rhizoma Preparata* (Zhi Gan Cao), *Citri Reticulatae Pericarpium* (Chen Pi), *Pinelliae Rhizoma* (Ban Xia), *Notopterygii Rhizoma seu Radix* (Qiang Huo), *Angelicae Sinensis Radix* (Dang Gui), *Wenyujin Rhizoma Concisum* (Pian Jiang Huang), *Glycyrrhizae Radix Et Rhizoma Preparata* (Zhi Gan Cao), *Atractylodis Macrocephalae Rhizoma* (Bai Zhu), *Piperis Kadsurae Caulis* (Hai Feng Teng), *Paeoniae Radix Rubra* (Chi Shao), *Zingiberis Rhizoma Recens* (Sheng Jiang).

常用药:人参、白术、茯苓、炙甘草、陈皮、半夏、羌活、当归、片姜黄、炙甘草、白术、海风藤、赤芍、生姜。

Modification: For rigidity of limbs, add *Polygonati Rhizoma* (Huang Jing), *Angelicae Sinensis Radix* (Dang Gui), and *Paeoniae Radix Albae* (Bai

加减:肢体强直者,加黄精、当归、白芍养血柔肝;食欲欠佳者,加陈皮、焦山楂、

Shao) to nourish blood and emolliate liver; for poor appetite, add *Citri Reticulatae Pericarpium* (Chen Pi), *Crataegi Fructus Ustus* (Jiao Shan Zha), and *Galli Endothelium Corneum Gigerii* (Ji Nei Jin) to fortify the spleen and digest food.

鸡内金健脾消食。

(4) Obstruction of phlegm and blood stasis in the channels

(4) 痰瘀阻络

Manifestations: Slow response after birth, low intelligence, squamous and dry skin, withered hair, salivation, difficulty in swallowing, stiff joints, flaccid muscles, involuntary movements, seizure of epilepsy, dark purple tongue, white and slimy tongue coating, hesitant and deep pulse.

证候: 自出生之后反应迟钝，智力低下，肌肤甲错，毛发枯槁，口流痰涎，吞咽困难，关节强硬，肌肉软弱，动作不自主，或有癫痫发作，舌质紫暗，苔白腻，脉沉涩。

Therapeutic method: To dissipate phlegm and open the orifices, activate blood and dredge the collaterals.

治法: 涤痰开窍，活血通络。

Main formula: *Orifice-Freeing Blood-Quickening Decoction* (Tong Qiao Huo Xue Tang) and *Two Matured Ingredients Decoction* (Er Chen Tang) with modification.

主方: 通窍活血汤合二陈汤加减。

Commonly used herbs: *Paeoniae Radix Rubra* (Chi Shao), *Chuanxiong Rhizoma* (Chuan Xiong), *Persicae Semen* (Tao Ren), *Fructus Jujubae* (Hong Zao), *Carthami Flos* (Hong Hua), *Pinelliae Rhizoma* (Ban Xia), *Citri Reticulatae Pericarpium* (Chen Pi), *Poria* (Fu Ling), *Glycyrrhizae Radix Rt Rhizoma* (Gan Cao).

常用药: 赤芍、川芎、桃仁、红枣、红花、半夏、陈皮、茯苓、甘草。

Modification: For rigid limbs, add *Angelicae Sinensis Radix* (Dang Gui) and *Spatholobi Caulis* (Ji Xue Teng) to nourish and activate blood; for convulsion, add *Os Draconis* (Long Gu), *Ostreae Concha* (Mu Li), *Gastrodiae Rhizoma* (Tian Ma), and *Uncariae ramulus Cum uncis* (Gou Teng) to extinguish wind and check convulsion.

加减: 肢体强直者，加当归、鸡血藤养血活血；抽搐者，加龙骨、牡蛎、天麻、钩藤息风止痉。

4 Other therapies

4.1 Acumoxatherapy

(1) Body acupuncture: For low intelligence, select Baihui (GV 20), Sishencong (EX-HN 1), and three intelligence acupoints (Shenting (GV 24), bilateral Benshen (GB 13)). For language disorders, select Tongli (HT 5), Lianquan (CV 23), Jinjin (EX 10), and Yuye (EX-HN 12). For flaccidity and paralysis of nape, select Tianzhu (BL 10), Dazhui (GV 14), and Lieque (LU 7). For salivation, select Shanglianquan (EX 12) and Dicang (ST 4). For difficulty in swallowing, select Lianquan (CV 23) and Tiantu (CV 22). For paralysis of upper limb, select Jianyu (LI 15), Quchi (LI 11), Shousanli (LI 10) and Sanjian (LI 3). For paralysis of lower limb, select Huantiao (GB 30), Zusanli (ST 36), Yanglingquan (GB 34) and Xuanzhong (GB 39). For paralysis of lumbus, select Shenshu (BL 23) and Yaoyangguan (GV 3). For scissor-like step, select Biguan (ST 31) and Fengshi (GB 31). For tiptoe step, select Jiexi (ST 41) and Taibai (SP 3). For strephenopodia, select Qiuxu (GB 40), Kunlun (BL 60), and spot one cun lateral to Chengshan (BL 57). For eversion of foot, select Shangqiu (SP 5), Taixi (KI 3), and spot one cun medial to Chengshan (BL 57). For urinary and fecal incontinence, select Shangliao (BL 31), Ciliao (BL 32), Zhongji (CV 3), and Guanyuan (CV 4), etc. According to different locations of limb paralysis, puncture the different segments of Huatuo Jiaji points (Extra). For sick children with poor muscle force, add moxibustion after acupuncture.

(2) Head acupuncture: Select Pt. Motor Zone,

4 其他疗法

4.1 针灸疗法

（1）体针：智力低下者，取百会、四神聪、智三针；语言障碍者，取通里、廉泉、金津、玉液；颈项软瘫者，取天柱、大椎、列缺；流涎者，取上廉泉、地仓；吞咽困难者，取廉泉、天突；上肢瘫者，取肩髃、曲池、手三里、三间；下肢瘫者，取环跳、足三里、阳陵泉、悬钟；腰部软瘫者，取肾俞、腰阳关；剪刀步者，取髀关、风市；尖足者，取解溪、太白；足内翻者，取丘墟、昆仑、承山外1寸；足外翻者，取商丘、太溪、承山内1寸；二便失禁者，取上髎、次髎、中极、关元等穴。根据肢体瘫痪部位不同，分别针刺华佗夹脊穴的不同节段。肌力低下患儿，针刺后加艾灸。

（2）头针：取运动区、足

Pt. Foot Motor Sensory Zone.

4.2 Tuina therapy

Apply the pressing, rubbing, pinching, and grasping method on the diseased limbs, with light and gentle manipulation for intense muscle tension, and with heavy manipulation for mild muscle tension. Apply the shaking, pulling and drawing method to alleviate contracture of tendon and to restore the functional positions of diseased limbs as much as possible. During Tuina treatment, it is necessary to press the major acupoints predominantly on purpose, such as Touwei (ST 8), Baihui (GV 20), and Sishencong (EX-HN 1) on the head, Yangxi (LI 5), Quchi (LI 11) and Jianzhen (SI 9) on the arm, and Qiuxu (GB 40), Taixi (KI 3), Shangqiu (SP 5), and Kunlun (BL 60) for strephenopodia and eversion of foot. It is usually advisable to apply the spine-knocking method, spine-pointing method and spine-pinching method on the Governor Vessel, Huatuo Jiaji points (Extra) and two lateral lines of the bladder meridian of the back. By Tuina treatment, it is possible to promote blood circulation, relieve spasm, strengthen the muscles, and reduce the muscle tension.

4.3 External therapy

Boil *Astragali Radix* (Huang Qi), *Angelicae Sinensis Radix* (Dang Gui), *Chuanxiong Rhizoma* (Chuan Xiong), *Spatholobi Caulis* (Ji Xue Teng), *Carthami Flos* (Hong Hua), and *Lycopodii Herba* (Shen Jin Cao) with water, pour the liquid into bathtub, soak and wash the diseased limbs in the medicated liquid at appropriate temperature, 20 minutes each time, once every day.

运感区。

4.2 推拿疗法

采取按、揉、捏、拿等手法作用于患肢。肌张力较高时手法宜轻柔；肌力较低时手法宜重。应用摇、扳、拔伸等手法改善肌腱的挛缩，使患肢尽量恢复于功能位。在推拿过程中配以点按穴位，头部取头维、百会、四神聪等穴；手部取阳溪、曲池和肩贞等穴；足部内、外翻分别取丘墟、太溪、商丘、昆仑等穴；背部的督脉、夹脊穴及膀胱经两条侧线多用扣脊法、点脊法和捏脊法等手法。通过推拿可促进血液的循环，缓解痉挛，增强肌力，降低肌张力。

4.3 外治疗法

将黄芪、当归、川芎、鸡血藤、红花、伸筋草等药加水煮沸，将药液倒入浴盆中，待温度适当时，用药液浸洗患肢，每次浸洗 20 分钟，每日 1 次。

Chapter 7 Common Psychological Disorders in Children

第7章 小儿常见心理障碍

Section 1 Attention Deficit and Hyperactivity Disorder

第1节 注意缺陷与多动障碍

Attention deficit and hyperactivity disorder, also known as "minimal brain dysfunction syndrome", and "hyperactive child syndrome", refer to a commonly-encountered abnormal behavior disorder during childhood, clinically characterized by distractibility, unstable emotion, hyperactivity, poor self-control ability beyond the age of the children, and possibly accompanied by cognitive disorder and learning difficulty, but with normal or basically normal intelligence. It frequently occurs in the age from 6 to 14 years old, higher ratio in the boys than in the girls, in an incidence ratio of (4～9)∶1. The majority of the sick children will gradually recover when they reach adolescence, but some cases would linger to the adulthood.

注意缺陷与多动障碍又称"轻微脑功能障碍综合征""儿童多动综合征"等，是儿童期常见的一种行为异常性疾患。以与年龄不相符的注意力涣散，情绪不稳，活动过多，自控能力差为主要临床特征，可伴有认知障碍和学习困难，但智力正常或基本正常。好发年龄为6～14岁，男孩明显多于女孩，约为(4～9)∶1，绝大多数患儿多动症状到青春期可逐渐好转而痊愈，但部分病例注意缺陷可延续到成年。

It belongs to the scope of "visceral agitation", "forgetfulness", "loss of hearing" in traditional Chinese medicine.

本病属于中医学"脏躁""健忘""失聪"等范畴。

1 Etiology and pathogenesis

1 病因病机

The etiological causes are mainly related to pre-

病因主要为先天禀赋不

natal insufficiency of the natural endowment, inappropriate postnatal care, improper nurture, and environmental influence, including other factors of blood stasis and stagnation due to traumatic injury or emotional disorders.

足，后天失于护养，教育不当，环境影响。其他如外伤瘀滞、情志失调等也可引起。

"The heart is often superabundant" and "the liver is often superabundant" in the infants. Improper education resulting in mental disharmony, emotional disorder resulting in fire formation of five minds, constitutional preponderance of heat with preference for fried and spicy food assisting heat to produce fire and harass the heart and liver, could present hyperactivity and impulsion, agitation and fidgetiness. The constitutionally fat infants, plus constitutional condition of phlegm and dampness, and predilection for rich, fatty and sweet food, or indulgence in hot, spicy and dry food, may induce the internal production of phlegm and fire, disturbing the mind and hence resulting in hyperactivity, impulsion and wilfulness. If the prenatal natural endowment is insufficient, the kidney yin would be insufficient, the water would fail to moisten wood, and the liver yang would be overabundant, presenting hyperactivity, difficulty to be quiet, and divergence of attention. If heart qi is insufficient, the heart would not be fully nourished, resulting in the failure of the heart in storing the spirit and mind, and there is divergency of attention. If the spleen is deficient due to lack of nourishment, there would be insufficient tranquility, changeable interests, speaking without due consideration, and poor memory. The deficiency of both the heart and spleen will cause distracted spirit, inconstant manner, and loss of self-control. The diseased location mainly lies in

小儿"心常有余""肝常有余"，若教育失当，心理失和；或情志失调，五志化火；或素体热盛，喜食油煎辛辣之品，助热生火，扰动心肝，而见多动冲动，烦躁不安。素体肥胖小儿，痰湿之体，平素喜食肥甘厚味之品，或偏食辛辣香燥之物，导致痰火内生，扰动心神，则见多动多语，冲动任性。若先天禀赋不足，肾阴不足，水不涵木，肝阳亢盛，则表现为多动难静，神思涣散。若心气不足，心失所养可致心神失守而精神涣散，注意力不集中。脾虚失养则静谧不足，兴趣多变，言语冒失，健忘；心脾两虚则神思不定，反复无常不能自制。病位主要责之于心、肝、脾、肾，其病机关键在于脏腑功能失常，阴阳平衡失调。

the heart, liver, spleen, and kidney. The key pathogenesis is related to dysfunction of the visceras, and imbalance between yin and yang.

2 Key to diagnosis

(1) Distracted concentration, absence of mind, frequent petty action, failure to finish homework on time, poor school records, but normal intelligence.

(2) Frequent restlessness, excessive action, unable to take part in actions quietly.

(3) Unstable emotion, impulsive and wilful, often fighting with others.

(4) Uncoordinated movements in the physical examination, positive in hand-turning test, finger-matching test, finger-nose test, and finger-to-finger test, and positive inattention test.

(5) The disease often starts before 7 years old, with its manifestations often unsuited to the developmental level, and the duration usually lasts over 6 months.

3 Pattern identification and treatment

Clinically, it is necessary to distinguish between bowels and visceras, deficiency and excess, yin and yang.

If the heart is involved, it can be manifested by distracted attention, unstable emotions, lots of dreams and agitation. If the liver is involved, it can be manifested by tendency to be impulsive, restlessness, difficulty to keep quiet, easy anger, and loss self-control. If the spleen is involved, it can be manifested by changeable interests, having a beginning but no end, and poor memory. If the kidney is

2 诊断要点

（1）注意力涣散，上课时思想不集中，常做小动作，作业不能按时完成，学习成绩差，但智力正常。

（2）多动不安，活动过度，不能安静地参加各种活动。

（3）情绪不稳，冲动任性，常与人打斗。

（4）体格检查动作不协调，翻手试验、对指试验、指鼻试验、指指试验可呈阳性。注意力测试常呈阳性。

（5）通常于7岁前起病，其表现与发育水平不相称，病程持续6个月以上。

3 辨证论治

临床辨证应注意辨脏腑、分虚实、判阴阳。

在心者，注意力不集中，情绪不稳定，多梦烦躁；在肝者，易于冲动，好动难静，容易发怒，常不能自控；在脾者，兴趣多变，做事有头无尾，记忆力差；在肾者，脑失精明，学习成绩低下，记忆力欠佳，或有遗尿、腰酸乏

involved, it can be manifested by loss of smart brain, poor school records, poor memory, or enuresis, aching lumbus and lack of strength.

力等。

Usually, the initial onset belongs to excess pattern, mostly characterized by fire exuberance in the heart and liver, and internal disturbance of phlegm and fire. The prolonged condition mostly belongs to deficiency pattern, mainly characterized by yin deficiency in the liver kidney and deficiency of both the heart and spleen, often in mixed pattern of deficiency and excess, or in pattern of deficiency in the constitution and excess in the symptoms.

一般初起多实证，以心肝火旺、痰火内扰为多；病久多虚证，以肝肾阴虚、心脾两虚为主。常虚实夹杂或本虚标实。

Lack of quietness due to insufficiency is manifested by distracted attention, poor self-control ability, unstable emotion, absence of mind. Agitation due to yang hyperactivity is manifested by restlessness, talkativeness, impulsion and willfulness, rashness, impatience, and irascibility.

阴静不足，表现为注意力不集中，自我控制差，情绪不稳，神思涣散；阳亢躁动，表现为多动不安，说话过多，冲动任性，急躁易怒。

The basic therapeutic principle is to subdue excess and rectify deficiency, harmonize bowels and viscera, and balance yin and yang. Fire hyperactivity in the heart and liver should be treated by clarifying the heart and balancing the liver. The internal disturbance by phlegm and fire should be treated by draining fire and dissipating phlegm. Yin deficiency in the liver and kidney should be treated by nourishing yin and subduing yang. The deficiency in the heart and spleen should be treated by supplementing and benefiting the heart and spleen.

以泻实补虚、调和脏腑、平衡阴阳为基本治则。心肝火旺者，治以清心平肝；痰火内扰者，治以泻火豁痰；肝肾阴虚者，治以滋阴潜阳；心脾两虚者，治以补益心脾。

(1) Fire hyperactivity in the heart and liver

（1）心肝火旺

Manifestations: Overactive, too talkative, impulsive and wilful, impatient and irascible, inattentive, rash, provoking and harassing the others, fighting with others, agitated with flushed face,

证候：多动多语，冲动任性，急躁易怒，注意力不集中，做事莽撞，或好惹扰人、常与人打闹，或面赤烦躁，大

constipation, yellow urine, red tongue or tongue tip, thin tongue coating or thin and yellow tongue coating, string-taut pulse or rapid pulse.

便秘结,小便色黄,舌质红或舌尖红,苔薄或薄黄,脉弦或弦数。

Therapeutic method: To clarify the heart, balance the liver, tranquilize the spirit and stabilize the mind.

治法:清心平肝,安神定志。

Main formula: *Spirit-tranquilizing and Mind-stabilizing Decoction* (An Shen Ding Zhi Tang) with modification.

主方:安神定志汤加减。

Commonly used herbs: *Bupleuri Radix* (Chai Hu), *Scutellariae Radix* (Huang Qin), *Cassiae Semen* (Jue Ming Zi), *Forsythiae Fructus* (Lian Qiao), *Bambusae Concretio Silicea* (Tian Zhu Huang), *Acori Rhizoma Tatarinowii* (Shi Chang Pu), *Curcumae Radix* (Yu Jin), *Angelicae Sinensis Radix* (Dang Gui), *Alpiniae Oxyphyllae Fructus* (Yi Zhi), *Polygalae Radix* (Yuan Zhi).

常用药:柴胡、黄芩、决明子、连翘、天竺黄、石菖蒲、郁金、当归、益智、远志。

Modification: For impatience and irascibility, add *Uncariae ramulus Cum uncis* (Gou Teng), and *Margaritifera Concha* (Zhen Zhu Mu); for impulsion, wilfulness, and restless agitation, add *Gardeniae Fructus* (Zhi Zi) and *Chloriti Lapis* (Qing Meng Shi); for constipation and defecation every several days, add *Rhei Radix Et Rhizoma* (Da Huang), *Aurantii Fructus Immaturus* (Zhi Shi), *Arecae Semen* (Bing Lang).

加减:急躁易怒者,加钩藤、珍珠母;冲动任性、烦躁不安者,加栀子、青礞石;大便干结、数日一行者,加大黄、枳实、槟榔。

(2) Internal disturbance of phlegm and fire

(2) 痰火内扰

Manifestations: Overactive, talkative, impulsive and wilful, difficult to control, changeable interests, inattentive, heat vexation in the chest, poor appetite, bitter taste in the mouth, constipation and brown urine, red tongue, yellow and slimy tongue coating, rapid and slippery pulse.

证候:多动多语,冲动任性,难于制约,兴趣多变,注意力不集中,胸中烦热,纳少口苦,便秘尿赤,舌质红,苔黄腻,脉滑数。

Therapeutic method: To clear away heat and

治法:清热泻火,化痰

drain fire, dissolve phlegm and quiet the heart.

Main formula: *Coptis Gallbladder-Warming Decoction* (Huang Lian Wen Dan Tang) with modification.

Commonly used herbs: *Coptidis Rhizoma* (Huang Lian), *Citri Reticulatae Pericarpium* (Chen Pi), *Pinelliae Rhizoma* (Ban Xia), *Arisaema Cum Bile* (Dan Nan Xing), *Bambusae Concretio Silicea* (Tian Zhu Huang), *Richosanthis Fructus* (Gua Lou), *Aurantii Fructus Immaturus* (Zhi Shi), *Acori Rhizoma Tatarinowii* (Shi Chang Pu), *Poria* (Fu Ling), *Margaritifera Concha* (Zhen Zhu Mu).

Modification: For vexation and irascibility, add *Uncariae ramulus Cum uncis* (Gou Teng), *Gentianae Radix Et Rhizoma* (Long Dan), and *Haliotidis Concha* (Shi Jue Ming); for constipation, add *Cassiae Semen* (Jue Ming Zi), and *Rhei Radix Et Rhizoma* (Da Huang); for poor appetite, add *Raphani Semen* (Lai Fu Zi), *Arecae Semen* (Bing Lang).

(3) Yin deficiency in the liver and kidney

Manifestations: Overactive, difficult to keep quiet, impatient and irascible, impulsive and wilful, undisciplined spirit and mind, difficult to sit quietly, poor memory, poor school records, feverish sensation in the chest, palms and soles, night sweating, dry mouth and throat, enuresis, constipation, red tongue, scanty tongue coating, thready and string-taut pulse.

Therapeutic method: To nourish yin and subdue yang, quiet the spirit and calm down the heart.

Main formula: *Lycium Berry, Chrysanthemum, and Rehmannia Pill* (Qi Ju Di Huang Wan) with modification.

宁心。

主方:黄连温胆汤加减。

常用药:黄连、陈皮、半夏、胆南星、天竺黄、瓜蒌、枳实、石菖蒲、茯苓、珍珠母。

加减:烦躁易怒者,加钩藤、龙胆、石决明;大便秘结者,加决明子、大黄;纳少者,加莱菔子、槟榔。

(3) 肝肾阴虚

证候:多动难静,急躁易怒,冲动任性,神思涣散,注意力不集中,难以静坐,记忆力欠佳,学习成绩低下,五心烦热,盗汗,口干咽燥,或有遗尿,大便秘结,舌质红,苔少,脉细弦。

治法:滋阴潜阳,宁神益智。

主方:杞菊地黄丸加减。

Commonly used herbs: *Hominis Placenta* (Zi He Che), *Lycii Fructus* (Gou Qi Zi), *Rehmanniae Radix Praeparata* (Shu Di Huang), *Corni Fructus* (Shan Zhu Yu), *Dioscoreae Rhizoma* (Shan Yao), *Poria* (Fu Ling), *Chrysanthemi Flos* (Ju Hua), *Moutan Cortex Radicis* (Mu Dan Pi), *Alismatis Rhizoma* (Ze Xie), *Dens Draconis* (Long Chi), *Carapax et Testudinis Carapax Et Plastrum* (Gui Jia).

常用药:紫河车、枸杞子、熟地黄、山茱萸、山药、茯苓、菊花、牡丹皮、泽泻、龙齿、龟甲。

Modification: For impatience and irascibility, add *Haliotidis Concha* (Shi Jue Ming), and *Paeoniae Radix Albae* (Bai Shao); for restless night sleep, add *Ziziphi Spinosi Semen* (Suan Zao Ren), and *Schisandrae Fructus Chinensis* (Wu Wei Zi); for night sweating, add *Tritici Levis Fructus* (Fu Xiao Mai), *Os Draconis Calcinata* (Duan Long Gu), *Ostreae Concha Calcinata* (Duan Mu Li); for constipation, add *Cannabis Fructus* (Huo Ma Ren), and *Angelicae Sinensis Radix* (Dang Gui).

加减:急躁易怒者,加石决明、白芍;夜寐不安者,加酸枣仁、五味子;盗汗者,加浮小麦、煅龙骨、煅牡蛎;大便秘结者,加火麻仁、当归。

(4) Deficiency of the heart and spleen

(4) 心脾两虚

Manifestations: Undisciplined spirit, inattentive, fatigued spirit and lack of strength, emaciation, puffiness, overactive without agitation, hasty end in doing things, rash speech, poor sleep, poor memory, spontaneous sweating and night sweating, food preference, poor appetite, lusterless facial complexion, pale tongue, white and thin tongue coating, weak pulse.

证候:神思涣散,注意力不能集中,神疲乏力,形体消瘦或虚胖,多动而不暴躁,做事有头无尾,言语冒失,睡眠不实,记忆力差,伴自汗盗汗,偏食纳少,面色无华,舌质淡,苔薄白,脉虚弱。

Therapeutic method: To nourish the heart and calm down the spirit, fortify the spleen and promote intelligence.

治法:养心安神,健脾睿智。

Main formula: *Spleen-Returning Decoction* (Gui Pi Tang) and *Licorice, Wheat, and Jujube Decoction* (Gan Mai Da Zao Tang) with modification.

主方:归脾汤合甘麦大枣汤加减。

Commonly used herbs: *Codonopsis Radix* (Dang Shen), *Astragali Radix* (Huang Qi), *Atractylodis Macrocephalae Rhizoma* (Bai Zhu), *Jujubae Fructus* (Da Zao), *Glycyrrhizae Radix Et Rhizomapraeparata* (Zhi Gan Cao), *Poria Cum Ligno Hospite* (Fu Shen), *Polygalae Radix* (Yuan Zhi), *Ziziphi Spinosi Semen* (Suan Zao Ren), *Longan Arillus* (Long Yan Rou), *Angelicae Sinensis Radix* (Dang Gui), *Tritici Levis Fructus* (Fu Xiao Mai).

常用药:党参、黄芪、白术、大枣、炙甘草、茯神、远志、酸枣仁、龙眼肉、当归、浮小麦。

Modification: For distraction, add *Alpiniae Oxyphyllae Fructus* (*Yi Zhi*), and *Os Draconis* (Long Gu); for poor sleep, add *Schisandrae Fructus Chinensis* (Wu Wei Zi), *Polygoni Multiflori Caulis* (Shou Wu Teng); for clumsy action, poor memory, slimy tongue coating, add *Pinelliae Rhizoma* (Ban Xia), *Citri Reticulatae Pericarpium* (Chen Pi), and *Acori Rhizoma Tatarinowii* (Shi Chang Pu).

加减:注意力不集中者,加益智仁、龙骨;睡眠不实者,加五味子、首乌藤;动作笨拙,记忆力差,舌苔腻者,加半夏、陈皮、石菖蒲。

4 Other therapies

4 其他疗法

4.1 Chinese Patent medicine

4.1 中成药

(1) *Quietness and Brightness Oral Liquid* (Jing Ling Kou Fu Ye) is used for a ttention deficit and hyperactivity disorder due to yin deficiency in the liver and kidney.

(1) 静灵口服液:适用于注意缺陷与多动障碍肝肾阴虚证。

(2) *Lycium Berry, Chrysanthemum, and Rehmannia Pill* (Qi Ju Di Huang Wan) is used for attention deficit and hyperactivity disorder due to yin deficiency in the liver and kidney.

(2) 杞菊地黄丸:适用于注意缺陷与多动障碍肝肾阴虚证。

(3) *Children's Intelligence Syrup* (Xiao Er Zhi Li Tang Jiang) is used for attention deficit and hyperactivity disorder, due to insufficiency in the heart and kidney, and blockage of orifices by phlegm and turbidity.

(3) 小儿智力糖浆:适用于注意缺陷与多动障碍心肾不足,痰浊阻窍证。

(4) *Spleen-Returning Pills* (Gui Pi Wan) is used

(4) 归脾丸:适用于注意

for attention deficit and hyperactivity disorder in pattern of deficiency in the heart and spleen.

缺陷与多动障碍心脾两虚证。

4.2 Acumoxatherapy

4.2 针灸疗法

(1) Body acupuncture: Main acupoints: Select Neiguan (PC 6), Taichong (LR 3), Dazhui (GV 14), Quchi (LI 11). For lack of attention, add Baihui (GV 20), Sishencong (EX-HN 1), Daling (PC 7); for hyperactivity, add Dingshen (Extra), Anmian (EX-HN 22), Xinshu (BL 15); for vexation, add Shenting (GV 24), Danzhong (CV 17), and Zhaohai (KI 6). Insert the needle by the twisting technique for sedation, without retaining the needle, once every day.

（1）体针：主穴取内关、太冲、大椎、曲池。注意力不集中者，配百会、四神聪、大陵；多动者，配定神、安眠、心俞；烦躁者，配神庭、膻中、照海。捻转进针，用泻法，不留针。每日 1 次。

(2) Ear acupuncture: Select ear points of Pt. Heart, Pt. Liver, Pt. Kidney, Pt. Ear-shenmen, Pt. Sympathetic, and Pt. Brain, puncture shallowly, without retaining the needle, once every day. Or embed and press *Semen Vaccariae* (Wang Bu Liu Xing Zi) on the acupoints, and use the same acupoints as above.

（2）耳针：取心、肝、肾、神门、交感、脑点。浅刺不留针，每日 1 次。或用王不留行子压穴，取穴同上。

Section 2 Tic Disorder

第 2 节 抽动障碍

Tic disorder is mainly manifested by repeated, involuntary, rapid movement tics or vocal tics of one or more parts of the muscle groups, often accompanied by emotional disorder or behavior disorder like hyperactivity, compulsion, inattention, etc. The disease can occur at any season, and often in children from 2 to 12 years old. The course of illness is long. The symptoms can be relieved or may be aggravated by themselves. The intelligence of the infants is not affected.

抽动障碍主要表现为反复的、不自主的、快速的一个部位或多部位肌群运动抽动或发声抽动，常伴有情绪障碍及多动、强迫、注意力不集中等行为障碍。发病无季节性，常在 2～12 岁之间起病。病程持续时间较长，病症可自行缓解或加重，患儿智力一般不受影响。

It belongs to scope of "chronic infantile convul-

本病属中医学"慢惊风"

sion", "tremor" in traditional Chinese medicine.

"抽搐"等范畴。

1 Etiology and pathogenesis

The causes of tic disorder are related to prenatal insufficiency of natural endowment, damage by food ingestion, infection of exogenous evils, impact from illness, emotional disorder, tension and fatigue.

The location of disease is mainly in the liver, often affecting the heart, spleen, and kidney, etc. The pathogenesis is deficiency in the Vital Energy and excess in the symptoms. The initial seizure mostly belongs to excessive pattern. The prolonged duration mostly belongs to deficient pattern. The causative reason is yin deficiency in the liver and kidney, and the clinical manifestations are upward stirring due to yang hyperactivity, wind and phlegm. It is often caused by wind engendering phlegm, phlegm engendering wind, coagulation of wind and phlegm, and stirring wind of liver qi stagnation.

1 病因病机

抽动症的病因与先天禀赋不足、饮食所伤、感受外邪、疾病影响、情志失调，以及紧张劳累等因素有关。

病位主要在肝，也常影响到心脾肾等其他脏腑。病机属性为本虚标实，病初多实，迁延日久多虚，以肝肾阴虚为本，阳亢风痰鼓动为标。常由风生痰，痰生风，风痰胶结，肝郁风动而发病。

2 Key to diagnosis

(1) If it starts before 18 years old, it is probally induced by past illness or emotional disorder or there is a family history.

(2) The involuntary rapid tic in the muscle groups of the eye, face, neck, shoulder, abdomen and upper and lower limbs occurs repeatedly in the fixed ways, with no rhythm, and disappears after sleep. In seizure of tic, there can be abnormal sound like giggling, coughing sound, groaning, or foul language. The above tic may attack by turns. Tic can be controlled by will power for a short while, and can stop temporarily.

2 诊断要点

（1）发病于 18 岁前，可有疾病及情志失调的诱因或有家族史。

（2）不自主的眼、面、颈、肩、腹及上下肢肌群快速抽动，以固定方式重复出现，无节律性，入睡后消失。在抽动时，可出现异常的发音，如咯咯、吭吭、咳声、呻吟声或粗言秽语。上述抽动可轮换发作。抽动也能受意志短暂控制，可暂时不发作。

(3) The mild cases, with duration within a year, belong to transient tic. The duration over one year, characterized by only one type of tic (either movement or vocal tic), belongs to chronic tic. The duration over one year, characterized by movement tic and vocal tic, belongs to multiple tic, with interval of no tic over 3 months.

(3) 病情轻者,病程在1年之内,属于短暂性抽动;病程超过1年,仅有一种抽动(或是运动抽动,或是发声抽动)属于慢性抽动;病程超过1年,既有运动抽动,又有发声抽动,属于多发性抽动,其无抽动间歇期不超过3个月。

(4) The disease develops in chronic procedure, with obvious fluctuation, and is often induced or aggravated by cold.

(4) 本病呈慢性过程,有明显波动性,常由感冒诱发或加重。

(5) There is no special abnormality by lab tests. The encephalogram shows normal or nonspecific abnormal. The intelligence test is basically normal.

(5) 实验室检查多无特殊异常,脑电图正常或非特异性异常。智力测试基本正常。

3 Pattern identification and treatment

3 辨证论治

It is necessary to identify the diseased location of viscera, the deficiency and excess. In those with winking and headshaking, vexation and irascibility, the illness mainly lies in the liver. In those with dreamful sleep, vexation and restlessness, foul language and tic, the illness mainly lies in the heart. In those with tic and lack of strength, poor appetite, anorexia, yellow face and fatigued body, the illness mainly lies in the spleen. In those with shaking limbs and twisting lumbus, feverish sensation in the palms and soles, red tongue and little tongue coating, the illness mainly lies in the kidney. In those with occasional infection of exogenous pathogens, abnormal sound in the throat and tic inducing, the illness mainly lies in the lung. Short duration, frequent and strong tic, loud voice, vexation, irascibility, dry stool, red tongue, and excessive pulse are

主要辨脏腑病位及虚实:眨眼摇头,烦躁易怒者,病主要在肝;夜眠多梦,心烦不宁,秽语抽动者,病主要在心;抽动无力,纳少厌食,面黄体倦者,病主要在脾;肢颤腰扭,手足心热,舌红苔少者,病主要在肾;时有外感,喉出异声,引发抽动者,病主要在肺。病程尚短,抽动频繁有力,发声响亮,伴烦躁易怒,大便干,舌质红,脉实者,辨证多属实证;病程较长,抽动较弱,发声较低,伴面色无华,懒言倦怠,舌淡苔薄,或潮热盗汗,舌红苔少者,辨证多属虚证。

mainly identified as excess pattern. Relatively long duration, relatively weak tic, low sound, lusterless facial complexion, reluctance to speak, fatigue, pale tongue, thin tongue coating, tidal feverish sensation and night sweat, red tongue and scanty tongue coating are mostly identified as deficiency pattern.

The excess pattern is mainly treated with methods to balance the liver and extinguish wind, dissipate phlegm and check tic. The deficiency pattern is mainly treated with nethods to nourish the kidney and supplement the spleen, soften the liver and extinguish wind. The pattern of mixed excess and deficiency is supposed to treat both the causative reason and clinical symptoms, jointly by the attacking and supplementing method.

治疗实证以平肝息风，豁痰定抽为主；虚证以滋肾补脾，柔肝息风为主，虚实夹杂治当标本兼顾，攻补兼施。

(1) Stirring wind due to liver hyperactivity

(1) 肝亢风动

Manifestations: Shaking head, shrugging shoulder, winking, pouting, kicking, frequent and forceful tic, occasional crying, loud voice, agitation and irascibility, poor self-control, accompanied by dizziness and headache, flushed face and eye, abdomen movement, hypochondriac pain, dry stool and yellow urine, red tongue, yellow tongue coating, rapid and string-taut pulse.

证候：摇头耸肩，挤眉眨眼，噘嘴踢腿，抽动频繁有力，不时喊叫，声音高亢，急躁易怒，自控力差，伴头晕头痛，面红目赤，或腹动胁痛，便干尿黄，舌红苔黄，脉弦数。

Therapeutic method: To balance the liver and extinguish wind, drain fire and check tic.

治法：平肝息风，泻火定抽。

Main formula: *Gastrodia and Uncaria Decoction* (Tian Ma Gou Teng Yin) with modification.

主方：天麻钩藤饮加减。

Commonly used herbs: *Gastrodiae Rhizoma* (Tian Ma), *Uncariae ramulus Cum uncis* (Gou Teng), *Haliotidis Concha* (Shi Jue Ming), *Gardeniae Fructus*(Zhi Zi), *Scutellariae Radix*(Huang Qin), *Cyathulae Radix* (Chuan Niu Xi), *Bupleuri*

常用药：天麻、钩藤、石决明、栀子、黄芩、川牛膝、柴胡、当归、茯神、远志。

Radix (Chai Hu), *Angelicae Sinensis Radix* (Dang Gui), *Poria Cum Ligno Hospite* (Fu Shen), *Polygalae Radix* (Yuan Zhi).

Modification: For agitation and irascibility, add *Prunellae Spica* (Xia Ku Cao), *Curcumae Radix* (Yu Jin), and *Paeoniae Radix Albae* (Bai Shao); for obvious tic, add *Chloriti Lapis* (Qing Meng Shi), *Antelopis Tataricae Cornu* (Ling Yang Jiao) (grind and take after infused with water); for nodding and head shaking, add *Puerariae Radix* (Ge Gen), *Viticis Fructus* (Man Jing Zi), *Cicadae Periostracum* (Chan Tui); for screaming and crying, add *Sophorae Tonkinensis Radix Et Rhizoma* (Shan Dou Gen), *Arctii Fructus* (Niu Bang Zi).

加减:急躁易怒者,加夏枯草、郁金、白芍;抽动明显者,加青礞石、羚羊角(研末冲服);点头摇头者,加葛根、蔓荆子、蝉蜕;喊叫声高者,加山豆根、牛蒡子。

(2) Harassment of Phlegm and heat

(2) 痰热扰动

Manifestations: Muscular spasm in the head and face, limbs and body, lots of quick and forceful twitching movement, constant crying and screaming, occasional foul language, vexation and thirst, easy fright in sleep or restless sleep, constipation, dried stool, scanty and yellow urine, red tongue, yellow tongue coating or thick and slimy tongue coating, slippery and string-taut pulse or rapid and slippery pulse.

证候:头面、四肢、躯体肌肉抽动,动作多、快、有力,呼叫不安,时说秽语,烦躁口渴,睡中易惊或睡眠不安,大便秘结,小便短黄,舌质红,苔黄或厚腻,脉弦滑或滑数。

Therapeutic method: To clear away heat and dissolve phlegm, extinguish wind and check tic.

治法:清热化痰,息风止抽。

Main formula: *Coptis Gallbladder-Warming Decoction* (Huang Lian Wen Dan Tang) with modification.

主方:黄连温胆汤加减。

Commonly used herbs: *Coptidis Rhizoma* (Huang Lian), *Pinelliae Rhizoma* (Ban Xia), *Citri Reticulatae Pericarpium* (Chen Pi), *Bambusae Caulis in Taenias* (Zhu Ru), *Aurantii Fructus Immaturus* (Zhi Shi), *Poria* (Fu Ling), *Bambusae*

常用药:黄连、半夏、陈皮、竹茹、枳实、茯苓、天竺黄、僵蚕、石菖蒲、远志。

Concretio Silicea (Tian Zhu Huang), *Bombyx Batryticatus* (Jiang Can), *Acori Rhizoma Tatarinowii* (Shi Chang Pu), *Polygalae Radix*(Yuan Zhi).

Modification: For frequent foul language, rale in the throat, add *Chloriti Lapis* (Qing Meng Shi), *Oroxyli Semen* (Mu Hu Die), and *Physalis Calyx seu Fructus* (Jin Deng Long); for frequent winking, add *Eriocauli Flos* (Gu Jing Cao), *Celosiae Semen* (Qing Xiang Zi), *Buddleja Flos* (Mi Meng Hua); for vexation and depression in the chest, add *Lophatheri Herba* (Dan Zhu Ye), *Forsythiae Fructus* (Lian Qiao), *Trichosanthis Pericarpium* (Gua Lou Pi).

(3) Spleen deficiency and liver hyperactivity

Manifestations: Weak tic, intermittent seizure, intermittent severity, winking and frown, pouting, nose twitching, abdominal tic, strange sound in the throat, fatigued spirit, sallow facial complexion, poor appetite, restless night sleep, irregular defecation, pale tongue, white and thin tongue coating or thin and slimy tongue coating, thready pulse or thready and string-taut pulse.

Therapeutic method: To support the earth and restrain the wood, harmonize the liver and spleen.

Main formula: *Liver-Relaxing and Spleen-Rectifying Decoction* (Shu Gan Li Pi Tang) with modification.

Commonly used herbs: *Codonopsis Radix*(Dang Shen), *Atractylodis Macrocephalae Rhizoma* (Bai Zhu), *Poria* (Fu Ling), *Dioscoreae Rhizoma* (Shan Yao), *Bupleuri Radix* (Chai Hu), *Paeoniae Radix Albae* (Bai Shao), *Angelicae Sinensis Radix* (Dang Gui), *Citri Reticulatae Pericarpium* (Chen Pi), *Ziziphi Spinosi Semen* (Suan Zao Ren), *Polygalae*

加减:秽语频出,喉中痰鸣者,加青礞石、木蝴蝶、锦灯笼;眨眼频繁者,加谷精草、青葙子、密蒙花;烦躁胸闷者,加淡竹叶、连翘、瓜蒌皮。

(3) 脾虚肝旺

证候:抽动无力,时发时止,时轻时重,眨眼皱眉,噘嘴搐鼻,腹部抽动,喉出怪声,精神倦怠,面色萎黄,食欲不振,夜卧不安,大便不调,舌质淡,苔薄白或薄腻,脉细或细弦。

治法:扶土抑木,调和肝脾。

主方:缓肝理脾汤加减。

常用药:党参、白术、茯苓、山药、柴胡、白芍、当归、陈皮、酸枣仁、远志、甘草。

Radix (Yuan Zhi), *Glycyrrhizae Radix Et Rhizoma* (Gan Cao).

Modification: For frequent tic, add *Puerariae Radix* (Ge Gen), and *Gastrodiae Rhizoma* (Tian Ma); for hyperactive liver qi, add *Uncariae ramulus Cum uncis* (Gou Teng), *Os Draconis Cruda* (Sheng Long Gu); for frequent twitching in the hand and foot, add *Chaenomelis Fructus*(Mu Gua), *Lycopodii Herba* (Shen Jin Cao), *Spatholobi Caulis* (Ji Xue Teng); for obvious abdominal tic, add *Chaenomelis Fructus*(Mu Gua), and *Aurantii Fructus* (Zhi Qiao), and *Paeoniae Radix Albae* (Bai Shao) and *Glycyrrhizae Radix Et Rhizoma* (Gan Cao) in high dose ; for twitching nose, add *Magnoliae Flos* (Xin Yi), *Xanthii Fructus* (Cang Er Zi); for poor appetite, add *Setariae Fructus Germinatus* (Gu Ya), *Crataegi Fructus Ustus* (Jiao Shan Zha), *Galli Endothelium Corneum Gigerii*(Ji Nei Jin); for restless sleep, add *Platycladi Semen*(Bai Zi Ren), and *Margaritifera Concha* (Zhen Zhu Mu).

加减:抽动频数者,加葛根、天麻;肝气亢旺者,加钩藤、生龙骨;手足蠕动频繁者,加木瓜、伸筋草、鸡血藤;腹部抽动明显者,加木瓜、枳壳,重用白芍、甘草;搐鼻者,加辛夷、苍耳子;食欲不振者,加谷芽、焦山楂、鸡内金;睡眠不安者,加柏子仁、珍珠母。

(4) Stirring wind due to yin deficiency

(4) 阴虚风动

Manifestations: Winking and frown, head shaking and lumbus twisting, limbs shaking, dry throat, hawking, emaciation, agitation, tidal flushed cheeks, feverish sensation in the chest, palms and soles, restless sleep, dry stool, red tongue with scanty fluid, scanty tongue coating or patchy peeled tongue coating, thready and rapid pulse or thready, weak and string-taut pulse.

证候:挤眉弄眼,摇头扭腰,肢体抖动,咽干清嗓,形体偏瘦,性情急躁,两颧潮红,五心烦热,睡眠不安,大便偏干,舌质红少津,苔少或花剥,脉细数或弦细无力。

Therapeutic method: To enrich the water to moisten wood, soften the liver and extinguish wind.

治法:滋水涵木,柔肝息风。

Main formula: *Major Wind-Stabilizing Pill* (Da Ding Feng Zhu) with modification.

主方:大定风珠加减。

Commonly used herbs: *Carapax et Testudinis*

常用药:龟甲、鳖甲、牡

Carapax Et Plastrum (Gui Jia), *Trionycis Carapax Et Rhizoma* (Bie Jia), *Ostreae Concha* (Mu Li), *Rehmanniae Radix Cruda* (Sheng Di Huang), *Colla Corii Asini* (E Jiao)(melted), *Ophiopogonis Radix* (Mai Dong), *Cannabis Fructus* (Huo Ma Ren), *Schisandrae Fructus Chinensis* (Wu Wei Zi), *Paeoniae Radix Albae* (Bai Shao), *Glycyrrhizae Radix Et Rhizoma*(Gan Cao).

蛎、生地黄、阿胶(烊化)、麦冬、火麻仁、五味子、白芍、甘草。

Modification: For obvious tic, add *Scorpio* (Quan Xie), *Scolopendra* (Wu Gong); for abnormal sound in the throat, add *Canarii Fructus* (Qing Guo), *Scrophulariae Radix* (Xuan Shen), *Platycodonis Radix* (Jie Geng); for feverish sensation in the chest, palms and soles, add *Lycii Cortex* (Di Gu Pi), *Moutan Cortex Radicis* (Mu Dan Pi), and *Artemisiae Annuae Herba* (Qing Hao); for restless sleep, add *Ziziphi Spinosi Semen Semen* (Suan Zao Ren), *Bulbus Lilii* (Bai He), *Polygoni Multiflori Caulis* (Shou Wu Teng); for restless spirit, and inattention, add *Acori Rhizoma Tatarinowii* (Shi Chang Pu), *Alpiniae Oxyphyllae Fructus* (Yi Zhi), *Ziziphi Spinosi Semen* (Suan Zao Ren); for dizziness, and pale tongue, add *Polygoni Multiflori Radix* (He Shou Wu), *Angelicae Sinensis Radix* (Dang Gui), and *Gastrodiae Rhizoma* (Tian Ma).

加减:抽动明显者,加全蝎、蜈蚣;喉发异声者,加青果、玄参、桔梗;五心烦热者,加地骨皮、牡丹皮、青蒿;睡眠不实者,加酸枣仁、百合、首乌藤;心神不定,注意力不集中者,加石菖蒲、益智、酸枣仁;头昏,舌质淡者,加何首乌、当归、天麻。

4 Other therapies

4 其他疗法

4.1 Chinese Patent medicine

4.1 中成药

(1) *Chinese Angelica, Gentian, and Aloe Pill* (Dang Gui Long Hui Wan) is used for tic disorder in pattern of stirring wind due to liver hyperactivity.

(1) 当归龙荟丸:适用于抽动障碍肝亢风动证。

(2) *Chlorite Phlegm-Dissipating Pill* (Meng Shi Gun Tan Wan) is used for harassing tic disorder in pattern of harassment of phlegm and heat.

(2) 礞石滚痰丸:适用于抽动障碍痰热扰动证。

(3) *Lycium Berry, Chrysanthemum, and Rehmannia Pill* (Qi Ju Di Huang Wan) is used for tic disorder in pattern of stirring wind due to yin deficiency.

(3) 杞菊地黄丸:适用于抽动障碍阴虚风动证。

(4) *Anemarrhena, Phellodendron, and Rehmannia Pill* (Zhi Bo Di Huang Wan) is used for tic disorder in pattern of stirring wind due to yin deficiency.

(4) 知柏地黄丸:适用于抽动障碍阴虚风动证。

4.2 Tuina Therapy

4.2 推拿疗法

Push Pt. Pitu, rub Pt. Pitu, rub Pt. Wuzijie, push Pt. Neibagua, knead the hand divergently, push Pt. Shangsanguan, rub Yongquan (KI 1), and Zusanli (ST 36).

推脾土,揉脾土,揉五指节,运内八卦,分手阴阳,推上三关,揉涌泉、足三里。

4.3 Acumoxatherapy

4.3 针灸疗法

(1) Body acupuncture: The main acupoints: Taichong (LR 3), Fengchi (GB 20), Baihui (GV 20). The additional acupoints: Yintang (EX-HN3), Yingxiang (LI 20), Sibai (ST 2), Dicang (ST 4), Neiguan (PC 6), Fenglong (ST 40), Shenmen (HT 7).

(1) 体针:主穴太冲、风池、百会。配穴印堂、迎香、四白、地仓、内关、丰隆、神门。

(2) Ear acupuncture: Select Pt. Subcortex, Pt. Ear-Shenmen, Pt. Heart, Pt. Liver, Pt. Kidney, two to three points each time, embed the ear points with the needle, twice a week. It is appropriate to press the ear acupoints for two to three times a day, 5 minutes each time.

(2) 耳针:皮质下、神门、心、肝、肾,每次选 2～3 穴。耳穴埋针,每周 2 次。每日可按压 2～3 次,每次 5 分钟。

Chapter 8 Endocrine Disease

第8章 内分泌疾病

Section 1 Sexual Precocity

第1节 性早熟

Sexual precocity refers to a type of endocrine disease of abnormal growth and development, manifested by advanced puberty characteristics in childhood. Internationally, the sexual development present before 9 years old in boys and 8 years old in girls is generally attributed to sexual precocity. The normal age for the sexual development is different in different races. Clinically, sexual precocity is one of the commonest endocrine diseases in children. The incidence of sexual precocity is around 0.6%～1.7%, because of different assessment of the data on growth and development in different countries, races and regions. The incidence of sexual precocity is obviously higher in girls than that in boys, in which the ratio of incidence of central sexual precocity (true sexual precocity) is about 1/23～1/5 between the boys and girls.

性早熟是指儿童青春期特征提早出现的一类生长发育异常的内分泌疾病，一般国际上把男孩 9 岁以前、女孩 8 岁以前出现性发育征象，归为性早熟。性发育开始的正常年龄在不同的种族之间可以有一定的差异。性早熟是小儿临床最常见的内分泌疾病之一，儿童性早熟的发病率在 0.6%～1.7%。性早熟的发生率女孩明显高于男孩，其中，中枢性性早熟(真性性早熟)的发生率男孩与女孩比率约为 1/23～1/5。

In ancient medical classics of traditional Chinese medicine, Chinese characters for "hypertrophy of breast" were used to describe the partial manifestations of girls' breast development.

古医籍中"乳疬"描述似包括女童乳房发育的部分表现。

1 Etiology and pathogenesis

1 病因病机

The etiological factors include both internal and

病因包括内因和外因两

external causes. In terms of internal cause, mostly it is related to transmission of yin deficiency and internal heat from the parents into the fetus. In terms of external cause, it is related to over ingestion of fat, sweet and greasy food, meat products, or long-term contact of hormones, or administration of tonic products or medicine. These may nourish the kidney qi too much, leading to early preponderance of Xiang-premier fire and imbalance of yin and yang, and hence early arrival of Tiangui-gonadotropin, and early appearance of gender attributes. The pathogenesis mainly lies in the liver and kidney, more predominantly in the kidney.

方面。内因多系父母阴虚内热体质传至胎儿。外因则或过食膏粱厚味、血肉有情之品，或长期接触类激素物，或因食补品、药品，过培肾气，相火早旺，阴阳失衡，“天癸”早至，性征早现。病机主要责之肝肾二脏，以肾为主。

2 Key to diagnosis

(1) Early appearance of secondary gender characters: before 8 years old in girls, and before 9 years old in boys.

(2) Stimulation test of GnRH (gonadotropin releasing hormone), stimulation peak of luteinizing hormone (LH) is >12 U/L in girls and >25 U/L in boys. The peak of LH/the peak of FSH is >0.6~1.0.

(3) Enlargement of sexual glands: Under ultrasonic scan, the ovarian volume is >1 ml in girls, and several ovarian follicles in diameter >4 mm can be seen, and the testicular volume is >4 ml in boys, progressive enlarged with the course of illness.

(4) Linear growth accelerates.

(5) The bone age is one year or over one year older than the age.

(6) Serum sex hormone levels rise to the level

2 诊断要点

（1）第二性征提前出现：女孩8岁前，男孩9岁前。

（2）促性腺激素释放激素（GnRH）激发试验：促黄体生成素（LH）激发峰值，女孩>12单位/升，男孩>25单位/升，LH峰值/FSH峰值>0.6~1.0。

（3）性腺增大：女孩在B超下见卵巢容积>1毫升，并可见多个直径>4毫米的卵泡；男孩则睾丸容积>4毫升，并随病程延长进行性增大。

（4）线性生长加速。

（5）骨龄超越年龄1年或1年以上。

（6）血清性激素水平升

of puberty. Of the above diagnostic basis, item 1, 2, and 3 are the most important and requisite. However, if the duration is quite short in the clinical visit, the stimulation value of GnRH may not reach the above diagnostic values, neither does the size of ovary. In such cases, follow-up visits are necessary, and when necessary, the above examinations should be carried out several months later.

高至青春期水平。以上诊断依据中 1、2、3 条是最重要而且是必具的。但是，如就诊时病程很短，则 GnRH 激发值有时可能达不到以上诊断值，卵巢大小亦然。对此类病例应进行随访，必要时在数月后复查以上检测。

3 Pattern identifications and treatment

3 辨证论治

It is necessary to distinguish between deficiency and excess. The deficiency is related to insufficiency of the kidney yin, and hyperactivity in the kidney yang. The excess is related to either accumulation of heat in the liver meridian, or transformation of accumulated liver qi into fire, or accumulation of phlegm and dampness due to spleen deficiency, or qi stagnation and blood stasis, affecting balance between yin and yang in the kidney and hence the problem. The sick children with true sexual precocity are mostly related to constant over-nutrition, over ingestion of fat, sweet and greasy food, constitution in internal heat due to yin deficiency, and constant yin deficiency in the kidney and preponderance of Xiang-premier fire, or mostly related to yin deficiency in the liver and kidney, and frenetic flow of Xiang-premier, or in complication with phlegm, or with dampness, or with fire, or with blood stasis, mostly identified as pattern of mixed deficiency and excess or excess pattern.

辨证需注意辨别其虚实，虚者为肾阴不足，肾阳偏亢；实者或肝经郁热，肝郁化火；或脾虚痰湿，气滞血瘀，累及肾之阴阳平衡失调而发病。真性性早熟者患儿多长期营养过剩，过食膏粱厚味，或体禀阴虚内热体质，肾阴虚相火旺持续存在，多肝肾阴虚，相火妄动，或夹痰、或夹湿、或夹火、或夹瘀，多为虚实夹杂或为实证。

(1) Pattern of fire hyperactivity due to yin deficiency

（1）阴虚火旺

Manifestations: Breast development accompanied by development of sexual charaters and inter-

证候：女孩乳房发育或伴其他性征及内外生殖器发

nal and external reproductive organs, even menstruation in girls, testis enlargement (≥4 ml), or accompanied by prominence of Adam's apple, voice change, or seminal emission in boys; or accompanied by aversion to heat, night sweating, feverish sensation in the chest, palms and soles, constipation, red tongue or red tongue tip, scanty tongue coating, rapid and thready pulse.

育,甚者月经来潮;男孩睾丸增大(大于等于4毫升),或伴喉结突出,变声,或有遗精。或伴有怕热、盗汗、五心烦热、便秘、舌红或尖红少苔,脉细数。

Therapeutic method: To enrich yin and supplement the kidney, drain and downbear deficient fire.

治法:滋阴补肾,降泄虚火。

Main formula: *Anemarrhena, Phellodendron, and Rehmannia Pill/Decoction* (Zhi Bo Di Huang Wan/Tang) with modification.

主方:知柏地黄丸(汤)加减。

Commonly used herbs: *Anemarrhenae Rhizoma* (Zhi Mu), *Phellodendri Cortex Chinensis* (Huang Bo), *Rehmanniae Radix Praeparata* (Shu Di Huang), *Corni Fructus* (Shan Zhu Yu), *Moutan Cortex Radicis* (Mu Dan Pi), *Dioscoreae Rhizoma* (Shan Yao), *Poria* (Fu Ling).

常用药:知母、黄柏、熟地黄、山茱萸、牡丹皮、山药、茯苓。

Modification: For feverish sensation in the chest, palms and soles, add *Nelumbinis Plumula* (Lian Xin); for night sweating, add *Lycii Cortex* (Di Gu Pi), and *Scrophulariae Radix* (Xuan Shen); for much vaginal fluid, add *Cortex Toonae Radicis* (Chun Gen Bai Pi).

加减:五心烦热者,可加莲心;盗汗者,可加地骨皮、玄参;阴道分泌物多者,可加椿根白皮。

(2) Pattern of accumulated heat in the liver meridian

(2) 肝经郁热

Manifestations: Development of gender attributes is the same as that of pattern of fire hyperactivity due to yin deficiency in girls and boys, probably accompanied by uncomfortable depression in the chest, distenting pain in the breast, vexation and irascibility, foul breathing, acne, constipation, red

证候:男女性征发育同阴虚火旺型,或伴胸闷不舒、乳房胀痛、心烦易怒、口臭、痤疮、便秘、舌红苔黄或黄腻,脉弦数或弦细数。

tongue and yellow tongue coating, or yellow and slimy tongue coating, rapid and string-taut pulse or thready and rapid pulse.

Therapeutic method: To enrich yin and downbear fire, soothe the liver and resolve accumulation.

治法：滋阴降火，疏肝解郁。

Main formula: *Anemarrhena, Phellodendron, and Rehmannia Pill* (Zhi Bo Di Huang Wan) and *Moutan and Gardenia Free Wanderer Powder* (Dan Zhi Xiao Yao San).

主方：知柏地黄丸合丹栀逍遥散。

Commonly used herbs: *Anemarrhenae Rhizoma* (Zhi Mu), *Phellodendri Cortex Chinensis* (Huang Bo), *Rehmanniae Radix Praeparata* (Shu Di Huang), *Corni Fructus* (Shan Zhu Yu), *Moutan Cortex Radicis* (Mu Dan Pi), *Dioscoreae Rhizoma* (Shan Yao), *Poria* (Fu Ling), *Atractylodis Macrocephalae Rhizoma* (Bai Zhu), *Bupleuri Radix* (Chai Hu), *Angelicae Sinensis Radix* (Dang Gui), *Glycyrrhizae Radix Et Rhizoma* (Gan Cao), *Gardeniae Fructus*(Shan Zhi), *Paeoniae Radix* (Shao Yao).

常用药：知母、黄柏、熟地黄、山茱萸、牡丹皮、山药、茯苓、白术，柴胡、当归、甘草、栀子、芍药。

Modification: For obvious distending pain in the breast, add *Cyperi Rhizoma* (Xiang Fu), and *Curcumae Radix*(Yu Jin); for yellow leucorrhea in profuse volume, add *Phellodendri Cortex Chinensis* (Huang Bo); for foul breath, add *Coptidis Rhizoma* (Huang Lian).

加减：乳房胀痛明显者，加香附、郁金；带下色黄量多者，加黄柏；口臭者，酌加黄连。

4　Other therapies

4　其他疗法

(1) *Anemarrhena, Phellodendron, and Rehmannia Pill* (Zhi Bo Di Huang Wan) is used for gender precocity in mild pattern of fire hyperactivity due to yin deficiency.

(1) 知柏地黄丸：适用于性早熟阴虚火旺型轻症。

(2) *Major Yin Supplementation Pill* (Da Bu Yin Wan) is used for gender precocity in mild pat-

(2) 大补阴丸：适用于性早熟阴虚火旺型轻症。

tern of fire hyperactivity due to yin deficiency.

(3) *Free Wanderer Pill* (Xiao Yao San) is used for gender precocity in pattern of accumulated heat in the liver meridian.

(3) 逍遥丸:适用于性早熟肝经郁热型轻症。

Section 2 Childhood Diabetes

第2节 儿童期糖尿病

Diabetes is a disease mainly characterized by metabolic disorders of glucose, and induced by metabolic disorders of glucide, fat, water and electrolytes, etc., due to a lack of or an insufficiency of insulin. Childhood diabetes refers to diabetes in children under 15 years old, predominantly in type 1 diabetes. In recent years, type 2 diabetes of children tends to increase like that of adults.

It belongs to the scope of "emaciation-thirst" in traditional Chinese medicine. Type 1 diabetes is mainly explained in this section.

糖尿病是一种以葡萄糖代谢失常为主的疾病,由于胰岛素缺乏或不足引起糖类、脂肪、水、电解质等一系列物质代谢紊乱。儿童期糖尿病是指15岁以下发生的糖尿病,以1型糖尿病为主,近年来,儿童2型糖尿病与成人一样有不断增多趋势。

本病属中医学"消渴"范畴。本节重点讲述1型糖尿病。

1 Etiology and pathogenesis

Visceral qi deficiency is the internal cause of the disease. If affected with exogenous evils, diet irregularity, emotion disorders, fatigue and internal injury, it tends to cause consumption of yin body fluid due to exuberance of internal dryness and heat in children. The pathological changes can involve the Upper, Middle and Lower Energizer. The diseased location mainly lies in the lung, stomach, spleen and kidney. In terms of pathogenesis, the causative reason is yin deficiency, while dryness and heat belong to pathogenic factors. The lung is loca-

1 病因病机

脏气虚弱是发病的内因,若兼感受外邪,饮食失节,情志失调,劳倦内伤等诸多影响,易致患儿燥热内盛,阴液亏耗。病变可涉及上、中、下三焦,病位则主要在肺、胃、脾、肾。病机以阴虚为本,燥热为标。肺居上焦,主治节,输布津液,燥热伤肺,肺津不布则口渴;治节无权,津液不能敷布而直趋下

ted in the Upper Energizer, governs management and regulation, transports and distributes body fluid. If dryness and heat damage the lung, the lung would fail to distribute body fluid, leading to thirst. If the lung fails to perform management and regulation, body fluid would fail to be distributed and would go downward directly, without separating the clear from the turbid, to the bladder, leading to frequent urination or sweet urine with creamy fat. The spleen and stomach are located in the Middle Energizer. If the spleen and stomach are damaged by dryness and heat, there would be quick digestion, easy hunger and frequent food ingestion. When the stomach fire flames upward, there would be thirst and polydipsia. If the spleen is deficient due to long-term illness and fails to perform its ascending and descending ability, the essentials and dregs would go down together, inducing urination, with polyuria and sweet urine. The kidney, located in the lower triple burner, is an organ of water and fire. If the kidney yin is deficient, fire due to deficiency will be produced internally, burning the heart and lung in the upper body and causing thirst and polydipsia, and burning the spleen and stomach in the middle body and leading to rapid digestion and easy hunger. If the kidney qi is deficient, it would be abnormal in qi transformation and in the opening and closing ability, and fail to perform the securing and containing function, presenting frequent urination and profuse urine.

行,清浊不分而直下膀胱,致小便频多或有膏脂而甜;脾胃同居中焦,脾胃受燥热所伤,则消谷善饥而多食,胃火上炎而口渴多饮;久病脾虚,升降失职,精华与糟粕皆下趋而溺,致多溺而尿甜。肾居下焦,为水火之脏,肾阴亏损则虚火内生,上灼心肺则烦渴多饮,中灼脾胃则消谷善饥。肾气亏损,气化失常,开合失司,固摄失权,致尿频量多。

2 Key to diagnosis

(1) Fasting blood glucose ≥ 7.0 mmol/L (126 mg/dl), plus symptoms of diabetes.

2 诊断要点

(1) 空腹血糖≥7.0 毫摩尔/升(126 毫克/分升),并有

(2) Random blood sugar ≥ 11. 1 mmol/L (200 mg/dl).

(3) In sugar tolerance test, two-hour blood sugar≥11.1 mmol/L (200mg/dl).

With any one of the above three items, it can be diagnosed as diabetes. In type 1 childood diabetes, if there are clinical symptoms, positive urine sugar, and fasting blood-glucose≥7.0mmol/L, random blood sugar≥11. 1mmol/L, the diagnosis can be conformed without sugar tolerance test. When sugar based hemoglobin increases, and insulin and c-peptide decreases, blood serum ICA, GAD, and IAA can be positive in children of type 1 diabetes.

糖尿病症状。

（2）随机血糖≥11.1 毫摩尔/升(200 毫克/分升)。

（3）糖耐量试验中 2 小时血糖 ≥ 11.1 毫摩尔/升(200 毫克/分升)。

凡符合上述任何一条即可诊断为糖尿病。儿童 1 型糖尿病一旦出现临床症状、尿糖阳性、空腹血糖达 7.0 毫摩尔/升以上和随机血糖在 11.1 毫摩尔/升以上，一般不需做糖耐量实验就能确诊。糖化血红蛋白增高、胰岛素和 C 肽水平降低，1 型糖尿病患儿血清胰岛细胞自身抗体(ICA)、抗谷氨酸脱羧酶抗体(GAD)及胰岛自身抗体(IAA)可呈阳性。

3 Pattern identification and treatment

According to the constitution, duration, and clinical manifestations of sick child, pattern identification based upon the eight principles should be done in combination with pattern identification based upon the theory of internal organs.

In pattern identification of diabetes, yin deficiency is regarded as a fundamental reason while dryness and heat as the inducing factors. Childhood diabetes is mainly in excess patterns, also in patterns of mixed deficiency and excess. It mostly occurs with an acute onset and is respectively treated by clearing away heat and moistening the lung, clarifying the stomach and draining heat, and concur-

3 辨证论治

根据患儿体质、病程和临床证候，采用八纲辨证结合脏腑辨证。

糖尿病辨证以阴虚为主、燥热为标。儿童糖尿病以实证为主，也有虚实夹杂，多急性起病，分别采用清热润肺、清胃泻热，同时结合临床兼用养阴保津、益气健脾、滋阴补肾等加减。

rently by nourishing yin and safeguarding body fluid, boosting qi and fortifying the spleen, enriching yin and supplementing the kidney, in accordance with the clinical symptoms.

(1) Injury of body fluid by lung heat

Manifestations: Thirst, polydipsia, thirst immediately after drinking, dry tongue and throat, frequent urination and profuse urine, red tongue tip, thin and yellow tongue coating with scanty fluid, rapid and surging pulse or rapid and thready pulse.

Therapeutic method: To clear away heat and moisten the lung, engender body fluid and check thirst.

Main formula: *Jade Lady Brew* (Yu Nu Jian) with modification.

Commonly used herbs: *Gypsum Fibrosum* (Shi Gao), *Rehmanniae Radix Praeparata* (Shu Di Huang), *Ophiopogonis Radix* (Mai Dong), *Anemarrhenae Rhizoma* (Zhi Mu), *Achyranthis Bidentatae Radix* (Niu Xi).

Modification: For continuous thirst, frequent urine, rapid and forceless pulse due to deficiency of qi and yin, add *Ginseng Radix* (Ren Shen), *Astragali Radix* (Huang Qi), *Ophiopogonis Radix* (Mai Dong) in high dose, *Trichosanthis Radix* (Tian Hua Fen), and *Anemarrhenae Rhizoma* (Zhi Mu) to boost qi and nourish yin, engender body fluid and check thirst.

(2) Exuberance of stomach heat

Manifestations: Rapid hunger, large portion of food intake, emaciation, dry and constipated stool, frequent urination, red tongue, yellow tongue coating, thready and rapid pulse.

Therapeutic method: To clarify the stomach and drain heat, nourish yin and generate body fluid.

Main formula: *White Tiger Decoction Plus*

(1) 肺热津伤

证候:口渴多饮,随饮随渴,舌燥咽干,尿频量多,舌尖红,苔薄黄少津,脉洪数或细数。

治法:清热润肺,生津止渴。

主方:玉女煎加减。

常用药:石膏、熟地黄、麦冬、知母、牛膝。

加减:若烦渴不止,小便频数,脉数乏力者为气阴两伤,加人参、黄芪,重用麦冬、天花粉、知母益气养阴、生津止渴。

(2) 胃热炽盛

证候:多食善饥,口渴多饮,形体消瘦,大便燥结,小便频数,舌红,苔黄,脉细数。

治法:清胃泻热,养阴生津。

主方:白虎加人参汤合

Ginseng (Bai Hu Jia Ren Shen Tang) and *Humor-Increasing Decoction* (Zeng Ye Tang) with modification.

增液汤加减。

Commonly used herbs: *Anemarrhenae Rhizoma* (Zhi Mu), *Gypsum Fibrosum* (Shi Gao), *Ginseng Radix* (Ren Shen), *Glycyrrhizae Radix Et Rhizoma* (Gan Cao), *Scrophulariae Radix* (Xuan Shen), *Radix Ophiopogonis* (Mai Dong), *Rehmanniae Radix Cruda* (Sheng Di Huang).

常用药:知母、石膏、人参、甘草、玄参、麦冬、生地黄。

Modification: Add *Coptidis Rhizoma* (Huang Lian) and *Gardeniae Fructus*(Zhi Zi) to clear away heat and drain fire.

加减:热盛者,加黄连、栀子清热泻火。

(3) Qi deficiency in the spleen and stomach

(3) 脾胃气虚

Manifestations: Prolonged duration, thirst with a little desire for drinks, withered and yellow facial complexion, fatigue and lack of strength, hunger but with inability to eat, or low spirit with just a little hunger, or ability to eat with sloppy stool, pale tongue, weak pulse.

证候:病程较久,渴饮不多,面色萎黄,倦怠乏力,饥不能食或稍饥则馁,或能食与便溏并见,舌淡,脉弱。

Therapeutic method: To boost qi and fortify the spleen, engender body fluid and check thirst.

治法:益气健脾,生津止渴。

Main formula: *Seven Ingredient White Atractylodes Powder* (Qi Wei Bai Zhu San) with modification.

主方:七味白术散加减。

Commonly used herbs: *Ginseng Radix* (Ren Shen), *Poria Alba* (Bai Fu Ling), *Atractylodis Macrocephalae Rhizoma* (Bai Zhu), *Agastachis Folium* (Huo Xiang Ye), *Aucklandiae Radix* (Mu Xiang), *Glycyrrhizae Radix Et Rhizoma*(Gan Cao), *Puerariae Radix* (Ge Gen).

常用药:人参、白茯苓、炒白术、藿香叶、木香、甘草、葛根。

Modification: For prolonged qi deficiency and collapse of center qi, add *Astragali Radix* (Huang Qi), and *Cimicifugae Rhizoma* (Sheng Ma) to boost qi and upbear yang.

加减:气虚日久,中气下陷者,加黄芪、升麻益气升阳。

(4) Deficiency and depletion of kidney yin

(4) 肾阴亏损

Manifestations: Frequent urination, profuse

证候:尿频量多,浊如脂

urine turbid like cream, dry mouth and tongue, thirst with preference of excessive drinking, feverish sensation in the chest, palms and soles, dizziness, lack of strength, sour and weak lumbus and knees, red tongue, scanty tongue coating, thready and rapid pulse.

膏,口干舌燥,或渴而多饮,五心烦热,头昏乏力,腰膝酸软,形体消瘦,舌红,苔少,脉细数。

Therapeutic method: To enrich yin and supplement the kidney, engender body fluid and clear away heat.

治法:滋阴补肾,生津清热。

Main formula: *Six-Ingredient Rehmannia Pill* (Liu Wei Di Huang Wan) with modification.

主方:六味地黄丸加减。

Commonly used herbs: *Rehmanniae Radix Praeparata* (Shu Di Huang), *Corni Fructus* (Shan Zhu Yu), *Dioscoreae Rhizoma* (Shan Yao), *Alismatis Rhizoma* (Ze Xie), *Cortex Moutan Radicis* (Dan Pi), *Poria* (Fu Ling).

常用药:熟地黄、山茱萸、山药、泽泻、丹皮、茯苓。

Modification: For agitation due to fire hyperactivity of yin deficiency, feverish sensation in the chest, palms and soles, night sweating and insomnia, add *Anemarrhenae Rhizoma* (Zhi Mu), and *Phellodendri Cortex Chinensis* (Huang Bo) to enrich yin and drain fire.

加减:阴虚火旺而烦躁,五心烦热,盗汗,失眠者,加知母、黄柏滋阴泻火。

4 Other therapies

4 其他疗法

4.1 Empirical formula

Decoct *Maydis Stigma* (Yu Mi Xu), and drink it as tea, 30g every day.

4.1 经验方

玉米须煎汤代茶,每日30克。

4.2 Dietary therapy

(1) Pumpkin powder: Take 30g per day, successively for 1～3 months.

(2) *Lycii Fructus* (Gou Qi Zi): Take 6～12g with meals.

(3) *Dioscoreae Rhizoma* (Shan Yao): 200g per day, decoct it and take the decoction.

4.2 饮食疗法

(1) 南瓜粉:每日30克,连服1～3月。

(2) 枸杞子:每日6～12克佐餐。

(3) 山药:每日200克,煎汤服。

Chapter 9 Allergic Disease and Rheumatic Disease

第9章 变态反应性疾病及风湿性疾病

Section 1 Child Rheumatic Fever

第1节 儿童风湿热

Rheumatic fever is an immune inflammatory disease of the general connective tissue, caused by infection of Group A β-hemolytic streptococcus, and mainly manifested by carditis, wandering arthritis, chorea, erythema circinatum and subcutaneous nodule in repeated seizure. Carditis is the most serious manifestation in this disease, and may threaten the life of sick child in the acute stage. Its repeated seizure may cause permanent cardiac valvular lesion. It may occur in any season, more common in the winter and spring. The age of first onset is mostly from 6 to 12 years old, and rare under 3 years old.

This belongs to the scope of "impediment pattern", "migratory arthralgia", or "heart impediment" in traditional Chinese medicine.

风湿热是A族β溶血性链球菌感染引起的全身性结缔组织免疫炎性病变。主要表现为心脏炎、游走性关节炎、舞蹈病、环形红斑和皮下小结，可反复发作。心脏炎是本病最严重的表现，急性期可威胁患儿生命，反复发作后可致永久性心脏瓣膜病变。四季均可发病，冬春多见。首次发病年龄多为6～15岁，3岁以下少见。

本病属中医学"痹证""历节""心痹"范畴。

1 Etiology and pathogenesis

The internal causes are related to failue of defensive ability due to weak constitution. The external causes are related to pathogenic wind, cold, dampness, and heat.

Yang qi has not been sufficiently developed and the body surface has not been fully secured in the in-

1 病因病机

内因为体质虚弱，卫外不固；外因则责之于风、寒、湿、热之邪。

小儿阳气未充，腠理不固，若长期居处潮湿，或感受

fants. When they live in a damp place for a long time or are infected with pathogenic cold and dampness, their meridians and collaterals can be obstructed, resulting in pattern of accumulation of pathogenic cold and dampness in the collaterals, manifested by soreness and pain in the joints, which do not turn red locally but are exacerbated by exposure to cold and relieved by warmth.

If there is infection of pathogenic wind and heat together with dampness or long-term accumulation of wind, cold and dampness turning into heat, which obstructs the meridians and collaterals, red, swollen, hot and painful joints and fever could be present. If the impediment pattern lingers, and the Vital Energy is deficient and the pathogens are persistent, the internal organs will be involved, leading to obstruction of the heart meridian, and causing palpitation and shortness of breath by failure of blood in nourishing the heart. If enduring illness enters the collaterals and damages yang qi, it would lead to yang deficiency in the heart and spleen, then water and fluid would spill over the whole body due to lack of warmth and transformation, presenting palpitation, anxiety, shortness of breathing by exertion, and edema. If the problem lingers and blood is not sufficient in transformation, qi and blood would be deficient and blood flow would be unsmooth, leading to blood stasis, manifested by fatigued spirit, lack of strength, and blue lips and nails. If wind evils lodge in skin and flesh interstices, and Ying-nutrient qi and Wei-defensive qi are disharmonious, there would be erythema circinatum on the skin. If dampness is accumulated and congealed in the muscles and skin, there would be small subcutaneous

寒湿之邪，则经络壅塞，而见关节酸痛，局部不红，遇寒加剧，得温痛减等寒湿阻络之证。若感受风热之邪与湿相并，或因风寒湿痹郁久化热，阻于经络而见关节红肿热痛、发热等。痹证迁延，正虚邪恋，波及脏腑，导致心脉痹阻，以致血不养心而心悸气短。久病入络，损伤阳气，导致心脾阳虚，水液失于温化而泛溢周身，出现心悸、怔忡、动则气短、水肿等证候。疾病日久，营血化生不足，气血亏虚，血行不畅，瘀血由之而生，出现神疲乏力，唇甲发绀等气虚血瘀之证。若风邪留于肌肤腠理之间，营卫不和，皮肤可见环形红斑；若湿邪蕴郁，凝结于肌肉筋脉之间可见皮下小结；若湿热久羁，郁火伤阴，引动肝风，或痰湿中阻，筋脉失养，以致手足舞蹈，挤眉眨眼，努嘴吐舌等。

nodule. If damp ness and heat linger for long time, the accumulated fire damages yin, stirring up the liver wind, or if phlegm and dampness obstruct the Middle Energizer, the meridians and tendons cannot be nourished, presenting dancing with hands and feet, eyebrow squeezing, eye blinking, pouting and wagging tongue.

2 Key to diagnosis

It is necessary to process a comprehensive analysis by reference to Jones' Diagnostic Criteria for rheumatic fever, revised in 1992, together with clinical history, symptoms, physical features and results of lab tests. Under the precondition of streptococcal infection, the diagnosis can be made, if there are two items of major manifestations or one item of major manifestation together with two items of subsidiary manifestations. It should be noted that in atypical and mild cases of rheumatic fever, it is requested to make the comprehensive analysis and judgement, and carry out follow-up observations when necessary, in order to avoid making missed diagnosis or misdiagnosis.

2 诊断要点

参照1992年修订的Jones风湿热诊断标准，结合病史、症状、体征和实验室检查结果进行综合分析。在确定有链球菌感染的前提下，有两项主要表现或一项主要表现加两项次要表现，即可作出诊断。但应注意不典型风湿热和轻症病例，应综合分析判断，必要时追踪观察，以免漏诊和误诊。

Diagnositic Criteria for Rheumatic Fever

Subsidiary manifestation	Subsidiary manifestation	Streptococcal infection
Carditis	fever	positive throat swab culture
Polyarthritis	painful knees	positive in rapid streptococcal antigen test
Chorea	past history of rheumatic fever	high titer of anti streptococcal Antibody
Erythema circinatum	higher ESR, positive CRP	recent history of scarlet fever
Small intradermal nodules	prolonged P-R intervals	

Note: when the major manifestation is arthritis, painful knees are no longer regarded as subsidiary manifestation. When the main manifestation is carditis, prolonged P-R intervals is not considered as subsidiary manifestation.

风湿热的诊断标准

主要表现	次要表现	链球菌感染依据
心脏炎	发热	咽拭子培养阳性
多关节炎	关节痛	快速链球菌抗原试验阳性
舞蹈病	风湿热既往史	抗链球菌抗体滴度升高

续表

主要表现	次要表现	链球菌感染依据
环形红斑	血沉增高、CRP 阳性	近期猩红热病史
皮下小结	P-R 间期延长	

注：主要表现为关节炎者，关节痛不再作为次要表现；主要表现为心脏炎者，P-R 间期延长不再作为次要表现。

3　Pattern identification and treatment

It is requested to idenfity the nature of pathogenic evils and deficiency or excess of disease.

If infected with pathogenic cold and dampness, there would be aching joints, without red color in the local area, exacerbated by cold and relieved by warmth. If infected with pathogenic dampness and heat or long-term accumulation of dampness turning into heat, there would be painful and swollen joints, scorching hot in the local area, red macules on the skin, yellow and brwon urine, and constipated stool. If pathogenic wind is combined with pathogenic dampness, there would be mobile joint pain, heavy sensation in the head and body. Dancing with hand and foot, squeezing eyebrows and blinking eyes, pouting and wagging tongue are related to obstruction of phlegm and dampness in the Middle Energizer. Those with blood stasis can be manifested by somber facial complexion, blue lips and nails, dark purple tongue or stasis macules on the tongue, deep unsmooth and string-taut pulse.

New disease mostly belongs to excessive pattern, and old disease mostly belongs to deficient pattern. Excessive pattern is manifested by relatively acute onset, severe pathological situation and excessive and forceful pulse. Deficient pattern is manifested by long condition, continuous pain, mild pain, and vacuous and forceless pulse.

In view of excessive patterns mostly at the on-

3　辨证论治

主要辨别病邪的性质和疾病的虚实。

感受寒湿之邪，则出现关节酸痛，局部不红，遇寒则甚，得热则缓；感受湿热之邪或湿痹郁久化热，可见关节肿痛，局部灼热，皮肤红斑，小便黄赤，大便秘结；风邪与湿邪相并，可见关节疼痛，呈游走性，头重身困。手足舞蹈，挤眉眨眼，努嘴吐舌等为痰湿中阻；瘀血者可见面色晦暗、唇甲发绀、舌质紫暗甚或瘀斑，脉沉弦涩。

新病多实，久病多虚。实者，发病较急，痛势较剧，脉实有力；虚者，病情较长，疼痛绵绵，痛势较缓，脉虚无力。后期多虚实夹杂。

本病初起以实证为多，

set, the treatment is given to attack the evils and deal with symptoms in priority, by different methods to dispel wind, disperse cold, remove dampness, and clear away heat, in accordance with different infected evils. If the lingering duration damages qi and blood, and involves the liver and kidney, the treatment is given to support the Vital Energy mainly, or to support the Vital Energy and dispel evils simultaneously. If illness prolongs for quite a long time, with the heart involved, there would be the manifestations like obstruction of blood stasis in the heart meridian, water overflow due to spleen deficiency, and consumption and damage of qi and yin. Therefore, the treatment should be given by priority, based upon the identification between the causative reasons and clinical symptoms, and between deficiency and excess.

治疗以攻邪治标为先，根据感邪的不同，分别施以祛风、散寒、利湿、清热等法；久病耗伤气血，损及肝肾，治疗当以扶正为主，或扶正祛邪并用；若病延日久，则可出现心脉瘀阻、脾虚水泛、耗伤气阴的证候，当明辨标本虚实之主次而治之。

(1) Obstruction of dampness and heat in the collaterals

（1）湿热阻络

Manifestations: Painful and swollen joints, scorching heat in the local area, fever, aversion to wind, no relief after sweating, thirst with desire to drink, nosebleed, red macules on the skin, yellow and brown urine, constipated stool, red tongue, yellow, thick and slimy tongue coating, rapid and slippery pulse.

证候：关节肿痛，局部灼热，发热恶风，汗出不解，口渴欲饮，可有鼻衄，皮肤红斑，小便黄赤，大便秘结，舌质红，苔黄厚腻，脉滑数。

Therapeutic method: To clear away heat, remove dampness, dispel wind and dredge the collaterals.

治法：清热利湿，祛风通络。

Main Formula: *Impediment-Diffusing Decoction* (Xuan Bi Tang) with modification.

主方：宣痹汤加减。

Commonly used herbs: *Stephaniae Tetrandrae Radix* (Fang Ji), *Armeniacae Semen Amarum* (Xing Ren), *Talcum* (Hua Shi), *Durantae* (Lian Qiao), *Gardeniae Fructus* (Zhi Zi), *Coicis Semen* (Yi Yi

常用药：防己、杏仁、滑石、连翘、栀子、薏苡仁、半夏。

Ren), *Pinelliae Rhizoma* (Ban Xia).

Modification: For severe heat, add *Gypsum Fibrosum* (Sheng Shi Gao), *Scutellariae Radix*(Huang Qin), and *Isatidis Radix* (Ban Lan Gen) to clear away heat and resolve toxin; for swelling and distention of joints, add *Clematidis Radix Et Rtrhizoma* (Wei Ling Xian), *Achyranthis Bidentatae Radix* (Niu Xi), and *Luffae Fructus Retinervus* (Si Gua Luo) to dredge the collaterals; for severe pain of the joints, add *Olibanum* (Ru Xiang), *Myrrha* (Mo Yao), *Corydalis Rhizoma* (Yan Hu Suo) to activate blood and relieve pain; for red macules on the skin, add *Moutan Cortex Radicis* (Mu Dan Pi), *Arnebiae Radix* (Zi Cao) to cool blood and melt macules; for thirst, add *Ophiopogonis Radix* (Mai Dong), and *Dendrobii Herba* (Shi Hu) to nourish yin and engender body fluid; for nosebleed, add fresh *Agrimoniae Herba* (Xian He Cao), and *Imperatae Rhizoma* (Bai Mao Gen) to cool blood and check bleeding.

加减:热重者,加生石膏、黄芩、板蓝根以清热解毒;关节肿胀者,加威灵仙、牛膝、丝瓜络以通络;关节痛剧者,加乳香、没药、延胡索活血止痛;皮肤红斑者,加牡丹皮、紫草以凉血化斑;口渴者,加麦冬、石斛以养阴生津;鼻衄者,加鲜仙鹤草、白茅根以凉血止血。

(2) Obstruction of cold and dampness in the collaterals

(2) 寒湿阻络

Manifestations: Aching pain in the joints, no red color in the local area, exacerbated by cold, relieved by warmth, shortness of breath, lack of strength, palpitation, anxiety, pale tongue, slimy and white tongue coating, soft and slow pulse.

证候:关节酸痛,局部不红,遇寒加剧,得温痛减,气短乏力,心悸怔忡,舌质淡,苔白腻,脉濡缓。

Therapeutic method: To disperse cold and eliminate dampness, nourish blood and dispel wind.

治法:散寒除湿,养血祛风。

Main Formulas: *Impediment-Alleviating Decoction* (Juan Bi Tang) and *Pubescent Angelica and Mistletoe Decoction* (Du Huo Ji Sheng Tang) with modification.

主方:蠲痹汤合独活寄生汤加减。

Commonly used herbs: *Notopterygii Rhizoma seu Radix* (Qiang Huo), *Angelicae Pubescentis*

常用药:羌活、独活、桂枝、秦艽、海风藤、桑枝、当

Radix(Du Huo), *Cinnamomi Ramulus* (Gui Zhi), *Gentianae Radix Et Rhizoma Macrophyllae* (Qin Jiao), *Piperis Kadsurae Caulis* (Hai Feng Teng), *Mori Ramulus* (Sang Zhi), *Angelicae Sinensis Radix* (Dang Gui), *Chuanxiong Rhizoma* (Chuan Xiong), *Olibanum* (Ru Xiang), *Aucklandiae Radix* (Mu Xiang), *Glycyrrhizae Radix Et Rhizoma*(Gan Cao), *Taxilli Herba* (Sang Ji Sheng), *Paeoniae Radix Albae* (Bai Shao), *Rehmanniae Radix Praeparata* (Shu Di Huang), *Achyranthis Bidentatae Radix* (Niu Xi), *Asari Radix Et Rhizoma* (Xi Xin), *Poria Alba* (Bai Fu Ling), *Ledebouriellae Radix* (Fang Feng).

归、川芎、乳香、木香、甘草、桑寄生、白芍、熟地黄、牛膝、细辛、白茯苓、防风。

Modification: For swollen joints, add *Stephaniae Tetrandrae Radix* (Fang Ji), *Chaenomelis Fructus* (Mu Gua), *Atractylodis Rhizoma* (Cang Zhu) to dispel dampness; for severe pain, add *Aconiti Lateralis Radix Praeparata* (Zhi Fu Pian) to warm up the channels and disperse cold.

加减:关节肿胀者,可加防己、木瓜、苍术以祛湿;疼痛剧烈者,可加制附片温经散寒。

(3) Invasion of wind and dampness into the heart

(3) 风湿淫心

Manifestations: Unbated fever, heavy sensation in the head and body, palpitation, shortness of breath, fatigue and lack of strength, poor appetite, nausea, pale tongue, slimy tongue coating, slippery and soft pulse.

证候:发热不退,头重身困,心悸气短,疲乏无力,纳呆泛恶,舌质淡,苔腻,脉濡滑。

Therapeutic method: To dispel wind and eliminate dampness, dredge the collaterals and tranquilize the heart.

治法:祛风除湿,通络宁心。

Main Formula: *Large-leaved Gentian Decoction* (Da Qin Jiao Tang) with modification.

主方:大秦艽汤加减。

Commonly used herbs: *Gentianae Radix Et Rhizoma Macrophyllae* (Qin Jiao), *Chuanxiong Rhizoma* (Chuan Xiong), *Angelicae Pubescentis Radix* (Du Huo), *Angelicae Sinensis Radix* (Dang Gui), *Paeoniae Radix Albae* (Bai Shao), *Gypsum Fibrosum*

常用药:秦艽、川芎、独活、当归、白芍、石膏、甘草、羌活、防风、白芷、黄芩、白术、茯苓、生地黄、熟地黄、细辛。

(Shi Gao), *Glycyrrhizae Radix Et Rhizoma* (Gan Cao), *Notopterygii Rhizoma seu Radix* (Qiang Huo), *Ledebouriellae Radix* (Fang Feng), *Angelicae Radix Dahuricae* (Bai Zhi), *Scutellariae Radix* (Huang Qin), *Atractylodis Macrocephalae Rhizoma* (Bai Zhu), *Poria* (Fu Ling), *Rehmanniae Radix Cruda* (Sheng Di Huang), *Rehmanniae Radix Praeparata* (Shu Di Huang), *Asari Radix Et Rhizoma* (Xi Xin).

Modifications: For palpitation and cold limbs, add *Cinnamomi Ramulus* (Gui Zhi), *Paeoniae Radix Albae* (Bai Shao), *Curcumae Radix* (Yu Jin) to warm up the channels and disperse cold; for poor appetite and nausea, add *Pinelliae Rhizoma Praeparatum* (Fa Ban Xia), *Crataegi Fructus Ustus* (Jiao Shan Zha) to downbear counterflow and check vomiting.

加减:心悸肢冷者,加桂枝、白芍、郁金以温经散寒;纳呆泛恶者,加法半夏、焦山楂以降逆止呕。

(4) Yang Deficiency in the heart and spleen

(4) 心脾阳虚

Manifestations: Palpitation, anxiety, shortness of breath by exertion, difficulty in lying flat, lusterless facial complexion, puffiness, scanty urine, lack of warmth in the extremities, pale and enlarged tongue, thin and white tongue coating, intermittent knotted pulse.

证候:心悸怔忡,动则气短,难以平卧,面色无华,浮肿尿少,手足不温,舌质淡胖,苔薄白,脉结代。

Therapeutic method: To warm up yang and disinhibit water.

治法:温阳利水。

Main Formula: *True Warrior Decoction* (Zhen Wu Tang) and *Golden Coffer Kidney Qi Pill* (Jin Gui Shen Qi Wan) with modification.

主方:真武汤合金匮肾气丸加减。

Commonly used herbs: *Poria* (Fu Ling), *Paeoniae Radix* (Shao Yao), *Atractylodis Macrocephalae Rhizoma* (Bai Zhu), *Zingiberis Rhizoma Recens* (Sheng Jiang), *Aconiti Lateralis Radix Praeparata* (Fu Zi), *Rehmanniae Radix Praeparata* (Shu Di

常用药:茯苓、芍药、白术、生姜、附子、熟地黄、山茱萸(酒润,去核)、干山药(微炒)、牡丹皮、泽泻、车前子、川牛膝、肉桂。

Huang), *Corni Fructus* (Shan Zhu Yu)(soaked in liquor, seedless), *Dioscoreae Rhizoma* (Shan Yao) (slightly processed); *Moutan Cortex Radicis* (Mu Dan Pi), *Alismatis Rhizoma* (Ze Xie), *Plantaginis Semen* (Che Qian Zi), *Cyathulae Radix* (Chuan Niu Xi), *Cinnamomi Cortex* (Rou Gui).

Modification: For panting with inability to lie, and spontaneous sweating, add *Ginseng Radix* (Ren Shen), *Schisandrae Fructus Chinensis* (Wu Wei Zi), *Ostreae Concha Calcinata* (Duan Mu Li), and *Os Draconis Calcinata* (Duan Long Gu) to boost qi, restrain sweating and check prostration; for severe palpitation, add *Ginseng Radix* (Ren Shen), *Ophiopogonis Radix* (Mai Dong), *Glycyrrhizae Radix Et Rhizoma praeparata* (Zhi Gan Cao) to boost qi, nourish yin and restore the meridian.

加减:喘息不得卧,自汗出者,加人参、五味子、煅牡蛎、煅龙骨益气敛汗固脱;心悸甚者,加人参、麦冬、炙甘草益气养阴复脉。

(5) Qi Deficiency and Blood Stasis

(5) 气虚血瘀

Manifestations: Prolonged duration, fatigued spirit and lack of strength, palpitation, shortness of breath, exacerbated by exertion, somber facial complexion, blue lips and nails, emaciation, dark purple tongue, thin tongue coating, weak and thready pulse or intermittent knotted pulse.

证候:病程日久,神疲乏力,心悸气短,动则尤甚,面色晦暗,唇甲发绀,形体瘦弱,舌质紫暗,苔薄,脉细弱或结代。

Therapeutic method: To nourish and activate blood, boost qi and dredge the collaterals.

治法:养血活血,益气通脉。

Main Formulas: *Supplementing Yang and Returning Five Decoction* (Bu Yang Huan Wu Tang) with modification.

主方:补阳还五汤加减。

Commonly used herbs: *Astragali Radix* (Huang Qi), *Paeoniae Radix Rubra* (Chi Shao), *Angelicae Sinensis Radix* (Dang Gui), *Glycyrrhizae Radix Et Rhizoma* (Gan Cao), *Chuanxiong Rhizoma* (Chuan Xiong), *Persicae Semen* (Tao Ren), *Carthami Flos* (Hong Hua), *Puerariae Radix* (Ge Gen),

常用药:黄芪、赤芍、当归、甘草、川芎、桃仁、红花、葛根、地龙、丹参、白芍。

Lumbricus (Di Long), *Salviae Miltiorrhizae Radix Et Rhizoma* (Dan Shen), *Paeoniae Radix Albae* (Bai Shao).

Modification: For poor appetite, fatigue and lack of strength, add judiciously *Codonopsis Radix* (Dang Shen), *Poria* (Fu Ling), *Atractylodis Macrocephalae Rhizoma* (Bai Zhu) to fortify the spleen and boost qi; for severe cough and panting, and sticky sputum, add *Perillae Fructus* (Zi Su Zi), *Armeniacae Semen Amarum* (Xing Ren), *Sinapis semen Albae* (Bai Jie Zi), *Pinelliae Rhizoma Praeparatum* (Fa Ban Xia) judiciously to expel phlegm, diffuse the lung qi and stop panting; for cough and severe hemoptysis, add *Notoginseng Radix Et Rhizoma* (San Qi) to disperse blood stasis and stanch bleeding.

加减：纳呆食少，疲乏无力甚者，可酌加党参、茯苓、白术以健脾益气；咳喘甚而有黏痰者，可酌加紫苏子、杏仁、白芥子、法半夏以祛痰宣肺平喘；咳嗽咯血甚者，可加三七以散瘀止血。

4　Other therapies

4　其他疗法

4.1　Chinese Patent Medicine

Mysterious Four Pill (Si Miao Wan) is applicable to pattern of obstruction of dampness and heat in the collaterals.

4.1　中成药

四妙丸：适用于儿童风湿热湿热阻络证。

4.2　Acumoxatherapy

(1) Acupuncture: Commonly used acupoints for aching joints are Jianyu (LI 15), Quchi (LI 11), Waiguan (TB 5), Houxi (SI 3), Huantiao (GB 30), Yanglingquan (GB 34), Juegu (GB 38), Zusanli (ST 36), Xiyan (EX-LE 5). Select 3 to 5 acupoints each time, and puncture by the medium and strong stimulation, with the needling technique for sedation. It is applicable to elder children. For carditis, the acupoints are Jianshi (PC 5), Shenmen (HT 7), Ximen (PC 4), Xinshu (BL 15), and Danzhong (CV 17).

4.2　针灸疗法

（1）针刺治疗：关节痛常用穴位为肩髃、曲池、外关、后溪、环跳、阳陵泉、绝骨、足三里、膝眼等，每次取3～5穴，中强刺激，以泻法为主，适用于较大儿童；心脏炎常用穴位为间使、神门、郄门、心俞、膻中等。

(2) Moxibustion: Use mild moxibustion for joints pain due to cold and dampness.

(2) 灸法:采用温和灸法,可用于寒湿性关节疼痛。

4.3 Tuina Therapy

4.3 推拿疗法

For severe fever, clarify Pt. Tianheshui, open Pt. Tianmen, push Pt. Kangong; for joint pain in the upper limb, rub Jianjing (GB 21), push Pt. Sanguan, rub Pt. Yiwofeng; for joint pain in the lower limb, press and rub Zusanli (ST 36), pinch Xiyan (EX-LE 5), knead Kunlun (BL 60) and grasp Weizhong (BL 40).

发热重者,清天河水、开天门、推坎宫;上肢关节痛者,揉肩井、推三关、揉一窝风;下肢关节痛者,按揉足三里、掐膝眼、揉昆仑、拿委中。

Section 2 Allergic Purpura

第2节 过敏性紫癜

Allergic purpura, or Henoch-Schoenlein Purpura syndrome, is the most common vascular inflammatory lesion characterized by small vessel vasculitis in childhood, and clinically manifested by purpura on the skin, painful and swollen joints, abdominal pain, bloody stool, bloody urine, and protein urine. This disease mostly occurs in preschool children or school children, more commonly in boys than in girls, in all seasons, but more frequently in the spring and autumn.

过敏性紫癜又称亨-舒综合征,是儿童时期最常见的以小血管炎为主的血管炎性病变。临床表现以皮肤紫癜、关节肿痛、腹痛、便血、血尿和蛋白尿为特征。本病多发生于学龄前及学龄期儿童,男多于女,四季均可发病,以春秋季发病较多。

In traditional Chinese medicine, it is categorized into the scope of "purpura", "blood pattern", "muscular bleeding", "grape pestilence", or "purple patches".

本病属中医学"紫癜""血证""肌衄""葡萄疫""紫癜风"等范畴。

1 Etiology and pathogenesis

1 病因病机

The disease is related to the factors like infection of exogenous evils, improper diet, obstruction and stagnation of blood stasis, and qi-blood defi-

与感受外邪、饮食失节、瘀血阻滞、久病气血亏虚等因素有关。

ciency and depletion of qi and blood due to lingering disease, etc.

It is mostly induced by internal retention of hidden heat plus infection of seasonal evils. The invasion of pathogenic heat into blood, forcing blood to flow frenetically, and the failure of blood to flow through the meridians, damaging the collaterals by preponderant heat, belong to its main pathogenesis. At the early stage, it is mostly related to damage of the collaterals by pathogenic wind and heat, and frenetic blood flow due to blood heat, mostly identified as yang pattern, heat pattern and excess pattern. If excess turns into deficiency due to prolonged illness, or body constitution is predominantly in deficiency, it is mostly in deficiency pattern or concurrence of deficiency and excess. The disease is closely related to the heart, lung and spleen, and may also involve the liver and kidney.

多为内有伏热兼感时邪而发病，邪热入血，迫血妄行，血不循经，热盛伤络是其主要病机。早期多为风热伤络，血热妄行，以阳证、热证、实证居多；病久由实转虚，或素体亏虚为主者，则多见虚证，或虚实并见。与心、肺、脾有密切关系，也可涉及肝、肾。

2　Key to diagnosis

(1) There is a history of frequent upper respiratory tract infection, 1 to 3 weeks before the onset of the disease.

(2) The disease is characterized by recurrent purple patches on the skin. The skin rash mostly appears on the limbs and buttocks, especially on the stretching side of the lower limbs, and near the joints of the knees and ankles, in symmetrical distribution, in patches, and in different size and shape, presented with red macules or papules at the beginning, then gradually develops with hemorrhagic condition, above the skin, with no change in color by pressure, and afterwards becomes purple in color several days later, and then turns brown and fades

2　诊断要点

（1）起病前 1～3 周常有上呼吸道感染史。

（2）反复出现皮肤紫癜为本病特征。皮疹多见于四肢、臀部，尤以下肢伸侧及膝、踝关节附近最多，呈对称分布，分批出现。皮疹大小、形态不一，初起呈红色斑丘疹，渐成为出血性，高出皮面，压之不褪色，数日后转为紫色，继而呈棕褐色而消退。2/3 病例可见阵发性剧烈腹痛，常位于脐周或腹下部，可

away. About two thirds of the cases would present severe paroxysmal abdominal pain, often around umbilicus, or in the lower abdomen, probably accompanied by vomiting. 30%～50% of the patients would present the clinical manifestation of the renal lesions.

伴呕吐。约 1/3 病例可出现膝、踝等大关节肿痛。30%～50%患儿出现肾脏损害的临床表现。

(3) White blood cells are normal or elevated. Eosinophile granulocyte may increase. Blood platelet count, clotting time, and clot retraction test are normal. Erythrocyte sedimentation rate (ESR) is normal or increased. In some cases, the capillary fragility test is positive. When the kidney is involved, there can be blood urine and protein urine under microscopic inspection, and blood urine by the naked eyes in severe cases. There can be elevated C reactive protein, and higher titer of anti-"O" antibody.

(3) 白细胞正常或增加，嗜酸性粒细胞可增加；血小板计数、出凝血时间、血块收缩试验均正常。血沉正常或增快。部分病例毛细血管脆性试验阳性。肾脏受累时可出现镜下血尿及蛋白尿，重症可有肉眼血尿。可有 C 反应蛋白升高，抗"O"抗体效价增高。

3 Pattern identification and treatment

3 辨证论治

It is necessary to identify between excess and deficiency by its onset, duration, and color of purple patches. Sudden onset, short duration, and bright purple color belong mostly to excess. Slow onset, recurrent condition, lingering duration, and pale color mostly belong to deficiency.

根据起病、病程、紫癜颜色等辨虚实。起病急，病程短，紫癜颜色鲜明者多属实；起病缓，病情反复，病程缠绵，紫癜颜色较淡者多属虚。

The therapeutic principle is supposed to resolve toxin, cool blood, and disperse blood stasis. For damage of the collaterals by wind and heat, it is appropriate to dispel wind, clear away heat, cool blood and tranquilize the collaterals. For damp-heat impediment pattern by dampness and heat, it is appropriate to clear away heat, dispel dampness, activate blood and dredge the collaterals. For accumulated heat in the stomach and intestines, it is appropriate to drain fire, resolve toxin, clarify the stom-

以解毒凉血化瘀为治疗原则。风热伤络，宜祛风清热，凉血安络；湿热痹阻，宜清热祛湿，活血通络；胃肠积热，宜泻火解毒，清胃化斑；血分热盛，宜清热解毒，凉血化瘀；恢复期气阴亏虚，常用益气摄血、滋阴凉血之法。

ach and melt patches. For preponderance of heat in Xue-blood system, it is appropriate to clear away heat, resolve toxin, cool blood and melt stasis. For qi and yin depletion at the recovery stage, it is appropriate to boost qi and contain blood, nourish yin and cool blood.

(1) Damage of the collaterals by wind and heat

Manifestations: Purple patches mostly on the stretching side of the lower limbs and on the buttocks, in symmetrical distribution and bright red color, in rash or red macules, and in different size and shape, propably fused in patches, accompanied by fever, slight aversion to wind or cold, cough, sore throat, joint pain, abdominal pain, bloody stool, bloody urine, red tongue, thin and yellow tongue coating, and rapid and floating pulse.

Therapeutic method: To dispel wind and clear away heat, cool blood and tranquilize the collaterals.

Main Formula: *Lonicera and Forsythia Powder* (Yin Qiao San) with modification.

Commonly used herbs: *Forsythia Fructus* (Lian Qiao), *Lonicerae Flos Japonicae* (Jin Yin Hua), *Platycodonis Radix* (Ku Jie Geng), *Menthae Haploalycis Herba* (Bo He), *Arctii Fructus* (Niu Bang Zi), *Lophatheri Folium* (Zhu Ye), *Schizonepetae Spica* (Jing Jie Sui), *Glycyrrhizae Radix Et Rhizoma Cruda* (Sheng Gan Cao), *Sojae Semen Praeparata* (Dan Dou Chi).

Modification: For itching skin, add *Kochiae Fructus* (Di Fu Zi), *Cicadae Periostracum* (Chan Tui) to dispel wind and relieve itching; for bloody urine, add *Imperatae Rhizoma* (Bai Mao Gen), *Cirsii Herba* (Xiao Ji), *Rubiae Radix Et Rhizoma*

（1）风热伤络

证候：紫癜以下肢伸侧和臀部为多，呈对称性，颜色鲜红，呈丘疹或红斑，大小形态不一，可融合成片，或有痒感，伴发热，微恶风寒，咳嗽，咽红，或见关节痛，腹痛，便血，尿血，舌质红，苔薄黄，脉浮数。

治法：祛风清热，凉血安络。

主方：银翘散加减。

常用药：连翘、金银花、苦桔梗、薄荷、牛蒡子、竹叶、荆芥穗、生甘草、淡豆豉。

加减：皮肤瘙痒者，加地肤子、蝉蜕祛风止痒；尿血者，加白茅根、小蓟、茜草凉血止血；关节痛者，加秦艽、防己、牛膝祛风通络；腹痛

(Qian Cao) to cool blood and stanch bleeding; for joint pain, add *Gentianae Radix Et Rhizoma Macrophyllae* (Qin Jiao), *Stephaniae Tetrandrae Radix* (Fang Ji), *Achyranthis Bidentatae Radix* (Niu Xi) to dispel wind and dredge the collaterals; for abdominal pain, add *Aucklandiae Radix* (Mu Xiang), and *Corydalis Rhizoma* (Yan Hu Suo) to circulate qi and relieve pain.

者,加木香、延胡索行气止痛。

(2) Frenetic Blood Flow due to Heat

（2）血热妄行

Manifestations: Rapid and sudden onset, red face and vigorous heat, dry throat, vexation, thirst with perference for cold drinks, dense or patchy static macules or spots on the skin, accompanied by nosebleed, bleeding gum, dry stool, yellow or brown urine, crimson tongue, dry and yellow tongue coating, rapid and string-taut pulse.

证候:起病急骤,壮热面赤,咽干,心烦,渴喜冷饮,皮肤瘀斑瘀点密集或成片,伴鼻衄、齿衄,大便干燥,小便黄赤,舌质红绛,苔黄燥,脉弦数。

Therapeutic method: To clear away heat, resolve toxin, cool blood and disperse blood stasis.

治法:清热解毒,凉血化瘀。

Main Formula: *Rhinoceros Horn and Rehmannia Decoction* (Xi Jiao Di Huang Tang) with modification.

主方:犀角地黄汤加减。

Commonly used herbs: *Bubali Cornu* (Shui Niu Jiao), *Rehmanniae Radix Cruda* (Sheng Di Huang), *Paeoniae Radix* (Shao Yao), *Moutan Cortex Radicis* (Mu Dan Pi).

常用药:水牛角、生地黄、芍药、牡丹皮。

Modification: For multiple purple patches on the skin, add *Nelumbinis Rhizomatis Nodus Carbonisatus* (Ou Jie Tan), *Sanguisorbae Radix Carbonisatus* (Di Yu Tan) to cool blood and melt macules; for much nosebleed, add fried *Gardeniae Fructus* (Zhi Zi), *Imperatae Rhizoma* (Bai Mao Gen) to cool blood and resolve toxin; for bloody urine, add *Cirsii japonica herba* (Da Ji), *Cirsii Herba* (Xiao Ji) to cool blood and stanch bleeding; for

加减:皮肤紫癜多者,加藕节炭、地榆炭凉血化斑;鼻衄量多者,加炒栀子、白茅根凉血解毒;尿血者,加大蓟、小蓟凉血止血;腹中痛者,加白芍、甘草缓急止痛。

pain in the abdomen, add *Paeoniae Radix Albae* (Bai Shao), *Glycyrrhizae Radix Et Rhizoma* (Gan Cao) to relax urgency and relieve pain.

(3) Impediment and obstruction by damp-heat

Manifestations: Purple patches mostly around the joints, scorching pain, swelling and distension of the joints affecting movements of the limbs, occasional pain in the abdomen, bloody urine, red tongue, slimy and yellow coating, rapid and slippery pulse or rapid and string-taut pulse.

Therapeutic method: To clear away heat and dispel dampness, activate blood and dredge the collaterals.

Main Formula: *Mysterious Four Powder* (Si Miao San) with modification.

Commonly used herbs: *Phellodendri Cortex Chinensis* (Huang Bo), *Atractylodis Rhizoma* (Cang Zhu), *Achyranthis Bidentatae Radix* (Niu Xi), *Coicis Semen* (Yi Yi Ren).

Modification: For pain and swelling of the joints and limited movements, add *Paeoniae Radix Rubra* (Chi Shao), *Spatholobi Caulis* (Ji Xue Teng) and *Caulis Lonicerae* (Ren Dong Teng) to clear away heat, remove dampness, and dredge the collaterals; for bloody urine, add *Cirsii Herba* (Xiao Ji), *Pyrrosiae Folium* (Shi Wei) to cool blood and stanch bleeding; for relatively severe pain in the abdomen, add *Peony and Licorice Decoction* (Shao Yao Gan Cao Tang) to relax urgency and relieve pain.

(4) Accumulated heat in the stomach and intestines

Manifestations: Stasis macules everywhere, mostly over the lower limbs, paroxysmal pain in the

(3) 湿热痹阻

证候:皮肤紫癜多见于关节周围,或关节肿胀灼痛,影响肢体活动,偶见腹痛、尿血,舌质红,苔黄腻,脉滑数或弦数。

治法:清热祛湿,活血通络。

主方:四妙散加减。

常用药:黄柏、苍术、牛膝、薏苡仁。

加减:关节肿痛,活动受限者,加赤芍、鸡血藤、忍冬藤清热利湿通络;尿血者,加小蓟、石韦凉血止血;腹痛较著者,则可配以芍药甘草汤缓急止痛。

(4) 胃肠积热

证候:瘀斑遍布,下肢多见,腹痛阵作,口臭纳呆,腹

abdomen, bad breath, poor appetite, abdominal distention, constipation, occasional bleeding gum, bloody stool, red tongue, yellow coating or slimy and yellow coating, rapid and slippery pulse.

胀便秘，或伴齿龈出血，便血，舌质红，苔黄或黄腻，脉滑数。

Therapeutic method: To drain fire, resolve toxin, clarify the stomach and melt macules.

治法：泻火解毒，清胃化斑。

Main Formula: *Pueraria, Scutellaria, and Coptis Decoction* (Ge Geng Huang Qin Huang Lian Tang) and *Minor Qi-Coordinating Decoction* (Xiao Chen Qi Tang).

主方：葛根黄芩黄连汤合小承气汤加减。

Commonly used herbs: *Puerariae Radix* (Ge Gen), *Glycyrrhizae Radix Et Rhizoma* (Gan Cao), *Scutellariae Radix* (Huang Qin), *Coptidis Rhizoma* (Huang Lian), *Rhei Radix Et Rhizoma* (Da Huang), *Magnoliae Officinalis Cortex* (Hou Pu), *Aurantii Fructus Immaturus* (Zhi Shi).

常用药：葛根、甘草、黄芩、黄连、大黄、厚朴、枳实。

Modification: For bloody stool, add *Flos Sophorae Carbonisatus* (Huai Hua Tan), *Sanguisorbae Radix Carbonisatus* (Di Yu Tan) to astringe and stanch bleeding; for severe pain in the abdomen, add *Paeoniae Radix Albae* (Bai Shao), *Salviae Miltiorrhizae Radix Et Rhizoma* (Dan Shen), *Corydalis Rhizoma* (Yan Hu Suo) to relax urgency and relieve pain; for preponderant heat toxin, add *Isatidis Folium* (Da Qing Ye), *Gardeniae Fructus Ustus* (Jiao Zhi Zi) to clear away heat and resolve toxin; for much bleeding, add *Bubali Cornu* (Shui Niu Jiao), *Moutan Cortex Radicis* (Mu Dan Pi) to cool blood and stanch bleeding.

加减：便血者，加槐花炭、地榆炭以收涩止血；腹痛甚者，加白芍、丹参、延胡索以缓急止痛；热毒盛者，加大青叶、焦栀子清热解毒；出血较多者，可加水牛角、牡丹皮凉血止血。

(5) Qi failing to contain the blood

(5) 气不摄血

Manifestations: Long duration, recurrent purple patches, faintly visible and scattered in light purple color, continuous pain in abdomen, low spirit and fatigue, pale and lusterless complexion,

证候：病程较长，紫癜反复发作，隐约散在，色泽淡紫，腹痛绵绵，神疲倦怠，面白少华，食少纳呆，头晕心

poor appetite, dizziness, palpitation, pale tongue, white and thin coating, thready and forceless pulse.

悸，舌质淡，苔薄白，脉细无力。

Therapeutic method: To fortify the spleen and boost qi, nourish and contain blood.

治法：健脾益气，养血摄血。

Main Formula: *Spleen-returning Decoction* (Gui Pi Tang) with modification.

主方：归脾汤加减。

Commonly used herbs: *Atractylodis Macrocephalae Rhizoma* (Bai Zhu), *Angelicae Sinensis Radix* (Dang Gui), *Poria Alba* (Bai Fu Ling), *Astragali Radix* (Huang Qi), *Longan Arillus* (Long Yan Rou), *Polygalae Radix* (Yuan Zhi), *Ziziphi Spinosi Semen* (Suan Zao Ren), *Aucklandiae Radix* (Mu Xiang), *Glycyrrhizae Radix Et Rhizoma* (Gan Cao).

常用药：白术、当归、白茯苓、黄芪、龙眼肉、远志、酸枣仁、木香、甘草。

Modification: For incessant bleeding, add *Spatholobi Caulis* (Ji Xue Teng), *Crinis Carbonisatus* (Xue Yu Tan), *Colla Corii Asini* (E Jiao) to nourish blood and stanch bleeding; for poor appetite, add *Setariae Fructus Germinatus* (Gu Ya), *Atractylodis Rhizoma* (Cang Zhu), *Massa Fermentata* Medicinalis (Shen Qu) to fortify the spleen and assist transportation; for pain in the abdomen and bloody stool, add *Ledebouriellae Radix Carbonisatus* (Fang Feng Tan), *Sanguisorbae Radix* (Di Yu) to harmonize blood and relieve pain.

加减：出血不止者，加鸡血藤、血余炭、阿胶以养血止血；纳差者，加炒谷芽、苍术、神曲健脾助运；腹痛便血者，加防风炭、生地榆和血止痛。

(6) Hyperactivity of fire due to yin deficiency

（6）阴虚火旺

Manifestations: Slow onset, intermittently visible purple patches, or lingering soreness and weakness in the lumbus and back after relief of purple patches, feverish sensation in the chest, palms and soles, tidal heat and night sweating, dry mouth and throat, dizziness, tinnitus, bloody urine, bloody stool, red tongue, scanty coating, thready and rapid pulse.

证候：起病缓慢，时发时隐，或紫癜已退，仍有腰背酸软，五心烦热，潮热盗汗，口干咽燥，头晕耳鸣，尿血，便血，舌质红，苔少，脉细数。

Therapeutic method: To enrich yin and down-

治法：滋阴降火，凉血止

bear fire, cool blood and stanch bleeding.

血。

Main Formula: *Major Yin Supplementation Pill* (Da Bu Yin Wan) with modification.

主方:大补阴丸加减。

Commonly used herbs: *Phellodendri Cortex Chinensis* (Huang Bo), *Anemarrhenae Rhizoma* (Zhi Mu), *Rehmanniae Radix Praeparata* (Shu Di Huang), *Testudinis Carapax Et Plastrum* (Gui Ban).

常用药:黄柏、知母、熟地黄、龟板。

Modification: For bloody urine, add *Succini Pulvis* (Hu Po Fen), *Notoginseng Radix Et Rhizoma Pulverata* (San Qi Fen) to cool blood and stanch bleeding; for kidney yin depletion, add *Lycii Fructus* (Gou Qi Zi), *Corni Fructus* (Shan Zhu Yu), *Ecliptae Herba* (Han Lian Cao), *Ligustri Lucidi Fructus* (Nu Zhen Zi) to enrich yin and supplement the kidney.

加减:尿血色红者,可另吞服琥珀粉、三七粉凉血止血;肾阴亏虚者,加枸杞子、山茱萸、旱莲草、女贞子滋阴补肾。

4 Other therapies

4 其他疗法

4.1 Chinese Patent Medicine

4.1 中成药

(1) *Lotus Leaf Pill* (He Ye Wan) can be used for allergic purpura in pattern of frenetic blood circulation due to heat.

(1) 荷叶丸:适用于过敏性紫癜血热妄行证。

(2) *Spleen-Returning Pill* (Gui Pi Wan) is used for allergic purpura in pattern of qi failing to contain the blood.

(2) 归脾丸:适用于过敏性紫癜气不摄血证。

4.2 Acumoxatherapy

4.2 针灸疗法

Main acupoints: Quchi (LI 11), Zusanli (ST 36). Additional acupoints: Hegu (LI 4), Xuehai (SP 10). Firstly puncture the main acupoints. If not effective, add the additional acupoints. For abdominal pain, add Sanyinjiao (SP 6), Taichong (LR 3), Neiguan (PC 6).

主穴:曲池、足三里。备穴:合谷、血海。先刺主穴,效果不好加刺备穴。有腹痛加刺三阴交、太冲、内关。

Section 3　Mucocutaneous Lymph Node Syndrome

第 3 节　皮肤黏膜淋巴结综合征

Mucocutaneous lymph node syndrome, also known as "Kawasaki disease", is an acute fever and rash disease, characterized by the main pathological change of generalized vasculitis, and clinically manifested by fever, skin rash, congestion of bulbar conjunctiva, strawberry-like tongue, swollen lymph node, stiff and swollen extremities.

皮肤黏膜淋巴结综合征又称"川崎病"，是一种以全身血管炎为主要病理改变的急性发热性出疹性疾病。临床表现以发热、皮疹、球结膜充血、杨梅舌、淋巴结肿大、手足硬肿为特征。

The disease frequently occurs in the infants and children, accounting for 80% to 90% under 5 years old, more common in boys, without apparent seasonality, and with duration in 6 to 8 weeks, and acute period in about 2 weeks. All the organs can be involved, but the cardiovascular lesions are most serious and may lead to coronary heart disease and pancarditis. Most sick childen can recover after positive treatment. The cardiovascular symptoms in sick children may last from several months to several years, and the cause of death is mainly related to rupture of aneurysm or myocardial infarction.

好发于婴幼儿，5 岁以下者占 80%～85%，男孩多见，无明显季节性。病程多为 6～8 周，急性期约 2 周。各脏器均可受累，但以心血管病变最严重，可致冠状动脉心脏病及全心炎。多数患儿经积极治疗可以康复，有些患儿的心血管症状可持续数月至数年，其死亡原因多为动脉瘤破裂或心肌梗死。

It can be categorized into the scope of "febrile diseases" in traditional Chinese medicine.

本病属中医学"温病"范畴。

1　Etiology and pathogenesis

1　病因病机

The etiological cause is related to infection of exogenous warm and heat evil. The invasion of the pathogenic warmth and heat through the mouth and nose can be manifested by a process of transmission and development in Wei-defensive system, Qi-energy system, Ying-nutrient system and Xue-blood system.

病因为外感温热毒邪。温热毒邪自口鼻入侵，表现为卫气营血的传变过程。

In invading through the mouth and nose, the pathogenic warmth and heat attack Wei-defensive qi of the lung first, and then stay in the interstices of the flesh and block the dispersing ability of the exterior, leading to pattern of Wei-defensive system, manifested by fever, red throat, cough, etc. While penetrating into the interior quickly, the pathogenic factors would turn into heat and fire, resulting in pattern of preponderance of heat in the lung and stomach with symptoms like strong feverish sensation, vexation and thirst. The preponderance of heat toxin transmits from Wei-defensive system and Qi-energy system to Ying-nutrient system, to smoke and steam Ying-nutrient system and Xue-blood system. Once the heat toxin goes and flows with Ying-nutrient system and Xue-blood system, it would spread in the interior and exterior, resulting in skin rash, red eyes, stiff and swollen extremities, painful and swollen lymph nodes. More severely, if it gets the heart involved, there would be pattern of insufficiency of the heart yang and pattern of obstruction and stagnation of blood stasis, manifested by pale facial complexion, green-blue or purple lips, palpitation and oppression in the chest. In the final stage, the long-term retention of heat evil would consume and damage yin. When yin fluid is consumed and damaged, the extremities cannot be sufficiently nourished, leading to skin decrustation on the tips of toes. When the lung yin is damaged, there would be dry throat and cracked lips. When the stomach yin is damaged, there would be thirst with preference for drinks, red tongue and scanty tongue coating. "The lung links with hundreds of meridians." Zong-pectoral qi governs breathing,

温热毒邪从口鼻入，初犯肺卫，蕴于肌腠，卫表不宣，则见发热，咽红，咳嗽等卫分证；然后迅速入里，化热化火，故有壮热烦渴，肺胃热炽之征。热毒炽盛，由卫气及营，熏蒸营血，热毒随营血走窜流注，充斥内外而见皮疹、目赤、手足硬肿、臖核肿痛，甚可内陷于心，出现面色苍白、口唇青紫、心悸胸闷等心阳不足，瘀血阻滞之证。病之后期，热邪久羁，耗气伤阴。阴津耗伤，肢末失养，则指端、趾端皮肤脱皮；肺阴伤，则咽干唇裂；胃阴伤，则口渴喜饮，舌红苔少；“肺朝百脉”，宗气司呼吸，贯心脉，气虚血脉瘀滞，故见疲乏少力，心悸，脉结代。

and passes through the heart meridian. When Qi is deficient and blood vessels are obstructed with blood stasis, there would be fatigue and lack of strength, palpitation, and intermittent irregular pulse.

2 Key to diagnosis

The diagnosis is based upon the diagnostic criteria for Kawasaki disease, recommended by the research group of Japanese Kawasaki Disease (revised in Feburary, 2002, the fifth edition)

(1) Fever lasts more than 5 days.

(2) There is conjunctival congestion in the bilateral eyeballs.

(3) Manifestations in the oral cavity: Wet and red lips, strawberry-like tongue, diffuse congestion in the mucosa of the mouth and throat.

(4) Amorphous skin rash.

(5) Change in the end of extremities: hard edema in the hands and feet, red macules on the palmoplantar part, tips of fingers and toes at the acute stage; film-like skin decrustation at the skin of nail bed at the recovery stage.

(6) Non-suppurative neck lymph node at the acute stage.

Over 5 items in conformity with the above symptoms can be diagnosed. 4 items in conformity with the above symptoms, but if coronary aneurysm (including artery widening) is confirmed by two dimensional echocardiography or cardiac angiography, can also be diagnosed.

3 Pattern identification and treatment

It is predominant to identify the pathological location and severity of the disease, mainly based upon pattern idenfitication in accordance with the

2 诊断要点

本病的诊断可根据日本川崎病研究班推荐的川崎病诊断标准(2002 年 2 月修订，第 5 版)。

(1) 发热持续 5 天以上。

(2) 双侧眼球结膜充血。

(3) 口腔表现：口唇潮红、杨梅舌，口腔咽部黏膜弥漫性充血。

(4) 不定形皮疹。

(5) 四肢末端变化：急性期手足硬性水肿，掌跖及指、趾端红斑；恢复期甲床皮肤移行处膜样脱皮。

(6) 在急性期非化脓性颈部淋巴结肿大。

符合上述症状 5 项以上者即可诊断，4 项符合，但在病程中经二维超声心动图或心血管造影证实有冠状动脉瘤(包括动脉扩张)者亦可诊断。

3 辨证论治

主要辨别病位及轻重：以卫气营血辨证为主。初犯肺卫，症见发热微恶风，轻咳

theory on Wei-defensive system, Qi-energy system, Ying-nutrient system and Xue-blood system.

In the initial attack of Wei-defensive ability of the lung, the symptoms could be manifested by fever, slight aversion to wind, mild cough, no sputum, red throat, and short duration. When it enters the interior and turns into heat quickly, burning Qi-energy system, there would be corresponding symptoms like strong heat, vexation and thirst, and early skin rashes. When it involves Ying-nutrient system and harasses blood, there can be hot sensation in the body, worse at night, and clustered papules and macules in bright red color, strawberry-like tongue, vexation and agitation, or somnolence. At the final stage, when both qi and yin are damaged, there could be the symptoms of fatigue, profuse sweating, skin decrustation at the tips of toes, palpitation and lack of strength. The disease tends to cause blood stasis. If the collaterals are obstructed by blood stasis, there could be multiple signs of cardiac pain, oppression in the chest, and lumps in the right hypochondriac region, etc. Lasting fever, accompanied by pale facial complexion, lack of strength, green-blue or purple lips, oppression in the chest, subcostal pain, rapid pulse or intermittent irregular pulse indicates severe condition.

无痰，咽红，一般较短暂；迅速入里化热，炽于气分，症见壮热烦渴，皮疹初显；及营扰血，可见身热夜甚，斑疹鲜红密集，杨梅舌，烦躁不宁或嗜睡；后期气阴两伤，则见疲乏多汗，指趾末端脱皮，心悸乏力。本病易于形成瘀血，若瘀阻脉络，可有心痛、胸闷、右胁下痞块等多种征象。高热持续不退，伴面色苍白，乏力，口唇青紫，胸闷，剑突下痛，脉数或结代提示病情较重。

The basic therapeutic principle is to clear away heat and resolve toxin, activate blood and disperse blood stasis. For the pathological condition of both Wei-defensive system and Qi-energy system, it is appropriate to clear away heat, resolve heat and expel evils. For flaring heat in both Qi-energy system and Ying-nutrient system, it is appropriate to clarify qi, cool blood and resolve toxin. At the later

以清热解毒，活血化瘀为基本治则。卫气同病，宜清热解毒透邪；气营两燔，宜清气凉营解毒；后期益气养阴。本病易于形成血瘀，且温邪最易伤阴，所以治疗时应注意活血化瘀和顾护阴津。

stage, it is appropriate to boost qi and nourish yin. The disease tends to cause blood stasis, moreover the pathogenic warmth may most easily damage yin. Therefore, during treatment, it is necessary to activate blood, disperse blood stasis, and protect yin fluid.

(1) Involvement of both Wei-defensive system and Qi-energy system

(1) 卫气同病

Manifestations: Rapid and sudden onset, fever or strong heat, slight cough no sputum, thirst with preference for drinks, red eyes and throat, wet and red color on the palmoplantar part or hard swelling, early papules, poor appetite, nausea, vomiting, swollen lymph nodes at the neck, red tongue tip and margin, thin and white or yellow coating, rapid and floating pulse, purple fingerprint.

证候:起病急骤,发热或壮热,轻咳无痰,口渴喜饮,目赤咽红,掌跖潮红,或见硬肿,皮疹初显,胃纳减退,可有吐泻,颈部臖核肿大,舌边尖红,舌苔薄白或黄,脉浮数,指纹紫。

Therapeutic method: To expel pathogens through the exterior by spicy and cool herbs, clear away heat and resolve toxin.

治法:辛凉透表,清热解毒。

Main Formula: *Lonicera and Forsythia Powder* (Yin Qiao san) and *White Tiger Decoction* (Bai Hu Tang) with modification.

主方:银翘散合白虎汤加减。

Commonly used herbs: *Lonicerae Flos Japonicae* (Jin Yin Hua), *Forsythia Fructus* (Lian Qiao), *Gypsum Fibrosum* (Sheng Shi Gao), *Anemarrhenae Rhizoma* (Zhi Mu), *Menthae Haploalycis Herba* (Bo He), *Arctii Fructus* (Niu Bang Zi), *Schizonepetae Herba* (Jing Jie), *Sojae Semen Praeparatum* (Dan Dou Chi), *Lophatheri Herba* (Dan Zhu Ye), *Phragmitis Rhizoma* (Lu Gen), *Platycodonis Radix* (Jie Geng), *Glycyrrhizae Radix Et Rhizoma* (Gan Cao).

常用药:金银花、连翘、生石膏、知母、薄荷、牛蒡子、荆芥、淡豆豉、淡竹叶、芦根、桔梗、甘草。

Modification: For severe red eye, add *Chrysanthemi Flos* (Ju Hua); for swollen lymph node at

加减:目赤甚者,加菊花;颈部臖核肿大者,加浙贝

neck, add *Bulbus Fritillariae Thumbergii* (Zhe Bei Mu), *Bombyx Batryticatus* (Jiang Can); for wet and red color on the palmoplantar part, add *Rehmanniae Radix Cruda* (Sheng Di Huang), *Scutellariae Radix*(Huang Qin), *Moutan Cortex Radicis* (Mu Dan Pi); for thirst and dry lips, add *Trichosanthis Radix* (Tian Hua Fen), *Ophiopogonis Radix* (Mai Dong); for vomiting, add *Bambusae Caulis in Taenias* (Zhu Ru), and *Citri Reticulatae Pericarpium* (Chen Pi); for diarrhea, add *Atractylodis Rhizoma* (Cang Zhu), *Plantaginis Semen* (Che Qian Zi); for hard edema in the extremities, add *Mori Ramulus* (Sang Zhi), *Caulis Lonicerae* (Ren Dong Teng), *Polygoni Cuspidati Rhizoma Et Radix* (Hu Zhang).

母、僵蚕；掌跖潮红者，加生地黄、黄芩、牡丹皮；口渴唇干者，加天花粉、麦冬；呕吐者，加竹茹、陈皮；腹泻者，加苍术、车前子；手足硬肿者，加桑枝、忍冬藤、虎杖。

(2) Flaring heat in both Qi-energy system and Ying-nutrient system

(2) 气营两燔

Manifestations: Persistent strong heat, vexation and agitation, somnolence, clustered macules and papules in bright red color, red and painful swollen throat, red eyes, painful swollen lymph nodes in the neck, wet and red color in the fingertips and palmoplantar part or around anus, hard edema in the extremities, dry and cracked lips, red or crimson tongue, strawberry-like tongue, purple and stagnated fingerprints, thready and rapid pulse or thready and forceful pulse, possibly pale facial complexion, green-blue or purple lips, oppression in the chest, subcostal pain, green-blue or purple fingerprints, rapid pulse or intermittent irregular pulse.

证候：壮热不已，烦躁不宁或嗜睡，斑疹鲜红密集，咽红肿痛，目赤，颈部臖核肿痛，掌跖指端或肛周潮红，手足硬肿，口唇干裂，舌质红绛，杨梅舌，指纹紫滞，脉细数或数而有力，或可见面色苍白，口唇青紫，胸闷，剑突下痛，指纹青紫，脉数或结代。

Therapeutic method: To clarify qi, cool Ying-nutrient system, resolve toxin and disperse blood stasis.

治法：清气凉营，解毒化瘀。

Main Formula: *Scourge-Clearing Toxin-Van-*

主方：清瘟败毒饮加减。

quishing Decoction (Qing Wen Bai Du Yin) with modification.

Commonly used herbs: *Bubali Cornu* (Shui Niu Jiao), *Rehmanniae Radix Cruda* (Sheng Di Huang), *Scrophulariae Radix* (Xuan Shen), *Scutellariae Radix* (Huang Qin), *Gardeniae Fructus* (Zhi Zi), *Platycodonis Radix* (Jie Geng), *Paeoniae Radix Rubra* (Chi Shao), *Forsythia Fructus* (Lian Qiao), *Lophatheri Herba* (Dan Zhu Ye), *Moutan Cortex Radicis* (Mu Dan Pi), *Gypsum Fibrosum* (Sheng Shi Gao), *Anemarrhenae Rhizoma* (Zhi Mu).

常用药:水牛角、生地黄、玄参、黄芩、栀子、桔梗、赤芍、连翘、淡竹叶、牡丹皮、生石膏、知母。

Modification: For severe sore throat, add *Isatidis Radix* (Ban Lan Gen), *Sophorae Tonkinensis Radix Et Rhizoma* (Shan Dou Gen); for painful swollen lymph nodes in the neck, add *Prunellae Spica* (Xia Ku Cao) and *Bombyx Batryticatus* (Jiang Can); for constipated stool and constipation, add *Rhei Radix Et Rhizoma (Da Huang)*; for bright red and clustered macules and papules, add *Arnebiae Radix* (Zi Cao), *Indigo Naturalis* (Qing Dai); for green-blue lips, pale facial complexion, oppression in the chest, substernal pain, intermittent irregular pulse, add *Pulse-Engendering Powder* (Sheng Mai San), *Salviae Miltiorrhizae Radix Et Rhizoma* (Dan Shen), and *Carthami Flos* (Hong Hua) in combination.

加减:咽喉肿痛甚者,加板蓝根、山豆根;颈部臀核肿痛者,加用夏枯草、僵蚕;大便秘结者,加大黄;皮疹鲜红密集者,加紫草、青黛。若见口唇青紫,面色苍白,胸闷,剑突下痛,脉结代等症时,可与生脉散加丹参、红花配合应用。

(3) Damage of both qi and yin

(3) 气阴两伤

Manifestations: Abatement in general feverish sensation, fatigue, lack of strength, spontaneous sweating and night sweating, diminished mculopapular eruption, film-like decrustation at the skin of toe nail bed, possibly decrustation around the anus, palpitation, thirst with preference for drinks, red

证候:身热已退,疲乏少力,自汗盗汗,斑疹消退,指、趾末端甲床皮肤移行处膜样脱皮,或见肛周脱皮,心悸,口渴喜饮,舌质红少津,苔少或无苔,脉细弱或结代等。

tongue with scanty fluid, scantyor no coating, thready and weak pulse or intermittent irregular pulse, etc.

Therapeutic method: To boost qi and nourish yin, clear away and resolve residual heat.

治法:益气养阴,清解余热。

Main Formula: *Pulse-Engendering Powder* (Shen Mai San) and *Glehnia and Ophiopogon Decoction* (Shan Shen Mai Dong Tang) with modifications.

主方:生脉散合沙参麦冬汤加减。

Commonly used herbs: *Pseudostellariae Radix* (Tai Zi Shen), *Ophiopogonis Radix* (Mai Dong), *Adenophorae Radix* (Sha Seng), *Trichosanthis Radix* (Tian Hua Fen), *Polygonati Odorati Rhizoma* (Yu Zhu), *Schisandrae Fructus Chinensis* (Wu Wei Zi), *Mori Folium* (Sang Ye), *Testa Lablab* (Bian Dou Yi), *Salviae Miltiorrhizae Radix Et Rhizoma* (Dan Shen), *Paeoniae Radix Rubra* (Chi Shao).

常用药:太子参、麦冬、沙参、天花粉、玉竹、五味子、桑叶、扁豆衣、丹参、赤芍。

Modification: For poor appetite, add *Eupatorii Herba* (Pei Lan), *Crataegi Fructus* (Shan Zha), *Massa Fermentata Medicinalis* (Liu Shen Qu); For persistent low heat, add *Lycii Cortex* (Di Gu Pi), *Cynanchi Atrati Radix Et Rhizoma* (Bai Wei); For lingering heat, use *Lophatherum and Gypsum Decoction* (Zhu Ye Shi Gao Tang) with modifications; For hard dry stool, add *Trichosanthis Semen* (Gua Lou Zi), *Cannabis Fructus* (Huo Ma Ren); For palpitation and intermittent irregular pulse, add *Astragali Radix* (Huang Qi), *Glycyrrhizae Radix Et Rhizoma* (Gan Cao), and *Moutan Cortex Radicis* (Mu Dan Pi).

加减:纳呆者,加佩兰、山楂、六神曲;低热不退者,加地骨皮、白薇;有邪热留恋者,可予竹叶石膏汤加减;大便硬结者,加瓜蒌子、火麻仁;心悸、脉结代者,加黄芪、甘草、牡丹皮。

4 Other therapies

4 其他疗法

4.1 Chinese Patent Medicine

4.1 中成药

(1) *Toxin-Dissolving Elixir* (Hua Du Dan) is used for mucocutaneous lymph node syndrome in

(1) 化毒丹:适用于皮肤黏膜淋巴结综合征卫气同

pattern of involvement of both Wei-defensive system and Qi-energy system.

病。

(2) *Clearing and Opening Efficacy Injection* (Qing Kai Ling Zhu She Ye) is used for mucocutaneous lymph node syndrome in pattern of flaring heat in both Qi-energy system and Ying-nutrient system.

(2) 清开灵注射液:适用于皮肤黏膜淋巴结综合征气营两燔证。

(3) *Pulse-Engendering Decoction* (Sheng Mai Ying) is used for mucocutaneous lymph node syndrome in pattern of flaring heat in both Qi-energy system and Ying-nutrient system.

(3) 生脉饮:适用于皮肤黏膜淋巴结综合征气阴两伤证。

(4) *Salvia Drop Pill* (Dan Shen Di Wan) is used for mucocutaneous lymph node syndrome present with pattern of blood stasis.

(4) 丹参滴丸:适用于皮肤黏膜淋巴结综合征出现血瘀证者。

4.2 Acumoxatherapy

4.2 针灸疗法

(1) For evils in Wei-defensive system and Qi-energy system, select Dazhui (GV 14), Quchi (LI 11), Hegu (LI 4), Yuji (LU 10), Waiguan (TB 5), and puncture with the needling technique for sedation, without retaining the needles. For sore throat, additionally bleed Shaoshang (LU 11) with a three-edged needle.

(1) 邪在卫气取大椎、曲池、合谷、鱼际、外关穴。针用泻法,不留针。咽喉肿痛者,加少商穴,用三棱针点刺出血。

(2) For preponderant heat in Qi-energy system, select Dazhui (GV 14), Quchi (LI 11), Shangyang (LI 1), Neiting (ST 44), Guanchong (TE 1), and Hegu (LI 4), and puncture with the needling technique for sedation, without retaining the needles. For continuous high fever, add Shixuan (EX 20); for thirst with preference for drinks, add Chize (LU 5), Jinjin (EX 10), Yuye(EX-HN 13).

(2) 气分热盛取大椎、曲池、商阳、内庭、关冲、合谷穴。针用泻法,不留针。高热不解者,加十宣穴;口渴引饮者,加尺泽、金津、玉液穴。

(3) For invasion of evils in Ying-nutrient system and Xue-blood system, select Quze (PC 3), Zhongchong (PC 9), Shaochong (HT 9), Weizhong (BL 40), Quchi (LI 11), and puncture with the

(3) 邪入营血取曲泽、中冲、少冲、委中、曲池穴。针用泻法,不留针。烦躁谵语者,加人中、十宣穴;斑疹多

needling technique for sedation, without retaining the needles. For vexation and agitation, and delirious speech, add Renzhong (GV 26), and Shixuan (EX 20); for many papules and macules, additionally bleed Xuehai (SP 10), Jing-well points, Shixuan (EX 20), with a three-edged needle.

者,加血海、井穴、十宣穴,用三棱针点刺出血。

(4) For lingering heat due to yin deficiency, select Taixi (KI 3), Zhaohai (KI 6), Yuji (LU 10), Futu (LI 18), puncture with the needling technique for supplementation, and puncture Yuji (LU 10) and Futu (LI 18) with the needling technique for sedation. For persistent low heat, add Jianshi (PC 5) and Dazhui (GV 14). For dry mouth and throat, add Lianquan (CV 23). For feverish sensation in the heart, palms and soles, add Shaofu (HT 8).

(4) 阴虚热恋取太溪、照海、鱼际、扶突穴。太溪、照海,用补法,鱼际、扶突用轻泻法。持续低热者,加间使、大椎穴;咽干口燥者,加廉泉穴;手足心热者,加少府穴。

Section 4 Bronchial Asthma

第4节 支气管哮喘

Bronchial asthma, short for asthma, is a chronic airway inflammatory disease involving a variety of cells (such as eosinophil, mast cells, T lymphocytes, neutrophil, epithelia) and cell components, clinically manifested by recurrent asthma, hasty breathing, oppression in the chest, cough, etc, and often present or aggravated at night and/or in the morning. Most patients will be relieved after treatment or be relieved naturally. It starts from infanthood and young childhood in most cases, and occurs more frequently in the fall and winter.

支气管哮喘简称哮喘,是由多种细胞(如嗜酸性粒细胞、肥大细胞、T淋巴细胞、中性粒细胞、气道上皮细胞)和细胞组分等参与的气道慢性炎症性疾病,以反复发作性的喘息、气促、胸闷、咳嗽等为临床表现,常在夜间和(或)清晨发作或加剧,多数患者可经治疗缓解或自然缓解。多数始于婴幼儿,以秋冬季多见。

This disease is categorized into the scope of "wheezing and panting", "wheezing pattern", and

本病属中医学"哮喘""哮证""齁喘"等范畴,"哮"

"rapid panting with phlegm rale in throat" in traditional Chinese medicine. "Wheezing" implies sound. "Panting" implies breathing. Wheezing is surely accompanied by panting. Therefore, it is generally called "wheezing and panting".

指声响言,"喘"指气息言,哮必兼喘,故通称哮喘。

1 Etiology and pathogenesis

1 病因病机

The internal causes are related to insufficiency of the lung, spleen and kidney, internal retention of phlegm and fluid, and genetic factor from the prenatal natural endowment, being the long-standing reasons of wheezing and panting. The inducing factors are infection of exogenous evils, contact with foreign matters, improper diet, emotional disorder, or over fatigue, etc. The internal causes and external causes interact with each other, and phlegm and qi obstruct the airway together, leading to repeated seizure.

内因责之于肺、脾、肾不足,痰饮内伏,以及先天禀赋遗传因素,成为哮喘之夙根;感受外邪、接触异物、饮食不慎、情志失调、以及劳倦过度等,是哮喘的诱发因素。内外因素交互,痰气交阻,阻塞气道,反复不已。

The attack stage is characterized by excessive evils, manifested by accumulation of in the lung, and obstruction of the airway by tangible phlegm, causing wheezing in the throat and rapid breathing. Due to differences in the pathogenic causes and personal constitution, the pathogenesis can evolve into cold nature and heat nature respectively. If wheezing and panting occur persistently, for days, or repeatedly, phlegm would be accumulated and panting would be worse by exertion, in those with deficiency in the Vital Energy, resulting in pattern of excess in the clinical symptoms and deficiency in the Vital Energy. The remission stage is mainly characterized by deficiency in the Vital Energy. If wheezing and panting occur repeatedly, the lung qi would be exhausted and dissipated and would not be restored for a long time. The mother illness would affect the

发作期以邪实为主,表现为痰邪壅肺,有形之痰阻于气道,形成喉中哮鸣,呼吸急促。由于病因不同,体质差异,病机演变有寒、热之分;若哮喘持续发作,经日持久,或反复多次发作,正气亏虚者,痰壅气喘,动则尤甚,可出现邪实正虚证。缓解期以正虚为主。哮喘反复发作,肺气耗散,久而不复,母病及子,子病又可及母,肺虚则脾气亦虚,脾虚不运,则停湿生痰,痰浊上阻,则呼吸不利,故本病往往表现为时发时止,反复不已。肺脾久虚,又可导致肾气虚弱,或患儿

child, and vice verse. The lung depletion will lead to spleen qi depletion, and the spleen deficiency will lead to its failure in transportion, resulting in retention of dampness and production of phlegm. When the phlegm turbidity is obstructed in the upper body, breathing would surely be difficult. Therefore, the disease is often characterized by intermittent and repeated seizure. The long-term deficiency in the lung and spleen can cause kidney qi deficiency. The insufficiency of prenatal kidney qi in the sick child can be manifested by yang depletion of the spleen and kidney, and dysfunction in the accepting and containing ability, leading to upward counterflow of qi and hence "panting and unable to breathe". Therefore, the remission stage can be characterized by mild signs of persistent wheezing and panting. Besides, due to constitutional yin deficiency in a few children, or injury of yin by the lung heat and by over ingestion of warm and heat foodstuffs, yin deficiency of the lung and kidney could be induced, losing the moistening and nourishing ability. The lung governs qi, and if it fails to perform its respiratory function, similarly it will lead to recurrence of wheezing and panting.

先天肾气未充，均可表现为脾肾阳虚，摄纳失职，气逆于上，产生“喘气不足以吸”，故在缓解时，也可表现有轻度持续性哮喘征象。另有少数患儿素体阴虚，或者肺热伤阴、过食温热之品伤阴，则致肺肾阴虚，失于润养，肺主气，司呼吸功能失职，同样可以使哮喘反复发作。

2 Key to diagnosis

(1) Mostly there is a history of allergic disease like eczema in infanthood, or a family history of wheezing and panting. Its seiaure is often related to some inducing causes like infection of exogenous evils or contact with allergy-causing substances.

(2) Recurrent panting and wheezing. It often occurs suddenly, and before seizure, there are often the premonitory signs like sneezing and cough, etc.

2 诊断要点

(1) 多有婴儿期湿疹等过敏性疾病史，家族哮喘史。发作多与某些诱发因素有关，如感受外邪、接触致敏物质等。

(2) 气喘哮鸣反复发作。常突然发作，发作之前多有喷嚏、咳嗽等先兆症状。发

When it occurs, there are hasty panting, rapid breathing, wheezing, cough, and even difficulty to lie down flat, vexation and agitation, restlessness, and green-blue or purple lips in severe cases.

作时喘促、气急、哮鸣、咳嗽，甚者不能平卧、烦躁不安、口唇青紫。

(3) In the attack stage, wheezing rale can be heard in the both lungs, obvious in exhalation and prolonged in inhalation. If there is secondary infection, medium or fine rales can be heard.

（3）发作时两肺可闻及哮鸣音，以呼气时明显，呼气延长。如继发感染，可闻及中、细湿啰音。

(4) Blood routine examinations could show an increase in eosinophils, and elevated serum IgE. The pulmonary function tests could show increased airway resistance, or positive bronchial provocation, and positive bronchial dilation test.

（4）血常规检查可见嗜酸性粒细胞增高，血清 IgE 增高，肺功能检查气道阻力增加，或支气管激发试验阳性、支气管舒张试验阳性。

3　Pattern identification and treatment

3　辨证论治

In the attack stage, it is necessary to identify cold and heat, deficiency and excess. The seizure of panting and wheezing, with clear, thin and white sputum or foamy sputum, accompanied by cold sensation in the body and limbs, or accompanied by wind-cold exterior pattern, mostly belongs to cold pattern. The seizure of panting and wheezing, with thick and yellow sputum, difficult expectoration, accompanied by vexation, constipation, red face and lips, mostly belongs to heat pattern. The seizure of wheezing, accompanied by panting, coughing and gushing sputum, loud voice and rough breathing, or new disease in the initial stage, mostly belongs to excess pattern. The enduring wheezing and panting, faint cough and panting, shortness of breath, hard to keep on, mostly belong to pattern of mixed deficiency and excess.

发作期辨寒热虚实。若哮喘发作痰白清稀或泡沫痰，伴形寒肢冷，或伴风寒表证者，多属寒证；若哮喘发作痰黄质稠难咯，伴心烦便秘，面赤唇红者，多属热证；哮作喘咳痰涌，声高息粗，或新病初起者，多属实证；哮喘久发不止，咳喘息微，气短难续者，多属虚实夹杂。

In the remission stage, it is necessary to identify the organs. Spontaneous sweating, recurrent

缓解期辨脏腑。自汗出，反复感冒，痰多、便溏，属

cold, profuse sputum, and sloppy stool are attributed to qi deficiency in the lung and spleen. Poor appetite, sloppy stool, shortness of breath by exertion, pale face, and cold limbs are attributed to yang deficiency in the spleen and kidney. Flushed facial complexion, emaciation, short of breath, dry cough, scanty sputum, red tongue and scanty coating, rapid and thready pulse are attributed to yin deficiency in the lung and kidney.

肺脾气虚；食少便溏，动则气短，面白肢冷，则属脾肾阳虚；面色潮红，消瘦气短，干咳少痰，舌红少苔，脉细数，属肺肾阴虚。

The treatment is designed and given based upon the attack stage and remission stage respectively. The attack stage is mainly treated by attacking the causastive evils for dealing with the clinical symptoms, and by downbearing qi and stoping panting in predominance. The remission is mainly treated by supporting the Vital Energy, supplementing the lung and secure the exterior, replenishing the spleen and benefiting the kidney. To regulate the functions of the organs is thereby to eliminate phlegm-engendering sources.

治疗按发作期和缓解期分别施治。发作期当攻邪以治其标，降气平喘为主；缓解期当扶正以治其本，以补肺固表，补脾益肾为主，调整脏腑功能，去除生痰之因。

3.1 Attack stage

3.1 发作期

(1) Wheezing and panting in cold nature

(1) 寒性哮喘

Manifestations: Coughing, hasty breathing, wheezing in the throat, coughing of clear sputum, running nose, clear snivel, nasal obstruction, sneezing, pale facial complexion, cold body, no sweating, slight red tongue, white coating, tight and floating pulse, red fingerprint.

证候：咳嗽气促，喉间哮鸣，咳痰清稀，鼻流清涕，鼻塞喷嚏，面色淡白，形寒无汗，舌质淡红，苔白，脉浮紧，指纹红。

Therapeutic method: To warm up the lung and disperse cold, dissolve phlegm and alleviate panting.

治法：温肺散寒，化痰定喘。

Main Formula: *Supplemented Minor Blue Dragon Decoction* (Xiao Qing Long Tang Jia Wei).

主方：小青龙汤加味。

Commonly used herbs: *Ephedrae Herba* (Ma

常用药：麻黄、桂枝、细

Huang), *Cinnamomi Ramulus* (Gui Zhi), *Asari Radix Et Rhizoma* (Xi Xin), *Zingiberis Rhizoma* (Gan Jiang), *Pinelliae Rhizoma* (Ban Xia), *Schisandrae Fructus Chinensis* (Wu Wei Zi), *Paeoniae Radix Albae* (Bai Shao), *Glycyrrhizae Radix Et Rhizoma* (Gan Cao).

辛、干姜、半夏、五味子、白芍、甘草。

Modification: For severe cough, add *Asteris Radix Et Rhizoma* (Zi Wan), *Farfarae Flos* (Kuan Dong Hua), *Inulae Flos* (Xuan Fu Hua). For hasty panting, add *Haematitum* (Zhe Shi).

加减: 咳嗽甚者,加紫菀、款冬花、旋覆花;喘促甚者,加赭石。

(2) Wheezing and panting in heat nature

(2) 热性哮喘

Manifestations: Cough, rapid panting, phlegm roaring and wheezing in the throat, thick and yellow expectoration, fever, flushed face, vexation, agitation, thirst, drystool, scanty yellow urine, red tongue, yellow coating or slimy and yellow coating, rapid and slippery pulse, purple fingerprint.

证候: 咳嗽喘促,喉间痰吼哮鸣,咯痰黄稠,发热面红,烦躁口渴,大便干结,小便黄少,舌质红,苔黄或黄腻,脉滑数,指纹紫。

Therapeutic method: To clarify the lung and dissolve phlegm, downbear qi and stop panting.

治法: 清肺化痰,降气平喘。

Main Formula: *Ephedra, Apricot Kernel, Licorice, and Gypsum Decoction* (Ma Xing Gan Shi Tang) plus *Perilla Seed and Descurainiae Pill* (Su Ting Wan) with modification.

主方: 麻杏甘石汤合苏葶丸加减。

Commonly used herbs: *Ephedrae Herba* (Ma Huang), *Gypsum Fibrosum* (Sheng Shi Gao), *Armeniacae Semen Amarum* (Ku Xing Ren), *Mori Cortex* (Sang Bai Pi), *Descurainiae Lepidii Semen* (Ting Li Zi), *Perillae Fructus* (Zi Su Zi), *Belamecandae Rhizoma* (She Gan), *Richosanthis Fructus* (Gua Lou), *Glycyrrhizae Radix Et Rhizoma* (Gan Cao).

常用药: 麻黄、生石膏、苦杏仁、桑白皮、葶苈子、紫苏子、射干、瓜蒌、甘草。

Modification: For rapid panting, add *Lumbricus* (Di Long), *Bombyx Batryticatus* (Jiang Can). For copious sputum, add *Arisaema Cum Bile* (Dan

加减: 喘急者,加地龙、僵蚕;痰多者,加胆南星、竹沥;咳甚者,加百部、款冬花;

Nan Xing), *Bambosae Succus* (Zhu Li). For severe cough, add *Stemonae Radix* (Bai Bu), *Farfarae Flos* (Kuan Dong Hua); for severe heat, add *Gardeniae Fructus* (Zhi Zi), *Houttuyniae Herba* (Yu Xing Cao), *Scutellariae Radix* (Huang Qin). For constipation, add *Trichosanthis Semen* (Gua Lou Zi), *Rhei Radix Et Rhizoma* (Da Huang).

热重者,加栀子、鱼腥草、黄芩;便秘者,加瓜蒌子、大黄。

(3) Cold and heat Complex

(3) 寒热错杂

Manifestations: Hasty panting, rapid breathing, cough, wheezing, aversion to cold, no sweating, nasal obstruction, clear snivel, thick, slimy and yellow sputum, thirst, yellow or brown urine, dry stool, sore throat, red tongue, thin and white or thin and yellow coating.

证候:喘促气急,咳嗽哮鸣,恶寒无汗,鼻塞清涕,咯痰黏稠色黄,口渴,小便黄赤,大便干结,咽红,舌质红,苔薄白或薄黄。

Therapeutic method: To disperse cold, clear away heat, downbear qi and alleviate panting.

治法:散寒清热,降气平喘。

Main Formula: *Major Blue Dragon Decoction* (Da Qing Long Tang) with modification.

主方:大青龙汤加减。

Commonly used herbs: *Ephedrae Herba* (Ma Huang), *Cinnamomi Ramulus* (Gui Zhi), *Paeoniae Radix Albae* (Bai Shao), *Asari Radix Et Rhizoma* (Xi Xin), *Schisandrae Fructus Chinensis* (Wu Wei Zi), *Pinelliae Rhizoma* (Ban Xia), *Gypsum Fibrosum* (Sheng Shi Gao), *Scutellariae Radix* (Huang Qin), *Descurainiae Lepidii Semen* (Ting Li Zi), *Perillae Fructus* (Zi Su Zi).

常用药:麻黄、桂枝、白芍、细辛、五味子、半夏、生石膏、黄芩、葶苈子、紫苏子。

Modification: For severe heat, add *Gardeniae Fructus* (Zhi Zi), *Mori Cortex* (Sang Bai Pi), *Houttuyniae Herba* (Yu Xing Cao), *Polygoni Cuspidati Rhizoma Et Radix* (Hu Zhang). For severe cough, add *Mori Cortex* (Sang Bai Pi), *Peucedani Radix* (Qian Hu), *Farfarae Flos* (Kuan Dong Hua). For severe hasty panting, add *Belamecandae Rhizoma* (She Gan) and *Lumbricus* (Di Long). For severe

加减:热重者,加栀子、桑白皮、鱼腥草、虎杖;咳嗽重者,加桑白皮、前胡、款冬花;喘促甚者,加射干、地龙;痰热重者,加黛蛤散、竹沥。

phlegm and heat, add *Indigo and Clamshell Powder* (Dai Ge San), *Bambosae Succus* (Zhu Li).

(4) Deficiency and excess complex

Manifestations: Long duration, continuous panting and wheezing, hasty panting and oppression in the chest, panting aggravated by exertion, cough, profuse sputum, gurgling in the throat, lusterless facial complexion, aversion to cold, cold limbs, fatigued spirit, poor appetite, profuse and clear urine, pale tongue, thin and white or slimy and white coating, thready and weak pulse, light and stagnated fingerprints.

Therapeutic method: To drain the lung fire and alleviate panting, supplement the kidney and promote qi acceptance.

Main Formula: *Belamcanda and Ephedra Decoction* (She Gan Ma Huang Tang) plus *Major Qi Pills* (Du Qi Wan) with modification.

Commonly used herbs: *Belamecandae Rhizoma* (She Gan), *Ephedrae Herba Mel* (Mi Ma Huang), *Pinelliae Rhizoma* (Ban Xia), *Schisandrae Fructus Chinensis* (Wu Wei Zi), *Asari Radix Et Rhizoma* (Xi Xin), *Farfarae Flos* (Kuan Dong Hua), *Rehmanniae Radix Praeparata* (Shu Di Huang), *Corni Fructus* (Shan Zhu Yu), *Dioscoreae Rhizoma* (Shan Yao), *Psoraleae Fructus* (Bu Gu Zhi).

Modification: For panting by exertion, add *Amethyst* (Zi Shi Ying), *Chebulae Fructus* (He Zi). For aversion to cold and cold limbs, add *Aconiti Lateralis Radix Praeparata* (Fu Zi), *Epimedii Folium* (Yin Yang Huo). For aversion to cold, and abdominal fullness, add *Zanthoxyli Semen* (Jiao Mu), *Magnoliae Officinalis Cortex* (Hou Pu). For incessant and copious white sputum, add *Ginkgo*

(4) 虚实夹杂

证候:病程较长,哮喘持续不已,喘促胸闷,动则喘甚,咳嗽痰多,喉中痰吼,面色少华,畏寒肢冷,神疲纳呆,小便清长,舌质淡,苔薄白或白腻,脉细弱,指纹淡滞。

治法:泻肺平喘,补肾纳气。

主方:射干麻黄汤合都气丸加减。

常用药:射干、蜜麻黄、半夏、五味子、细辛、款冬花、熟地黄、山茱萸、山药、补骨脂。

加减:动则气喘者,加紫石英、诃子;畏寒肢冷者,加附子、淫羊藿;畏寒腹满者,加椒目、厚朴;痰多色白,屡吐不绝者,加白果、芡实;发热咯痰黄稠者,加黄芩、冬瓜子、金荞麦。

Semen (Bai Guo), *Euryales Semen* (Qian Shi). For fever and yellow and thick sputum, add *Scutellariae Radix* (Huang Qin), *Benincasae Semen* (Dong Gua Zi), *Fagopyri Dibotryis Rhizoma* (Jin Qiao Mai).

3.2 Remission stage

(1) Qi deficiency in the lung and spleen

Manifestations: Pale and lusterless facial complexion, shortness of breath, spontaneous sweating, forceless coughing, fatigued spirit, reluctance to speak, emaciation, poor appetite, sloppy stool, susceptible to cold, pale tongue, white and thin coating, thready and pulse, pale fingerprints.

Therapeutic method: To supplement the lung and secure the exterior, fortify the spleen and boost qi.

Main Formula: *Jade Wind-Barrier Powder* (Yu Ping Feng San) plus *Ginseng and Schisandra Decoction* (Ren Shen Wu Wei Zi Tang) with modification.

Commonly used herbs: *Astragali Radix* (Huang Qi), *Codonopsis Radix* (Dang Shen), *Poria* (Fu Ling), *Atractylodis Macrocephalae Rhizoma* (Bai Zhu), *Pinelliae Rhizoma* (Ban Xia), *Schisandrae Fructus Chinensis* (Wu Wei Zi), *Ledebouriellae Radix* (Fang Feng), *Glycyrrhizae Radix Et Rhizoma Praeparata* (Zhi Gan Cao).

Modification: For severe qi deficiency, add *Pseudostellariae Radix* (Tai Zi Shen), and *Polygonati Rhizoma* (Huang Jing). For copious sweating, add *Os Draconis Calcinata* (Duan Long Gu), *Ostreae Concha Calcinata* (Duan Mu Li), *Oryzae Glutinosae Radix Et Rhizoma* (Nuo Dao Gen). For reduced food intake, add *Amomi Fructus* (Sha Ren), and *Crataegi Fructus* (Shan Zha). For sloppy stool,

3.2 缓解期

（1）肺脾气虚

证候：面白少华，气短自汗，咳嗽无力，神疲懒言，形瘦纳差，大便溏薄，易于感冒，舌质淡，苔薄白，脉细，指纹淡。

治法：补肺固表，健脾益气。

主方：玉屏风散合人参五味子汤加减。

常用药：黄芪、党参、茯苓、白术、半夏、五味子、防风、炙甘草。

加减：气虚甚者，加太子参、黄精；汗出多者，加煅龙骨、煅牡蛎、糯稻根；食纳减少，加砂仁、山楂；便溏，加山药、白扁豆。

add *Dioscoreae Rhizoma* (Shan Yao), and *Lablab Semen Album* (Bai Bian Dou).

(2) Yang deficiency in the spleen and kidney

Manifestations: Pale facial complexion, cold body, cold limbs, panting, coughing by exertion, shortness of breath, palpitation, flaccid and weak legs, abdominal distention, poor appetite, sloppy stool, profuse and clear urine, pale tongue, white and thin coating, thready and weak pulse, light fingerprint.

Therapeutic method: To warm up and supplement the spleen and kidney, to accept qi and build up the origin.

Main Formula: *Golden Coffer Kidney Qi Pill* (Jin Gui Shen Qi Wan) with modification.

Commonly used herbs: *Aconiti Lateralis Radix Praeparata* (Fu Zi), *Cinnamomi Cortex* (Rou Gui), *Corni Fructus* (Shan Zhu Yu), *Rehmanniae Radix Praeparata* (Shu Di Huang), *Dioscoreae Rhizoma* (Shan Yao), *Epimedii Folium* (Yin Yang Huo), *Poria* (Fu Ling), *Atractylodis Macrocephalae Rhizoma* (Bai Zhu), *Juglandis Semen* (He Tao Ren), *Schisandrae Fructus Chinensis* (Wu Wei Zi).

Modification: For obvious vacuous panting, add *Gecko* (Ge Jie) and *Cordyceps* (Dong Chong Xia Cao). For severe cough, add *Farfarae Flos* (Kuan Dong Hua) and *Asteris Radix Et Rhizoma* (Zi Wan). For frequent urination at night, add *Alpiniae Oxyphyllae Fructus* (Yi Zhi), *Cuscutae Semen* (Tu Si Zi), and *Psoraleae Fructus* (Bu Gu Zhi).

(3) Yin deficiency in the lung and kidney

Manifestations: Flushed complexion, night sweating, emaciation, shortness of breath, feverish

(2) 脾肾阳虚

证候:面色苍白,形寒肢冷,动则喘咳,气短心悸,脚软无力,腹胀纳差,大便溏薄,小便清长,舌质淡,苔薄白,脉细弱,指纹淡。

治法:温补脾肾,纳气培元。

主方:金匮肾气丸加减。

常用药:附子、肉桂、山茱萸、熟地黄、山药、淫羊藿、茯苓、白术、核桃仁、五味子。

加减:虚喘明显者,加蛤蚧、冬虫夏草;咳甚者,加款冬花、紫菀;夜尿多者,加益智、菟丝子、补骨脂。

(3) 肺肾阴虚

证候:面色潮红,夜间盗汗,消瘦气短,手足心热,干

Chapter 10 Infectious Diseases

第 10 章 感染性疾病

Section 1 Measles

第 1 节 麻疹

Measles is an acute infectious respiratory disease caused by measles virus, clinically characterized by fever, cough, running nose, conjunctivitis, oral measles mucous patches, and skin papules on the whole body. The source of infection is sick children. The disease spreads by droplets in the air and mostly occurs in the winter and spring. Children over 6 months and under 5 years old are susceptible to it. After recovery, most patients will be immune to it for the rest of their life.

麻疹是麻疹病毒引起的急性呼吸道感染病，临床表现以发热、咳嗽、流涕、结膜炎、口腔麻疹黏膜斑及全身皮肤斑丘疹为主要特征。患者为主要的传染源，传播方式为空气飞沫传播，冬春季节发病多，6 个月以上、5 岁以下小儿更易罹患，病后多数可获终身免疫。

In traditional Chinese medicine, it is called "measles papules", or "papules", "rash" in Chinese language.

中医称之"麻疹"，俗称"麻子""痧子""疹子"等。

1 Etiology and pathogenesis

1 病因病机

It is caused by infection of Seasonal measles virus. In the winter and spring, measles virus, seasonal pathogens and pathogenic wind invade Wei-defensive ability of the lung and accumulate in the spleen; when discharged outward to the skin, there is eruption of measles.

由感受麻毒时邪所致。冬春之季，麻毒时邪与风邪相合，侵袭肺卫，郁阻于脾而外泄于肌肤，发为麻疹。

In the initial stage, measles virus and seasonal pathogen invade Wei-defensive ability of the lung, causing disharmony between the exterior and Wei-

麻疹初起，麻毒时邪侵犯肺卫，表卫失和，肺气不宣，则见发热、咳嗽、流涕等

defensive ability of the lung and the failure of lung in its diffusing ability, manifested by exterior pattern of Wei-defensive ability of lung, such as fever, cough, running nose, etc. When the seasonal evils and measles virus penetrate to the interior from the exterior and to the spleen and stomach from the lung, the heat would be preponderant in the lung and spleen, resulting in the symptoms of high fever and thirst, etc. When the evils outthrust to the skin, measles would occur, and gradually spread over the whole body and reach the end of four extremities. After eruption, measles toxin is discharged with eruption of measles, and fever would decline and papules would disappear. However, measles is regarded as a yang toxin, and tends to damage yin fluid. Often yin damage in the lung and stomach would be present and needs to recover gradually.

肺卫表证。麻毒时邪由表入里，由肺而入脾胃，肺脾热炽，则见高热、口渴等症。外透肌肤，则见出疹，疹子依次出于全身，达于四末。疹透之后，麻毒随疹而泄，热退疹回。但麻为阳毒，易伤阴津，常见肺胃阴伤，需逐渐康复。

Due to abundance of evil toxin, or weak constitution of sick child, or inappropriate nursing and treatment, or infection of new evils, if measles toxin cannot be discharged smoothly and penetrate inward instead, various unfavorable or critical conditions would occur. When measles toxin is abundant and accumulated in the lung, it would burn body fluid into phlegm. If the lung is obstructed by phlegm and heat, the lung qi would be blocked, forming the pattern of blockage of the lung by measles toxin. If measles toxin is abundant and attacks the throat along the meridian, then the throat would be troubled and the airways would be blocked, leading to pattern of measles toxin attacking the throat. If the Vital Energy is deficient and unable to resist the pathogens, the pathogenic toxin

若邪毒炽盛，或年幼体弱，或调治失宜，或复感新邪等因素，麻毒不能顺利向外透达，而内陷入里，则发生各种逆证、险证。麻毒炽盛，内闭于肺，灼津炼液为痰，痰热阻肺，肺气郁闭，则形成麻毒闭肺证。麻毒炽盛，循经上攻咽喉，咽喉不利，气道痹阻，则形成麻毒攻喉证。正虚不抵邪，邪毒内陷厥阴，蒙闭心窍，引动肝风，形成毒陷心肝证。

would penetrate into Jueyin, misting the heart and stirring up the liver wind, and further forming the pattern of penetration of toxin into the heat and liver.

The invasion of seasonal measles toxin into the lung and spleen, abundant flaming heat in the lung and spleen, and external eruption on the skin are the main etiology and pathogenesis. In accordance with different pathomechanical changes in the different stages, there are invasion of pathogens into Wei-defensive ability of the lung, flaming abundance in the lung and spleen, and yin injury in the lung and stomach. Of these, flaming abundance in the lung and spleen is an evolving center of pathomechanical changes. If the Vital Energy fails to defeat the evil and measles toxin penetrates inward, there will be unfavorable or critical patterns, such as measles toxin blocking the lung, measles toxin attacking the throat, or measles toxin penetrating into the heart and liver, etc, in which measles toxin blocking the lung is the most common.

麻毒时邪侵犯肺脾,肺脾热炽,外发肌肤为主要病因病机。按其不同阶段又有邪犯肺卫、肺脾热炽、肺胃阴伤不同病机变化,肺脾热炽为病机演变中心。若正不胜邪,麻毒内陷,则可见麻毒闭肺、麻毒攻喉、毒陷心肝等逆证、险证,尤其麻毒闭肺最多见。

2 Key to diagnosis

(1) An epidemiologic history: It mostly occurs in the susceptible children in the seasons of the winter and spring, when measles occurs or prevails in the local region or there is recent contact history. The latent period usually lasts for 10 to 14 days.

(2) Clinical manifestations: Typical measles is divided clinically into three stages.

1) The initial heat stage: It lasts for 2～4 days, manifested by fever, conjunctival congestion, photophoby, lacrimation, running nose, sneezing, cough, visible white spots in a diameter of 0.5～1 mm on the bilateral buccal mucosa, surrounded by

2 诊断要点

(1) 流行病学史:多在冬春季节,常为易感儿童,当地有麻疹发生或流行,近期有接触史。潜伏期大多为10～14日。

(2) 临床表现:典型麻疹临床分三期。

1) 初热期:持续2～4日。表现为发热、眼结膜充血、畏光、流泪、流涕、喷嚏、咳嗽等症状,两侧颊黏膜可见0.5～1毫米直径大小的白

flushes, in varying number, termed Koplik's spots, and simultaneously there may be accompanied poor appetite, diarrhea and vomiting, etc.

色斑点,周围有红晕,为数不一,此为麻疹黏膜斑。同时可伴食欲不振,腹泻,呕吐等症。

2) The eruption stage: It lasts for 3～5 days. The skin rash usually breaks out 3～4 days later after fever, first behind the ears and at the hairline, then gradually onto the face, neck and body, onto the whole body in two to three days, and finally onto the palms and soles, and tip of the nose. Initially the skin rashs are light red maculopapules in a diameter of 2～5 mm. With the increase in number, the color of skin rashes will get darker, and converge into irregular patches, but the skin between the skin rashes is normal.

2) 出疹期:持续 3～5 日。一般于发热 3～4 日后出疹,初见于耳后、发际,依次向面、颈、躯干蔓延,约 2～3 日内遍布全身,最后达手足心、鼻准部。皮疹初为淡红色斑丘疹,直径 2～5 毫米不等,随着皮疹增多,颜色加深,融合成不规则片状,但疹间皮肤正常。

3) The recovery stage: It occurs 3～4 days after eruption. The high fever abates, the general condition gets better, and the skin rashes gradually disappear in the order of appearance, presenting bran-like desquamation and light brown pigmentation, which will completely fade away within 2 to 3 weeks.

3) 恢复期:出疹后 3～4 日。高热开始下降,全身情况好转,皮疹按出疹顺序逐渐隐退,出现糠麸样脱屑并见淡褐色的色素沉着,在 2～3 周完全消失。

(3) Laboratory Examinations

(3) 实验室检查

1) Blood routine examination: In the prodromal period, total white cell count is normal or decreases.

1) 血常规检查:前驱期白细胞总数正常或降低。

2) Cytologic examination and viral antigen examination: Polykaryocyte, eosinophilic inclusion, and measles virus antigen can be detected.

2) 细胞学和病毒抗原检查:可见多核巨细胞、嗜酸性包涵体和麻疹病毒抗原。

3) Serum antibody detection: Serum measles IgM antibody can be detected three days later after the acute stage. The positive rate reaches highest within 5 to 20 days. In the recovery stage (2 to 4 weeks after illness), if IgM antibody titer increases in 4 time-folds, it is significant for diagnosis, and

3) 血清抗体检测:血清麻疹 IgM 抗体在急性期发病后 3 日即可检出,5～20 日阳性率最高。恢复期(病后 2～4 周)IgM 抗体滴定度如大于 4 倍增长,有诊断价值,可作

Armeniacae Semen Amarum (Ku Xing Ren). For poor appetite, add *Setariae Fructus Germinatus* (Gu Ya) and *Hordei Fructus Germinatus* (Mai Ya). For slow shrinking of papules, add *Paeoniae Radix Rubra* (Chi Shao) and *Moutan Cortex Radicis* (Mu Dan Pi). For dry stool, add *Richosanthis Fructus* (Gua Lou) and *Cannabis Fructus*(Huo Ma Ren).

子回收迟缓者,加赤芍、牡丹皮;大便干结者,加瓜蒌、火麻仁。

3.2 Unfavorable pattern

3.2 逆证

(1) Blockage of Measles toxin in the lung

(1) 麻毒闭肺

Manifestations: Persistent high fever, cough, hasty breathing, phlegm rale in the throat, flaring nostrils, blue-purple face and lips, vexation and agitation, unsmooth eruption, dense and dark purple papules, red tongue, yellow tongue coating, rapid pulse, stagnant and purple fingerprints.

证候:高热不退,咳嗽气促,喉中痰鸣,鼻翼煽动,甚则面唇青紫、烦躁不安,疹出不畅,或疹稠紫暗,舌质红,舌苔黄,脉数,指纹紫滞。

Therapeutic method: To clear away heat, resolve toxin, open the lung and dissolve phlegm.

治法:清热解毒,开肺化痰。

Main formula: *Ephedra, Apricot Kernel, Gypsum and Licorice Decoction* (Ma Xing Shi Gan Tang) with modification.

主方:麻杏石甘汤加味。

Commonly used herbs: *Ephedrae Herba* (Ma Huang), *Gypsum Fibrosum* (Sheng Shi Gao), *Armeniacae Semen Amarum* (Ku Xing Ren), *Glycyrrhizae Radix Et Rhizoma*(Gan Cao), *Peucedani Radix*(Qian Hu), *Eriobotryae Folium* (Pi Pa Ye), *Schizonepetae Herba* (Jing Jie), *Ledebouriellae Radix* (Fang Feng), *Bulbus Fritillariae Cirrhosae* (Chuan Bei Mu).

常用药:麻黄、生石膏、苦杏仁、甘草、前胡、枇杷叶、荆芥、防风、川贝母。

Modification: For persistent high fever, add *Scutellariae Radix*(Huang Qin), *Lonicerae Flos Japonicae* (Jin Yin Hua), *Forsythia Fructus* (Lian Qiao), *Houttuyniae Herba* (Yu Xing Cao). For restless and hasty wheezing, excessive phlegm and salivation, add *Descurainiae Lepidii Semen* (Ting Li

加减:高热不退者,加黄芩、金银花、连翘、鱼腥草;喘促不安、痰涎壅盛者,加葶苈子、鲜竹沥、瓜蒌;腹胀便秘者,加大黄、玄明粉;面唇青紫者,加丹参、红花;疹出不

Zi), fresh *Bambosae Succus* (Zhu Li) and *Richosanthis Fructus* (Gua Lou). For abdominal distention and constipation, add *Rhei Radix Et Rhizoma* (Da Huang) and *Natrii Sulfas Exsiccatus* (Xuan Ming Fen). For green-blue or purple lips, add *Salviae Miltiorrhizae Radix Et Rhizoma* (Dan Shen) and *Carthami Flos* (Hong Hua). For unsmooth eruption, add *Puerariae Radix* (Ge Gen) and *Cimicifugae Rhizoma* (Sheng Ma). For dense eruption and dark purple papules, add *Moutan Cortex Radicis* (Mu Dan Pi), and *Arnebiae Radix* (Zi Cao).

畅者，加葛根、升麻；疹出稠密紫暗者，加牡丹皮、紫草。

(2) Measles toxin attacking the throat

（2）麻毒攻喉

Manifestations: Persistent heat sensation in the body, sore throat, cough like dog barking, hoarse voice, phlegm rale in the throat, even difficult inhalation, vexation and agitation, green-blue or purple lips, dense and dark purple papules, red tongue, yellow tongue coating, rapid pulse, stagnant and purple fingerprints.

证候：身热不退，咽喉肿痛，咳如犬吠，声音嘶哑，喉间痰鸣，甚则吸气困难，烦躁不安，面唇青紫，疹点稠密紫暗，舌质红，舌苔黄，脉数，指纹紫滞。

Therapeutic method: To clear away heat, resolve toxin, benefit the throat and diminish swelling.

治法：清热解毒，利咽消肿。

Main formula: *Arctium, Licorice and Platycodon Decoction* (Niu Bang Gan Jie Tang) with modification.

主方：牛蒡甘桔汤加减。

Commonly used herbs: *Arctii Fructus* (Niu Bang Zi), *Forsythia Fructus* (Lian Qiao), *Belamecandae Rhizoma* (She Gan), *Radix Tinosporae* (Jin Guo Lan), *Scrophulariae Radix* (Xuan Shen), *Platycodonis Radix* (Jie Geng), *Glycyrrhizae Radix Et Rhizoma* (Gan Cao), *Sophorae Tonkinensis Radix Et Rhizoma* (Shan Dou Gen), *Lonicerae Flos Japonicae* (Jin Yin Hua), *Scutellariae Radix* (Huang Qin), *Coptidis Rhizoma* (Huang Lian), *Gardeniae Fructus*

常用药：牛蒡子、连翘、射干、金果榄、玄参、桔梗、甘草、山豆根、金银花、黄芩、黄连、栀子。

(Zhi Zi).

Modification: For sore throat and phlegm rale in the throat, add *Richosanthis Fructus* (Gua Lou), *Bulbus Fritillariae Thumbergii* (Zhe Bei Mu). For dense and dark purple papules, add *Rehmanniae Radix Cruda* (Sheng Di Huang), *Moutan Cortex Radicis* (Mu Dan Pi) and *Arnebiae Radix* (Zi Cao). For dry stool, add *Rhei Radix Et Rhizoma* (Da Huang) and *Natrii Sulfas Exsiccatus* (Xuan Ming Fen). For difficult inhalation, green-blue face, purple lips and suffocation, it is appropriate to treat with integrated therapy of Chinese medicine and Western medicine.

加减：咽喉肿痛，喉间痰鸣者，加瓜蒌、浙贝母；疹点稠密紫暗者，加生地黄、牡丹皮、紫草；大便秘结者，加大黄、玄明粉；吸气困难，面青唇紫，出现窒息者，宜采用中西医结合治疗措施。

(3) Evil penetrating into the heart and liver

（3）邪陷心肝

Manifestations: Persistent high fever, vexation and agitation, delirious speech, coma, convulsion, phlegm rale in the throat, dense and dark purple papules, crimson tongue, coarse and yellow tongue coating, rapid pulse, stagnant and purple finger-prints.

证候：高热不退，烦躁谵语，神昏抽搐，喉间痰鸣，疹点密集紫暗，舌质红绛，舌苔黄糙，脉数，指纹紫滞。

Therapeutic method: To clear away heat, cool down Ying-nutrient system, extinguish wind and open the orifices.

治法：清热凉营，息风开窍。

Main formula: *Clear-Construction Decoction* (Qing Yin Tang) plus *Antelope Horn and Uncaria Decoction* (Ling Jiao Gou Teng Tang) with modification.

主方：清营汤合羚角钩藤汤加减。

Commonly used herbs: *Bubali Cornu* (Shui Niu Jiao), *Rehmanniae Radix Cruda* (Sheng Di Huang), *Moutan Cortex Radicis* (Mu Dan Pi), *Scrophulariae Radix* (Xuan Shen), *Antelopis Tataricae Cornu* (Ling Yang Jiao), *Uncariae Ramulus Cum Uncis* (Gou Teng), *Chrysanthemi Flos* (Ju Hua), *Paeoniae Radix Albae* (Bai Shao), *Glycyrrhizae*

常用药：水牛角、生地黄、牡丹皮、玄参、羚羊角、钩藤、菊花、白芍、甘草、石菖蒲、郁金、紫草。

Radix Et Rhizoma (Gan Cao), *Acori Rhizoma Tatarinowii* (Shi Chang Pu), *Curcumae Radix* (Yu Jin), *Arnebiae Radix* (Zi Cao).

Modification: For high fever, coma and convulsion, add *Purple Snow Elixir* (Zi Xue Dan) and *Peaceful Palace Bovine Bezoar Pill* (An Gong Niu Huang Wan). For dry stool, add *Rhei Radix Et Rhizoma* (Da Huang), and *Natrii Sulfas Exsiccatus* (Xuan Ming Fen).

加减:高热、神昏、抽搐者,可配合应用紫雪丹、安宫牛黄丸;大便干结,加大黄、玄明粉。

4　Other therapies

4　其他疗法

4.1　Chinese Patent medicine

4.1　中成药

(1) *Lonicera and Forsythia Toxin Resolving Pill* (Yin Qiao Jie Du Pian) is appropriate for measles in the initial stage and the stage of early formation.

(1) 银翘解毒丸:适用于麻疹初热期、见形早期。

(2) *Five Grains Return-of-Spring Elixir* (Wu Li Hui Chun Dan) is appropriate for measles in the stage of early formation.

(2) 五粒回春丹:适用于麻疹见形期。

(3) *Arnebia Pill for Child* (Xiao Er Zi Cao Wan)is appropriate for measles at the stage of early formation.

(3) 小儿紫草丸:适用于麻疹见形期。

4.2　External Therapy

4.2　外治疗法

Wrap and decoct the following herbs in cloth: *Ephedrae Herba* (Ma Huang), *Spirodelae Herba* (Fu Ping), *Herba Coriandri* (Yan Sui), *Tamaricis Cacumen* (Xi He Liu), 15g, each, then add rice wine of 250g, keep boiling to warm up and moisten air in the room. After the decoction cools down a bit, use it to wipe forehead, face, neck, chest, back, limbs and the back of hand to help promote eruption. Two to three of the above ingredients can also be selected and used in the same method.

麻黄、浮萍、芫荽、西河柳各 15 克,布包水煎,加黄酒 250 克,煮沸,使室内空气温暖湿润,待药液稍温,揩额面、颈部、胸背、四肢、手背等部位,以助透疹。亦可取其中2～3 味,同上法用之。

4.3　Diet therapy

4.3　饮食疗法

(1) Celery, non-glutinous rice, 50g each: Wash celery clean and chop it after blanching it in boiling

(1) 芹菜、粳米各 50 克。取芹菜洗净,沸水焯过切碎,

water. When the porridge is half done, put in celery till the porridge is done. Take warm porridge 1～2 times a day. It is used for those with unsmooth eruption.

(2) 50～100g of carrot, and 50g of non-glutinous rice, Wach carrot clean, and cut it into thin slices, and put into the rice, and cook porridge. Take the porridge once in the morning and once in the evening. It is used for those in the recovery stage of measles.

待粥至半熟时加入芹菜，同煮至粥熟为度，每日食1～2次，温服，用于麻疹透发不畅者。

（2）胡萝卜50～100克，粳米50克。将胡萝卜洗净，切成薄片，加入粳米中，一同加水煮粥。每日早、晚各食1次。适用于麻疹恢复期。

Section 2 Rubella

第2节 风疹

Rubella is an acute infectious disease of the respiratory tract, caused by rubella virus and clinically characterized by fever, skin rash, enlarged lymph nodes at the back of ears, at the posterior occipital region and in the neck. If the pregnant woman is infected with rubella within three months of pregnancy, virus can be transmitted to the fetus through placenta and results in a variety of congenital defects, called congenital rubella syndrome (CRS). It is more commonly seen in the infants at the age from 1 to 5 years old, and can occur in all seasons, more often in the winter and spring. It is often epidemic in the kindergarten and nursery. After sick with the disease, the sick children can obtain persistent immunity.

In traditional Chinese medicine, it is called "wind rash".

风疹是由风疹病毒引起的急性呼吸道感染病，临床表现以发热，皮疹及耳后、枕后、颈部淋巴结肿大为特征。孕妇在妊娠3个月内患风疹，病毒可通过胎盘传给胎儿而致各种先天缺陷，称为先天性风疹综合征。发病年龄以1～5岁小儿多见，四季均可发生，以冬春季节多见，常在幼托机构造成流行，患病后可获得持久性免疫。

中医学称之为"风痧"。

1 Etiology and pathogenesis

The disease is caused by seasonal toxin of rubella. After entering from the mouth and nose, the

1 病因病机

由感受风疹时毒所致。邪毒从口鼻而入，主要侵犯

evil toxin mainly invades and attacks Wei-defensive ability of the lung, and spreads onto the skin, causing the disease. This evil toxin is relatively mild, so it usually will only damage Wei-defensive ability of the lung and cause disharmony between the exterior and Wei-defensive ability, impairing the distributing ability of the lung qi, manifested by mild fever, cough, running nose, etc. The lung governs the skin and hair. When the evil is discharged outward to the exterior, it would induce sparse papules in light red color and tiny size. After the eruption, fever would fade away and the disease would be alleviated. In a few cases, exuberant evil toxin would penetrate inwards, affecting Qi-energy system and Ying-nutrient system, resulting in high fever, vexation and thirst, dense papules in bright red or dark purple color. Occasionally, the evil toxin would penetrate into the heart and liver, resulting in transmuted pattern of coma and convulsion.

肺卫，外透肌肤而发病。由于邪毒较轻，一般只伤及肺卫，表卫失和，肺气失宣，则见轻度发热、咳嗽、流涕等。肺主皮毛，邪从外泄，则见疹点稀疏、淡红细小。疹出之后，热退病解。个别邪毒炽盛，可内传入里。波及气营，则见高热、烦渴、疹点稠密、颜色鲜赤或紫暗。偶有邪陷心肝，出现神昏、抽搐变证。

The invasion of seasonal pathogenic wind and heat, attacking Wei-defensive ability of the lung and spreading outward onto the skin, is regarded as the main etiology and pathogenesis. Because the evils are mild and disease is shallow, Wei-defensive ability of the lung is a center of pathomechanic evolution. In some cases, exuberant evil toxin may involve Qi-energy system and Ying-nutrient system, and occasionally the evils may penetrate into the heart and liver or damage other organs.

风热时邪侵犯肺卫，外发肌肤为主要病因病机。由于邪轻病浅，以肺卫为病机演变中心，个别毒盛可波及气营，偶有邪陷心肝或伤他脏。

2 Key to diagnosis

2 诊断要点

(1) The disease tends to occur in the winter and spring, usually in the susceptible children. There may be contact history before the onset, and it

（1）好发于冬春季节，儿童普遍易感，发病可有接触史，幼儿园及学校等人员密

tends to spread in densely populated places like kindergartens or schools.

集场所易造成流行。

(2) Clinically, typical rubella is divided into the preeruptive stage and eruptive stage. In the preeruptive stage: the duration lasts short, about 0.5 to 1 day, only manifested by exterior pattern of Wei-defensive ability of the lung, and swollen and tender lymph nodes behind the ear, at the back of the neck and in the occipital region. In the eruption stage: the eruption occurs 1 to 2 days after fever, and spreads to the whole body in a day, manifested by fine and itching papules in skin rash. The skin rash would disappear 2 or 3 days after eruption, without desquamation and pigmentation.

(2) 典型的风疹临床有疹前期和出疹期。疹前期:时间较短,约 1/2～1 日,仅见肺卫表证及耳后、颈后、枕部臀核肿大触痛;出疹期:发热第 1～2 日出疹,1 日内布满全身,皮疹呈淡红色细小丘疹,有痒感。出疹后 2～3 日皮疹消退,无脱屑,无色素沉着。

(3) Routine blood test could show normal or slightly low total count in white blood cell, relative increase in lymphocyte, and abnormal lymphocyte.

(3) 血常规可见白细胞总数正常或稍低,淋巴细胞相对增多,可出现异常淋巴细胞。

3 Pattern identification and treatment

3 辨证论治

It is necessary to differentiate the severity of the disease. Mild fever, good spirit, light red and tiny skin rash in even and sparse distribution belong to mild pattern of retention of evils in Wei-defensive ability of the lung. High fever, vexation and agitation, bright red or dark purple skin rash in dense distribution or melted into patches belong to severe pattern of the pathogens attacking Qi-energy system and Ying-nutrient system.

主要辨轻重:发热不高,精神良好,皮疹淡红细小,分布稀疏均匀,属邪郁肺卫轻证;发热高,烦躁,皮疹鲜赤或紫暗,分布密集或融合成片,属邪犯气营重证。

The treatment is mainly designed to expel wind, clear away heat and resolve toxin. For the evils attacking Qi-energy system and Ying-nutrient system, the treatment is supposed to clarify qi, cool down Ying-nutrient system and resolve toxin.

治疗以疏风清热解毒为主,邪犯气营宜清气凉营解毒。

(1) Retentions of evils in Wei-defensive ability

(1) 邪郁肺卫

of the lung

Manifestations: Mild fever, cough, runny nose, light red and tiny papules, scanty in number and even in distribution, itching, swollen lymph nodes behind the ears, in the neck and occipital region, red tongue, thin white or slight yellow tongue coating, rapid and floating pulse, floating and purple fingerprints.

证候:轻度发热,咳嗽,流涕,疹点淡红细小,稀疏均匀,有痒感,耳后、颈后、枕部臖核肿大触痛,舌质偏红,舌苔薄白或微黄,脉浮数,指纹浮紫。

Therapeutic method: To expel wind, clear away heat and resolve toxin.

治法:疏风清热解毒。

Main formula: *Lonicera and Forsythia Powder* (Yin Qiao San) with modification.

主方:银翘散加减。

Commonly used herbs: *Lonicerae Flos Japonicae* (Jin Yin Hua), *Forsythia Fructus* (Lian Qiao), *Schizonepetae Herba* (Jing Jie), *Menthae Haploalycis Herba* (Bo He), *Sojae Semen Praeparatum* (Dan Dou Chi), *Arctii Fructus* (Niu Bang Zi), *Platycodonis Radix* (Jie Geng), *Cicadae Periostracum* (Chan Tui), *Glycyrrhizae Radix Et Rhizoma* (Gan Cao), *Phragmitis Rhizoma* (Lu Gen).

常用药:金银花、连翘、荆芥、薄荷、淡豆豉、牛蒡子、桔梗、蝉蜕、甘草、芦根。

Modification: For obvious sore throat, add *Bombyx Batryticatus* (Jiang Can), *Oroxyli Semen* (Mu Hu Die). For swollen lymph nodes, add *Prunella Spica* (Xia Ku Cao), and *Taraxaci Herba* (Pu Gong Ying). For severe itching skin, add *Dictamni Cortex* (Bai Xian Pi), and *Fructus Tribuli* (Bai Ji Li).

加减:咽红肿痛明显者,加僵蚕、木蝴蝶;臖核肿大者,加夏枯草、蒲公英;皮肤痒甚者,加白鲜皮、白蒺藜。

(2) Invasion of evils into Qi-energy system and Ying-nutrient system

(2) 邪犯气营

Manifestations: High fever, vexation and thirst, bright red or dark purple papules, dense or in patches, relative severe itching sensation, obvious swollen and tender lymph nodes behind the ears, in the neck and occipital region, red tongue, coarse and yellow tongue coating, rapid and surging

证候:高热,烦渴,疹点鲜赤或紫暗,密集或融合成片,瘙痒较重,耳后、颈后、枕部臖核肿大触痛明显,舌质红,舌苔黄糙,脉洪数,指纹紫滞。

pulse, stagnant and purple fingerprints.

Therapeutic method: To clear away heat, cool down Ying-nutrient system and resolve toxin.

治法:清热凉营解毒。

Main formula: *Eruption-Promoting and Cool Resolving Decoction* (Tou Zhen Lian Jie Tang) with modification.

主方:透疹凉解汤加减。

Commonly used herbs: *Mori Folium* (Sang Ye), *Menthae Haploalycis Herba* (Bo He), *Arctii Fructus* (Niu Bang Zi), *Cicadae Periostracum* (Chan Tui), *Lonicerae Flos Japonicae* (Jin Yin Hua), *Forsythia Fructus* (Lian Qiao), *Scutellariae Radix* (Huang Qin), *Violae Herba* (Zi Hua Di Ding), *Paeoniae Radix Rubra* (Chi Shao), *Carthami Flos*(Hong Hua).

常用药:桑叶、薄荷、牛蒡子、蝉蜕、金银花、连翘、黄芩、紫花地丁、赤芍、红花。

Modification: For severe thirst, add *Dendrobii Herba* (Shi Hu), and *Phragmitis Rhizoma* (Lu Gen). For dark purple and dense papules, add *Rehmanniae Radix Cruda* (Sheng Di Huang), *Moutan Cortex Radicis* (Mu Dan Pi), and *Arnebiae Radix* (Zi Cao). For constipated stool, add *Rhei Radix Et Rhizoma* (Da Huang), and *Natrii Sulfas* (Mang Xiao). For severe condition, treat with *Scourge-Clearing Toxin-Vanquishing Decoction* (Qing Wen Bai Du Yin) in modification.

加减:口渴甚者,加石斛、芦根;疹点密集紫暗,加生地黄、牡丹皮、紫草;大便秘结,加大黄、芒硝。本证重者,亦可用清瘟败毒饮加减治疗。

4 Other therapies

4 其他疗法

4.1 Chinese Patent medicine

4.1 中成药

(1) *Isatidis Radix Granules* (Ban Lan Gen Chong Ji) is appropriate for rubella in pattern of retentions of evils in Wei-defensive ability of the lung.

(1) 板蓝根冲剂:适用于风疹邪郁肺卫证。

(2) *Three Yellow Pills* (San Huang Pian) is appropriate for rubella in pattern of invasion of evils into Qi-energy system and Ying-nutrient system.

(2) 三黄片:适用于风疹邪犯气营证。

(3) *Child Papule Golden Pill* (Xiao Er Sha Zhen Jin Wan) is appropriate for rubella in pattern of evils into Qi-energy system and Ying-nutrient system.

(3) 小儿痧疹金丸：适用于风疹邪犯气营证。

4.2 External therapy

Heat 50g of peanut oil, and after it cools down slightly, add 30g of mint leaves into it. After it cools down completely and the dregs are filtered out, apply it on the itchy skin to relieve itch.

4.2 外治疗法

花生油 50 克，煮沸后稍冷加入薄荷叶 30 克，完全冷却后过滤去渣，外涂皮肤痒处，有止痒作用。

Section 3　Chicken Pox

第 3 节　水痘

Chicken pox is an infectious disease caused by varicella-zoster virus, clinically characterized by fever, itchy macules, papules, blister-papule, and crusting present on the skin and mucosa in patches or jointly. It mostly occurs in the winter and spring, in the susceptible population, and mainly in children, with the highest incidence at the age from 2 to 6 years old. Generally, its prognosis is good.

In traditional Chinese medicine, it is categorized into the scope of "chicken pox", "water sore", "water joyness" and "water flower".

水痘是水痘-带状疱疹病毒引起的感染性疾病，临床特征为发热，皮肤黏膜分批出现并同时存在的瘙痒性斑、丘疹，疱疹及结痂。冬春季节多见，人群普遍易感，主要见于儿童，以 2～6 岁为高峰。一般预后良好。

本病属中医学"水痘""水疮""水喜""水花"范畴。

1　Etiology and pathogenesis

It is caused by infection of seasonal chicken pox toxin. After entering through the mouth and nose, the seasonal toxin would be retained in the lung and stomach (spleen), and struggle with internal dampness, spreading outward onto the skin and hence the disease. The evil toxin is relatively mild and mainly invades and attacks Wei-defensive ability of the lung, resulting in disharmony between the exterior and Wei-defensive ability of the lung and imparing the distributing ability of the lung qi, manifested by

1　病因病机

由感受水痘时毒所致。时毒自口鼻而入，郁于肺胃(脾)，与内湿相搏，外透肌肤而发病。邪毒较轻，主要侵犯肺卫，表卫失和，肺气失宣，则见发热、咳嗽、流涕；累犯脾胃，与湿相搏，外透肌肤，水痘布露，表现较轻。少数患者邪毒炽盛，毒热内犯气营，则见壮热、烦渴；甚则

fever, cough, and running nose. When it repeatedly invades the spleen and stomach and struggles with dampness, it would spread outward onto the skin, causing water sores in mild condition. In a few of the patients, if evil toxin is abundant, the toxin and heat would attack Qi-energy system and Ying-nutrient system, manifested by strong fever, vexation and thirst. In severe condition, toxin and heat would turn into fire and penetrate into the heart and liver, leading to coma and convulsion.

毒热化火,内陷心肝,而见神昏、抽搐。

The main etiology and pathogenesis are related to the retention of seasonal chicken pox toxin in the lung and stomach (spleen), struggling with internal dampness, and spreading outward onto the skin.

水痘时毒郁于肺胃(脾),与内湿相搏,外发肌肤为主要病因病机。

2 Key to diagnosis

(1) It mostly occurs in the winter and spring, and can be epidemic. The infants may have a contact history.

(2) Typical chicken pox can be divided into the preeruptive stage and eruptive stage. The preeruptive stage: The duration is short, usually less than 24 hours, probally manifested by exterior pattern of Wei-defensive ability of the lung of fever, runny nose and slight cough, etc. The eruption stage: The eruption occurs on the same day or on the second day of fever. Initially it appears on the body and head, then spreads onto face and four limbs. The skin rash is red macule-papule firstly, and shortly afterwards it turns into blisters, in oval shape and different size, with transparent fluid inside, and surrounded by flushed color, with thin blister wall, easy to break and itchy, forming dry scabs laterly. The scabs would fall off without leaving any scar.

2 诊断要点

(1) 多在冬春季节发病,可造成流行,患儿近期可有接触史。

(2) 典型水痘可分为疹前期和出疹期。疹前期:时间较短,一般不超过 24 小时,可有发热、流涕、轻咳等肺卫表证;出疹期:发热当日或第 2 日透发皮疹,首见于躯干和头部,以后延及面部和四肢。皮疹初为红色斑丘疹,很快变为疱疹,呈椭圆形,大小不一,内含透明浆液,周围红晕,壁薄易破,有痒感,继而干燥结痂,然后痂盖脱落,不留瘢痕。起病后皮疹分批出现,此起彼落,参差不齐,同一时期,丘疹、疱

After onset, the skin rash will appear in batches, here and there intermittently and irregularly. Simultaneously, there may be papules, blisters, and crusts. The skin rash would spread centripetally, mainly on the body trunk, then onto the face and head, but seldom onto the far ends of four limbs. The skin rash may also appear in the oral, pharyngeal and laryngeal, conjunctival, and vulvar mucosa. Blisters are easy to break, and may cause ulcer.

疹、结痂同时存在。皮疹呈向心性分布，主要位于躯干，次为头面部，四肢远端较少。口腔、咽喉、眼结膜、外阴黏膜亦可见疹，疱疹易破，形成溃疡。

(3) Routine blood test could show normal or slight increase in the total count of white blood cell, relative increase in lymphocyte. In examining the scrapings from the root of fresh blisters, there may be multinucleated giant cells and intranuclear inclusion.

(3) 血常规可见白细胞总数正常，偶有轻度增多，淋巴细胞相对增多。新鲜疱疹底部刮取物检查，可见多核巨细胞和核内包涵体。

3　Pattern identification and treatment

3　辨证论治

To differentiate its severity: Mild fever, scanty poxes in ruddy color, clear pox fluid, obscure flushed color at the bottom of pox, no other accompanying symptoms, all these belong to mild pattern of retention of evils in Wei-defensive ability of the lung. Lingering high fever, dense poxes in dark purple color, turbid pox fluid, and obvious flushed color at the bottom of pox, existence of accompanying symptoms, all these belong to severe pattern of flaring abundance in Qi-energy system and Ying-nutrient system.

主要辨别轻重：轻度发热，痘疹稀疏，颜色红润，疱浆清亮，根脚红晕不著，无其他兼症，为邪郁肺卫轻证；壮热不解，痘疹稠密，颜色紫暗，疱浆混浊，根脚红晕显著，或有兼证，为气营两燔重证。

The basic therapeutic principle is supposed to clear away heat, resolve toxin, and to remove dampness assistantly. For retention of evils in Wei-defensive ability of the lung, it is appropriate to expel wind, clear away heat and resolve toxin mainly. For flaring abundance in Qi-energy system and Ying-nutrient system, it is appropriate to clear away

以清热解毒，佐以利湿为基本治则。邪郁肺卫，治宜疏风清热解毒为主；气营两燔，治宜清热凉营解毒为主，佐以利湿。

heat, cool down Ying-nutrient system, resolve toxin mainly, and remove dampness assiatantly.

(1) Retention of evils in Wei-defensive ability of the lung

(1) 邪郁肺卫

Manifestations: Slight fever, nasal obstruction, runny nose, sneezing, scanty poxes in ruddy appearance, clear pox fluid, unclear flushed color at the bottom of poxes, thin, white slight greasy tongue coating, floating and rapid pulse, floating and purple fingerprints.

证候:轻度发热,鼻塞流涕,喷嚏,咳嗽,痘疹稀疏,疹色红润,疱浆清亮,根脚红晕不著,舌苔薄白微腻,脉浮数,指纹浮紫。

Therapeutic method: To expel wind, clear away heat, resolve toxin, and remove dampness assistantly.

治法:疏风清热解毒,佐以利湿。

Main formula: *Lonicera and Forsythia Powder* (Yin Qiao San) with modification.

主方:银翘散加减。

Commonly used herbs: *Lonicerae Flos Japonicae* (Jin Yin Hua), *Forsythia Fructus* (Lian Qiao), *Schizonepetae Herba* (Jing Jie), *Menthae Haploalycis Herba* (Bo He), *Lophatheri Herba* (Dan Zhu Ye), *Arctii Fructus* (Niu Bang Zi), *Platycodonis Radix* (Jie Geng), *Glycyrrhizae Radix Et Rhizoma* (Gan Cao), *Talcum* (Hua Shi), *Plantaginis Semen* (Che Qian Zi).

常用药:金银花、连翘、荆芥、薄荷、淡竹叶、牛蒡子、桔梗、甘草、滑石、车前子。

Modification: For severe itchy poxes, add *Cicadae Periostracum* (Chan Tui), *Bombyx Batryticatus* (Jiang Can), and *Fructus Tribuli* (Ji Li).

加减:痘疹痒甚者,加蝉蜕、僵蚕、蒺藜。

(2) Flaring abundance in Qi-energy system and Ying-nutrient system

(2) 气营两燔

Manifestations: Persistent high fever, vexation and agitation, thirst with preference for drinks, flushed face and lips, dense poxes in dark purple color, turbid pox fluid, obvious flush at the bottom of poxes, constipated stool, yellow and brown urine, crimson tongue, thick and yellow tongue coat-

证候:壮热不解,烦躁不安,口渴欲饮,面红唇赤,痘疹稠密,颜色紫暗,疱浆混浊,根脚红晕显著,大便干结,小便黄赤,舌质红绛,舌苔黄厚,脉洪数有力,指纹紫

ing, rapid and surging pulse, purple and stagnant fingerprints.

滞。

Therapeutic method: To clear away heat, cool down Ying-nutrient system, resolve toxin, and remove dampness assistantly.

治法:清热凉营解毒,佐以利湿。

Main formula: *Clear-Stomach and Resolving-Toxin Decoction* (Qing Wei Jie Du Tang) with modification.

主方:清胃解毒汤加减。

Commonly used herbs: *Lonicerae Flos Japonicae* (Jin Yin Hua), *Forsythia Fructus* (Lian Qiao), *Isatidis Radix* (Ban Lan Gen), *Scutellariae Radix* (Huang Qin), *Gypsum Fibrosum* (Sheng Shi Gao), *Rehmanniae Radix Cruda* (Sheng Di Huang), *Moutan Cortex Radicis* (Mu Dan Pi), *Paeoniae Radix Rubra* (Chi Shao), *Arnebiae Radix* (Zi Cao), *Lophatheri Herba* (Dan Zhu Ye), *Talcum* (Hua Shi).

常用药:金银花、连翘、板蓝根、黄芩、生石膏、生地黄、牡丹皮、赤芍、紫草、淡竹叶、滑石。

Modification: For constipated stool, add *Rhei Radix Et Rhizoma* (Da Huang), and *Natrii Sulfas* (Mang Xiao). For coma and convulsion, add *Peaceful Palace Bovine Bezoar Pill* (An Gong Niu Huang Wan), and *Purple Snow Elixir* (Zi Xue Dan). For severe condition, use *Scourge-Clearing and Toxin-Vanquishing Decoction* (Qing Wen Bai Du Yin) in modification.

加减:大便干结者,加大黄、芒硝;神昏抽搐者,加安宫牛黄丸、紫雪丹。病情严重者,亦可用清瘟败毒饮加减治疗。

4 Other therapies

4 其他疗法

4.1 Chinese Patent medicine

4.1 中成药

(1) *Isatidis Radix Granules* (Ban Lan Gen Chong Ji) is appropriate for chicken pox in pattern of retention of evils in Wei-defensive ability of the lung.

(1) 板蓝根冲剂:适用于水痘邪郁肺卫证。

(2) *Lonicera and Forsythia Toxin Resolving Pill* (Yin Qiao Jie Du Wan) is appropriate for chicken pox in pattern of retention of evils in Wei-defensive

(2) 银翘解毒丸:适用于水痘邪郁肺卫证。

ability of the lung.

(3) *Five Happinesses Toxin-Transforming Exilir* (Wu Fu Hua Du Wan) is appropriate for chicken pox in pattern of flaring abundance in Qi-energy system and Ying-nutrient system.

（3）五福化毒丸：适用于水痘气营两燔证。

4.2 External therapy

4.2 外治疗法

(1) Decoct 30g of *Sophorae Flavescentis Radix* (Ku Shen), 30g of *Natrii Sulfas* (Mang Xiao), and 15g of *Spirodelae Herba* (Fu Ping) for topical wash, twice a day, appropriate for dense poxes and obvious itching.

（1）苦参 30 克，芒硝 30 克，浮萍 15 克，煎水外洗，每日 2 次。用于皮疹稠密、瘙痒明显者。

(2) Mix *Indigo Powder* (Qing Dai San) with sesame oil, for topical application, orce or twice a day, appropriate for suppurative and ulcerative poxes.

（2）青黛散麻油调后外敷，每日 1～2 次。用于疱疹破溃化脓者。

(3) *Tin-like Powder* (Xi Lei San), *Borneol and Borax Powder* (Bing Peng San), *Pearl and Bezoar Powder* (Zhu Huang San), select any one of them to insufflate into the mouth, 2 to 3 times a day, appropriate for ruptured and ulcerative blisters in the oral mucosa.

（3）锡类散、冰硼散、珠黄散，任选一种吹口，每日 2～3 次。用于口腔黏膜水疱破溃成溃疡者。

Section 4 Mumps

第 4 节 流行性腮腺炎

Mumps is an acute infectious disease of respiratory tract, caused by mumps virus and clinically characterized by swollen and painful parotid glands. In addition to the parotid glands, mumps virus can also cause meningitis, testitis, ovaritis, and pancreatitis, etc. It may occur in all seasons, and is easy to spread in the winter and spring. The patients in the early stage and the carriers with inapparant infection are the source of infection. It tends to be epi-

流行性腮腺炎是由腮腺炎病毒引起的急性呼吸道传染病，临床表现以腮腺肿胀、疼痛为主要特征。腮腺炎病毒除侵犯腮腺外，尚能引起脑膜炎、睾丸炎、卵巢炎和胰腺炎等。一年四季均可发生，冬春两季较易流行。早期患者及隐性感染者为传染

demic in children group. The route of transmission is mainly related to direct contact or transmission by droplets. It is mostly seen in the patients at the age from 5 to 15 years old, very seldom in the infants at the age below 2 years old. After infection, persistent immunity can be obtained.

源，易在儿童集体中流行，其传播途径主要通过直接接触或飞沫传播。5～15 岁患者较为多见，2 岁以下小儿少见。感染后可获持久免疫。

In traditional Chinese medicine, it is categorized into the scope of "mumps", "cormorant-like pestilence", or "toad pestilence".

本病属中医学"痄腮"范畴，又称为"鸬鹚瘟""蛤蟆瘟"。

1　Etiology and pathogenesis

1　病因病机

The retention and obstruction of the seasonal evils in Shaoyang meridian and in the cheeks are regarded as the main etiology and pathogenesis in mumps.

腮腺炎时邪壅阻少阳经脉，凝滞腮部为主要病因病机。

In infection of exogenous seasonal evil of mumps, initially it would invade Wei-defensive ability and exterior, leading to disharmony between Wei-defensive ability and exterior, manifested by fever, slight aversion to wind and cold, and headache. If the evil invades the Gallbladder Meridian of Foot Shaoyang, because the gallbladder meridian starts from the outer canthus of the eye, goes upward to the corners of the head, behind the ear, and then goes around the ear, the evil would go along and through the pathway of the meridian to attack cheeks upward, leading to obstruction in the meridian and poor circulation of qi and blood and further diffusive swelling and pain in the cheeks under the ears. If the evil is abundant and penetrates into the interior, there will be high fever, thirst, and severe swollen cheek. Shaoyang and Jueyin are related in a relationship of the exterior and interior. The meridian of Foot Jueyin goes through the lower abdomen and links with the genital organ. If the

外感腮腺炎时邪，初期邪犯卫表，表卫失和，则见发热、微恶风寒、头痛等症。邪犯足少阳胆经，胆经之脉起于目外眦，上行至头角，下耳后，绕耳而行；邪毒循经上攻腮颊，使经脉阻滞，气血不行，故耳下腮部漫肿疼痛。邪毒炽盛，内传入里，则见高热、口渴、腮肿加重。少阳与厥阴互为表里，足厥阴之脉循少腹络阴器，邪毒较重传入厥阴，故较大儿童可并发少腹痛、睾丸痛。若邪毒内陷心肝，肝风内动，心神蒙蔽，可出现壮热、神昏、抽搐等危重变证。

evil is relatively severe and is transmitted into Jueyin meridian, the elder children may be complicated with pain in the lower abdomen and testicle pain. If the evil penetrates into the heart and liver, the liver wind would be stirred upward to mist the heart and spirit, presenting the critical transmuted pattern of high fever, coma and convulsion, etc.

2 Key to diagnosis

(1) The disease is more likely to occur in the winter and spring. There can be a contact history 2 to 3 weeks before the onset.

(2) In the initial stage, there could be fever and headache, etc. One to two days later, swelling and pain could be present in the cheeks, usually on one side first and then on the opposite side. The swelling in the cheeks spreads centrifugally from the earlobe, unclear in the margin and not red in the skin, but tender. The orifices of the parotid gland are red and swollen, and no pus flows out from the orifices of the gland by pressure. The swelling of the parotid glands reaches the peak in 3 to 4 days, together with high fever, and then it gradually disappears. If no complication is present, it would last for about 1 to 2 weeks. The complicated testitis, epididymitis, and ovaritis are often seen in the sick post-adolescent children, manifested by swollen and painful testicle, or pain in the lower abdomen. Those complicated with meningocerebritis may suffer from fever, headache, vomit, somnolence, and stiff neck, and even coma, convulsion due to fright in a few cases. There may be pancreatitis, carditis, and nephritis, etc.

(3) Routine blood test could show normal or in-

2 诊断要点

（1）好发于冬春季，发病前2～3周有接触史。

（2）病初可有发热、头痛等，1～2日后，出现腮部肿胀疼痛，通常先见一侧，继而对侧。腮部肿胀以耳垂为中心漫肿，边缘不清，表皮不红，有压痛；腮腺管口红肿，按压腮腺时无脓液自腮腺管口流出。腮腺肿大3～4日达高峰，同时出现高热，以后逐渐消退，若无并发症，整个病程约1～2周。并发睾丸炎、副睾炎或卵巢炎者多见于青春期后患儿，常有睾丸肿痛或少腹疼痛；并发脑膜脑炎者可见发热、头痛、呕吐、嗜睡、颈项强直，少数病例可有昏迷、惊厥；还可引起胰腺炎、心肌炎、肾炎等。

（3）血常规可见白细胞

creased total count in white blood cell, relatively increase in leukomonocyte. Serum amylase and amylase in urine increase and serum specific antibody increases. Mumps virus can be isolated from their saliva, urine, cerebrospinal fluid or blood sample in the patients of the early stage.

总数多在正常或有增多,淋巴细胞相对增多;血清淀粉酶和尿淀粉酶增高;血清特异性抗体增高;发病早期患者唾液、尿液、脑脊液或血液标本可分离出病毒。

3 Pattern identification and treatment

3 辨证论治

It is necessary to differentiate the severity, ordinary pattern or transmuted pattern of the disease.

主要辨别疾病的轻、重及常证、变证。

Low fever or no fever, soft mumps, and warm toxin in the exterior mostly belong to mild pattern. Continuous high fever, hard swollen cheeks, aggravated by pressure, are mostly related to retention of heat toxin and belong to severe pattern. Swollen and painful testicles, pain in the lower abdomen or in the upper abdomen, nausea, vomiting, coma and convulsion mostly belong to transmuted pattern.

发热不高或无热,腮肿不坚硬,为温毒在表,多属轻症;高热不退,腮肿坚硬拒按,多为热毒蕴结,属重症;若见睾丸肿痛、少腹或上腹疼痛,或恶心呕吐、神昏抽搐者,为变证。

The basic therapeutic principle is to clear away heat, resolve toxin, diminish swelling and disperse retention. For warm toxin in the exterior, it is appropriate to expel wind and dispel the evil assistantly and jointly. For heat toxin penetrating into the interior, it is necessary to clear away heat and resolve toxin mainly. If the evil toxin changes and passes through testicles to the abdomen, it is necessary to clarify the liver and drain fire additionally. If it penetrates into the heart and liver, it is necessary to extinguish wind and open the orifices assistantly. The treatments are used together with external therapies.

以清热解毒,消肿散结为基本治则。温毒在表者,配以疏风散邪;热毒入里者,重用清热解毒。邪毒传变,窜睾入腹者,佐以清肝泻火;内陷心肝者,佐以息风开窍。常配合外治疗法。

3.1 Ordinary patterns

3.1 常证

(1) Warm toxin in the exterior

(1) 温毒在表

Manifestations: Slight fever, headache, diffu-

证候:轻微发热,或头

sive swelling and pain in the cheeks under the ears, difficult to open mouth, and inconvenient in chewing, red tongue, thin and white or thin and yellow coating, rapid and floating pulse.

痛，耳下腮部漫肿疼痛，张口不利，咀嚼不便，舌质红，苔薄白或薄黄，脉浮数。

Therapeutic method: To expel wind, clear away heat, diminish swelling and disperse retention.

治法：疏风清热，消肿散结。

Main formula: *Bupleurum and Pueraria Decoction* (Chai Hu Ge Gen Tang) with modification.

主方：柴胡葛根汤加减。

Commonly used herbs: *Bupleuri Radix* (Chai Hu), *Trichosanthis Radix* (Tian Hua Fen), *Puerariae Radix* (Ge Gen), *Scutellariae Radix* (Huang Qin), *Platycodonis Radix* (Jie Geng), *Forsythia Fructus* (Lian Qiao), *Arctii Fructus* (Niu Bang Zi), *Gypsum Fibrosum* (Sheng Shi Gao), *Glycyrrhizae Radix Et Rhizoma* (Gan Cao), *Cimicifugae Rhizoma* (Sheng Ma).

常用药：柴胡、天花粉、葛根、黄芩、桔梗、连翘、牛蒡子、生石膏、甘草、升麻。

Modification: For obvious swellon cheeks, add *Prunella Spica* (Xia Ku Cao). For sore throat, add *Lasiosphaera Calvatia* (Ma Bo), and *Isatidis Radix* (Ban Lan Gen).

加减：腮肿明显者，加夏枯草；咽喉红肿者，加马勃、板蓝根。

(2) Retention of heat toxin

(2) 热毒蕴结

Manifestations: High fever, vexation and thirst, sore throat, headache, vomiting, swelling and painful cheeks, aggravated by pressure, difficult to open mouth and chew, red tongue, yellow coating, rapid and surging pulse.

证候：高热，烦渴，咽红肿痛，或头痛、呕吐，腮部肿胀疼痛，坚硬拒按，张口、咀嚼困难，舌质红，苔黄，脉洪数。

Therapeutic method: To clear away heat, resolve toxin, soften stiffness and disperse retention.

治法：清热解毒，软坚散结。

Main formula: *Universal Salvation Toxin-Dispersing Decoction* (Pu Ji Xiao Du Yin) with modification.

主方：普济消毒饮加减。

Commonly used herbs: *Scutellariae Radix* (Huang Qin), *Coptidis Rhizoma* (Huang Lian), *Forsythia Fructus* (Lian Qiao), *Scrophulariae Radix*

常用药：黄芩、黄连、连翘、玄参、马勃、板蓝根、牛蒡子、僵蚕、升麻、柴胡、陈皮、

(Xuan Shen), *Lasiosphaera Calvatia* (Ma Bo), *Isatidis Radix* (Ban Lan Gen), *Arctii Fructus* (Niu Bang Zi), *Bombyx Batryticatus* (Jiang Can), *Cimicifugae Rhizoma* (Sheng Ma), *Bupleuri Radix* (Chai Hu), *Citri Reticulatae Pericarpium* (Chen Pi), *Platycodonis Radix* (Jie Geng), *Ginseng Radix* (Ren Shen), *Glycyrrhizae Radix Et Rhizoma* (Gan Cao).

桔梗、人参、甘草。

Modification: For high fever and thirst, add *Gypsum Fibrosum* (Sheng Shi Gao), and *Anemarrhenae Rhizoma* (Zhi Mu). For swollen and stiff cheeks, add *Salviae Miltiorrhizae Radix Et Rhizoma* (Dan Shen), and *Paeoniae Radix Rubra* (Chi Shao). For constipated stool, add *Rhei Radix Et Rhizoma* (Da Huang), and *Natrii Sulfas* (Mang Xiao).

加减:壮热、口渴者,加生石膏、知母;腮肿坚硬者,加丹参、赤芍;大便秘结者,加大黄、芒硝。

3.2 Transmuted pattern

3.2 变证

(1) Evils penetrating into the testicles and abdomen

(1) 邪窜睾腹

Manifestations: Gradual decline of swollen cheeks, repeated fever, unilateral or bilateral swollen and painful testicles, or pain in the lower abdomen, red tongue, yellow tongue coating, rapid and string-taut pulse.

证候:腮肿渐消,又见发热,一侧或两侧睾丸肿痛,或见少腹疼痛,舌质红,苔黄,脉弦数。

Therapeutic method: To clarify the liver, drain fire, activate blood and diminish swelling.

治法:清肝泻火,活血消肿。

Main formula: *Gentian Liver-Draining Decoction* (Long Dan Xie Gan Tang).

主方:龙胆泻肝汤加减。

Commonly used herbs: *Gentianae Radix Et Rhizoma* (Long Dan), *Gardeniae Fructus* (Zhi Zi), *Scutellariae Radix* (Huang Qin), *Bupleuri Radix* (Chai Hu), *Alismatis Rhizoma* (Ze Xie), *Angelicae Sinensis Radix* (Dang Gui), *Plantaginis Semen* (Che Qian Zi), *Rehmanniae Radix Cruda* (Sheng Di Huang), *Glycyrrhizae Radix Et Rhizoma* (Gan

常用药:龙胆、栀子、黄芩、柴胡、泽泻、当归、车前子、生地黄、甘草。

Cao).

Modification: For pain in the lower abdomen, add *Toosendan Fructus* (Chuan Lian Zi), and *Curcumae Radix* (Yu Jin). For painful and swollen testicles, add *Litchi Semen* (Li zhi He), *Corydalis Rhizoma* (Yan Hu Suo), *Persicae Semen* (Tao Ren), and *Paeoniae Radix Rubra* (Chi Shao).

加减：少腹疼痛者，加川楝子、郁金；睾丸肿痛者，加荔枝核、延胡索、桃仁、赤芍。

(2) Evils penetrating into the heart and liver

(2) 邪陷心肝

Manifestations: Swollen cheeks, together with lingering high fever, vexation and agitation, headache, stiff neck, vomiting, somnolence, coma, convulsion in the limbs, red tongue, yellow coating, rapid string-taut pulse.

证候：多在腮肿的同时，出现高热不退，烦躁不安，头痛项强，呕吐，嗜睡神昏，四肢抽搐，舌质红，苔黄，脉弦数。

Therapeutic method: To clear away heat, cool down Ying-nutrient system, extinguish wind and open the orifices.

治法：清热凉营，息风开窍。

Main formula: *Ying-Nutrient System-Clarifying Decoction* (Qing Ying Tang) and *Antelope Horn and Uncaria Decoction* (Ling Jiao Gou Teng Tang).

主方：清营汤合羚角钩藤汤加减。

Commonly used herbs: *Bubali Cornu* (Shui Niu Jiao), *Rehmanniae Radix Cruda* (Sheng Di Huang), *Scrophulariae Radix* (Xuan Shen), *Lophatheri Herba* (Dan Zhu Ye), *Ophiopogonis Radix* (Mai Dong), *Salviae Miltiorrhizae Radix Et Rhizoma* (Dan Shen), *Coptidis Rhizoma* (Huang Lian), *Lonicerae Flos Japonicae* (Jin Yin Hua), *Forsythia Fructus* (Lian Qiao), *Antelopis Tataricae Cornu* (Ling Yang Jiao), *Uncariae Ramulus Cum uncis* (Gou Teng), *Mori Folium* (Sang Ye), *Chrysanthemi Flos* (Ju Hua), *Paeoniae Radix Albae* (Bai Shao), *Bulbus Fritillariae Cirrhosae* (Chuan Bei Mu), *Bambusae Caulis in Taenias* (Zhu Ru), *Glycyrrhizae Radix Et Rhizoma* (Gan Cao).

常用药：水牛角、生地黄、玄参、淡竹叶、麦冬、丹参、黄连、金银花、连翘、羚羊角、钩藤、桑叶、菊花、白芍、川贝母、竹茹、甘草。

Modification: For high fever, coma and rela-

加减：高热、神昏、抽搐

tively severe convulsion, *Peaceful Palace Bovine Bezoar Pills* (An Gong Niu Huang Wan), *Purple Snow Elixir* (Zi Xue Dan) can be used in combination.

较甚者,可配合用安宫牛黄丸、紫雪丹。

4 Other therapies

4 其他疗法

4.1 Chinese Patent medicine

4.1 中成药

(1) *Isatidis Radix Granules* (Ban Lan Gen Chong Ji) is appropriate for epidemic mumps in pattern of warm toxin in the exterior.

(1) 板蓝根冲剂:适用于流行性腮腺炎温毒在表证。

(2) *Gentian Liver-Draining Pills* (Long Dan Xie Gan Wan) is appropriate for epidemic mumps in pattern of evils penetrating into the testicles and abdomen.

(2) 龙胆泻肝丸:适用于流行性腮腺炎邪窜睾腹证。

4.2 External therapy

4.2 外治疗法

(1) Select one of the followings: *Indigo Powder* (Qing Dai San), *Purple Gold Ingot* (Zi Jin Ding), *Agreeable Golden Yellow Powder* (Ru Yi Huang Jin San), mix it with vinegar or water, for topical application on the affected part, once or twice a day.

(1) 青黛散、紫金锭、如意金黄散,任选一种以食醋或清水调匀,外敷患处,每日1~2次。

(2) Select and smash one of Fresh *Taraxaci Herba* (Pu Gong Ying), fresh *Portulacae Herba* (Ma Chi Xian), fresh *Folium Hibisci Mutabilis* (Fu Rong Ye) or fresh *Hibisci Mutabilis Flos* (Fu Rong Hua), fresh *Opuntiae Radix et Caulis* (Xian Ren Zhang), for topical application on the affected area, once or twice a day.

(2) 鲜蒲公英、鲜马齿苋、鲜芙蓉叶或花、鲜仙人掌,任选一种捣烂外敷患处,每日1~2次。

Section 5 Infectious Mononucleosis

第5节 传染性单核细胞增多症

Infectious mononucleosis is an infectious disease caused by EB virus, clinically manifestated by fever, isthmitis, enlarged lymph nodes, enlarged liver and spleen, increased leukomonocytes in peripheral

传染性单核细胞增多症是由 EB 病毒引起的急性传染病,临床表现以发热,咽峡炎,淋巴结及肝脾肿大,外周

blood, and a large number of abnormal leukomonocytes.

血中淋巴细胞增多并出现大量异常淋巴细胞为特征。

The patients and those with latent infection are the resource of infection. The disease is transmitted through oral and throat secretion, occasionally by blood transfusion. The disease mostly occurs randomly, and may occur in all seasons. The susceptible group is mostly children or teenagers. The children under 6 years old are usually characterized by latent infection or mild infection. The elder children would present relatively severe symptoms, and even suffer from serious complications. The persistent immunity can be obtained after infection. The second infection is rare.

患者和隐性感染者为传染源，通过口咽分泌物接触传染，偶可经输血传播。多呈散发，四季均有，春秋季节较多。易感人群多为儿童或青少年，6岁以下儿童常表现为隐性感染或轻症，年长儿症状较重，甚至发生严重并发症。病后可获持久免疫力，第二次发病罕见。

In traditional Chinese medicine, it is categorized into the scope of "warm pestilence" in febrile disease.

本病属中医学温病"温疫"的范畴。

1 Etiology and pathogenesis

1 病因病机

The cause is related to infection of the seasonal warm evil, which enters through the mouth and nose, and invades Wei-defensive ability of the lung, causing disharmony between the exterior and Wei-defensive ability of the lung and further aversion to cold, fever, and sore throat. If the seasonal evil invades the stomach, the stomach qi would ascend reversely, leading to nausea and vomiting. If the evil toxin enters Qi-energy system and Ying-nutrient system, both Qi-energy system and Ying-nutrient system would flare abundantly, leading to high fever, vexation and thirst. If heat evil scorches and condenses body fluid into phlegm, phlegm and heat would be converged, leading to swollen lymph nodes. Exuberant heat, qi stagnation and blood sta-

病因为感受温疫时邪，时邪从口鼻而入，侵于肺卫，表卫失和，则恶寒发热，咽红肿痛；时邪犯胃，胃气上逆，见恶心呕吐。邪毒传入气营，气营两燔，则壮热烦渴；热邪灼津炼液成痰，痰热瘀结，故臀核肿大；热毒炽盛，气血瘀滞，可见腹中痞块；热毒夹湿，湿热蕴郁肝胆，可发为黄疸；热毒内窜营血，迫血妄行，可见皮下紫癜；热毒内陷心肝，可见昏迷、抽搐；痹阻脑络，故有口眼㖞斜、失语、吞咽困难、肢体瘫痪等症

sis may be manifested by palpable lumps in the abdomen. If heat toxin is mixed with dampness, dampness and heat would be accumulated in the liver and gallbladder, causing jaundice. If the heat toxin penetrates into Ying-nutrient system and blood internally, blood would be forced to flow frenetically, presenting subcutaneous purpura. If the heat toxin penetrates into the heart and liver, there may be coma and convulsion. If the collaterals of the brain are obstructed, there would be deviated eyes and mouth, aphasia, and body paralysis, etc. In the later stage, when yin is damaged and qi is exhausted, but the residual evil is not eliminated, there would be continuous low heat, dry mouth with less drinkings, flushed cheeks and night sweating, in pattern of yin damage due to lingering heat or pattern of damage of both qi and yin.

状。病至后期，阴伤气耗，而余邪未清，故低热缠绵，口干少饮，颧红盗汗，呈现热恋伤阴或气阴两伤之证。

The disease is caused by invasion of the seasonal warm evil into the lung and stomach and is transmitted and evolved based upon the rules of Wei-defensive system, Qi-energy system, Ying-nutrient system and Xue-blood system. The flaring abundance in Qi-energy system and Ying-nutrient system, scorching preponderance of heat toxin, and accumulation of phlegm and heat are the basic pathogenesis.

本病为温疫时邪，侵犯肺胃，并按卫气营血规律传变，以气营两燔、热毒炽盛、痰热瘀结为基本病机。

2　Key to diagnosis

(1) It mostly occurs in the spring and autumn. There could be a contact history.

(2) The onset is either acute or slow. The premonitory symptoms are general discomfort, headache, dizziness, poor appetite, nausea and vomiting, and mild diarrhea, etc. The typical symptoms are: ① Fever: body temperature between 38° C～

2　诊断要点

(1) 春秋季多见，可有接触史。

(2) 起病缓急不一，前驱症状为全身不适，头痛头昏，食纳不佳，恶心呕吐，轻度腹泻等。典型症状为：①发热，体温在 38～40 ℃，热型不

40°C, undefined fever type, duration of fever mostly in one to two weeks, and in several months in a few cases, not severe poisoning symptoms in most cases. ② Swollen lymph nodes: superficial swollen lymph nodes in most cases, in different size, no adhesion, present in the first week, and gradually fading away in two weeks, or lasting for months or years in some cases. ③ Isthmitis: sore throat, antiadoncus, congestion of throat, or tiny bleeding spots and ulcers in the throat. ④ Enlargement of the liver and spleen: mild enlargement of the spleen in about half of the cases, accompanied by pain and tenderness, and occasionally rupture of the spleen. Those with enlarged liver may have abnormal liver function, accompanied by the upper gastrointestinal symptoms of acute hepatitis, and mild jaundice in some cases. ⑤ Rash: Maculae, papules, cutaneous bleeding spots, or scarlet fever-like maculopapular eruption all over the body. ⑥ In the involvement of the lung, kidney, heart and brain, there may be the symptoms like cough, wheezing, bloody urine, convulsion due to fright, paralysis and aphasia.

定，热程大多 1～2 周，少数可达数月。中毒症状多不严重。②淋巴结肿大，大多数患者有浅表淋巴结肿大，大小不等，无粘连，在病程第 1 周即可出现，2 周后逐渐消退，少数持续数月甚至数年。③咽峡炎，有咽痛、扁桃体肿大、咽部充血或有小出血点及溃疡。④肝脾肿大，约半数有轻度脾肿大，伴疼痛及压痛，偶可发生脾破裂。肝大者可有肝功能异常，伴有急性肝炎的上消化道症状，部分有轻度黄疸。⑤皮疹，全身出现斑疹、丘疹、皮肤出血点或猩红热样斑疹。⑥累及肺、肾、心、脑时，可出现咳喘、血尿、惊厥、瘫痪失语等症状。

(3) Routine blood tests show total count of white blood cell mostly within the normal or slightly low range; one week after onset, there is increase in lymphocyte and monocyte, accounting for 50% or more. Atypical lymphocyte is over 10% or over 1.0×10^9/L. In serum, heterophile IgM antibody titer is higher than 1:64, or positive specific antibody of EB virus is of diagnostic value.

（3）血常规早期白细胞总数多在正常范围或稍低，发病 1 周后，白细胞总数增多，淋巴及单核增多，占 50%或以上，异型淋巴细胞超过 10%或 1.0×10^9/升以上。血清中嗜异性 IgM 抗体效价高于 1∶64，或 EB 病毒特异性抗体阳性有诊断意义。

3 Pattern identification and treatment

The key is to differentiate the different phases

3 辨证论治

辨证的关键在于分清

of stages of Wei-defensive system, Qi-energy system, Ying-nutrient system and Xue-blood system, to seize the pathomechanic nature of pathogenic heat, toxin, phlegm and blood stasis, and the mutual transfer and complication between excess pattern and deficiency pattern.

卫、气、营、血的不同阶段，抓住热、毒、痰、瘀的病机本质，以及实证、虚证的相互转化和兼夹。

When the evils linger in Wei-defensive system and Qi-energy system, fever, isthmitis, swollen lymph nodes and enlargement in the liver and spleen could usually be present, belonging to mild pattern. When the evils linger in Qi-energy system and Ying-nutrient system, cough, wheezing, jaundice, and stirring wind of preponderant heat would be accompanied, belonging to severe pattern. In the initial stage, the evils lingering in Wei-defensive system, Qi-energy system, and Ying-nutrient system belong to excess pattern. In the later stage, damage of body fluid, consumption of qi, deficiency in the Vital Energy, lingering of evils, and protracted duration belong to deficiency pattern. In pattern identification, it is necessary to grasp this basic pathologic feature of heat toxin, phlegm and blood stasis. The accumulation of phlegm could be manifested by swollen lymph nodes in the whole body. Blood stasis could be manifested by enlargement in the liver and spleen. The protracted duration could be manifested by patterns of deficiency complicated with excess.

邪在卫分气分，常以发热，咽峡炎、淋巴结及肝脾肿大为主，属轻症；邪在气营（血）分，常伴咳喘，黄疸，热盛动风，为重症。病初中期，邪在卫、气、营分，属实证；后期，津伤气耗，正虚邪恋，迁延不愈，属虚证。辨证时要抓住热毒痰瘀这一基本病理特征，痰结者可见全身淋巴结肿大，血瘀则可见肝脾肿大，病程迁延反复不愈者，可呈现虚中夹实证候。

The basic therapeutic principle is to clear away heat, resolve toxin, dissolve phlegm and expel blood stasis. If the evils stay in Wei-defensive system, it is appropriate to expel wind and alleviate the exterior. If in Qi-energy system, it is appropriate to clarify qi, discharge heat, dissolve phlegm, and disperse stagnation. If toxin enters Ying-nutrient system and

以清热解毒，化痰祛瘀为基本治则。在卫宜疏风解表，在气则清气泄热、化痰散结，毒入营血宜清营凉血，后期气阴耗伤则需益气养阴、兼清余邪，若兼湿邪夹杂，则应化湿通络。

Xue-blood system, it is appropriate to clarify Xue-blood system and the blood. In the later stage, consumption of qi and injury of yin should be treated by boosting qi and nourishing yin, and eliminating the residual evil. If complicated with damp evil, it is necessary to remove dampness and dredge the collaterals.

(1) Accumulation of evils in the lung and stomach

(1) 邪郁肺胃

Manifestations: Fever, slight aversion to wind and cold, sore throat, scrofula in the neck, poor appetite, vomiting and nausea, red tongue tip and margin, thin and white tongue coating or thin and yellow tongue coating, rapid and floating pulse.

证候:发热,微恶风寒,咽红疼痛,颈部瘰疬,纳差,恶心呕吐,舌边尖红,苔薄白或薄黄,脉浮数。

Therapeutic method: To expel wind, clear away heat, clarify the lung and benefit throat.

治法:疏风清热,清肺利咽。

Main formula: *Lonicera and Forsythia Powder* (Jia Jian Yin Qiao San) with modification.

主方:银翘散加减。

Commonly used herbs: *Lonicerae Flos Japonicae* (Jin Yin Hua), *Forsythia Fructus* (Lian Qiao), *Sojae Semen Praeparatum* (Dan Dou Chi), *Cremastrae seu Pleiones Pseudobulbus* (Shan Ci Gu), *Richosanthis Fructus* (Gua Lou), *Arctii Fructus* (Niu Bang Zi), *Schizonepetae Herba* (Jing Jie), *Menthae Haploalycis Herba* (Bo He), *Phragmitis Rhizoma* (Lu Gen), *Platycodonis Radix* (Jie Geng), *Glycyrrhizae Radix Et Rhizoma* (Gan Cao).

常用药:金银花、连翘、淡豆豉、山慈姑、瓜蒌、牛蒡子、荆芥、薄荷、芦根、桔梗、甘草。

Modification: For sore throat, add *Lasiosphaera Calvatia* (Ma Bo), *Scrophulariae Radix* (Xuan Shen), *Belamecandae Rhizoma* (She Gan), and *Sophorae Tonkinensis Radix Et Rhizoma* (Shan Dou Gen). For large scrofula, add *Prunella Spica* (Xia Ku Cao), *Bulbus Fritillariae Thumbergii* (Zhe Bei Mu), *Taraxaci Herba* (Pu Gong Ying), *Paeoniae Radix Rubra* (Chi Shao). For red skin rash, add *Arnebiae Radix* (Zi Cao), *Dictamni Cortex* (Bai

加减:咽喉肿痛者,加马勃、玄参、射干、山豆根;瘰疬较大者,加夏枯草、浙贝母、蒲公英、赤芍;皮疹色红者,加紫草、白鲜皮、蝉蜕。

Xian Pi), *Cicadae Periostracum* (Chan Tui).

(2) Flaring abundance in Qi-energy system and Ying-nutrient system

Manifestations: High fever, vexation and thirst, sore throat, swollen or even ulcerative tonsil, foul breathing, constipation, red face and lips, visible papules, scrofula, red tongue, lumps in the rib-side, red tongue, coarse and yellow coating, rapid and surging pulse.

Therapeutic method: To clarify qi, cool down Ying-nutrient system, resolve toxin and benefit the throat.

Main formula: *Scourge-clearing and Toxin-Vanquishing Decoction* (Qing Wen Bai Du Yin) with modification.

Commonly used herbs: *Gypsum Fibrosum* (Sheng Shi Gao), *Anemarrhenae Rhizoma* (Zhi Mu), *Glycyrrhizae Radix Et Rhizoma* (Gan Cao), *Coptidis Rhizoma* (Huang Lian), *Scutellariae Radix* (Huang Qin), *Gardeniae Fructus* (Zhi Zi), *Bubali Cornu* (Shui Niu Jiao), *Rehmanniae Radix Cruda* (Sheng Di Huang), *Paeoniae Radix Rubra* (Chi Shao), *Moutan Cortex Radicis* (Mu Dan Pi), *Forsythia Fructus* (Lian Qiao), *Scrophulariae Radix* (Xuan Shen), *Platycodonis Radix* (Jie Geng).

Modification: For lumps in the rib-side, add *Liver-Clarifying and Phlegm-Dissolving Pill* (Qing Gan Hua Tan Wan) with modifications. For fever, yellow color in the eyes and the skin, add *Virgate Wormwood Decoction* (Yin Chen Hao Tang) with modifications. For cough, rapid breathing, flaring nostrils, and blue lips, add *Ephedra, Apricot Kernel, Gypsum, and Licorice Decoction* (Ma Xing Shi Gan Tang) with modification. For rigidity of neck

(2) 气营两燔

证候:壮热烦渴,咽喉红肿疼痛,乳蛾肿大,甚则溃烂,口臭便秘,面红唇赤,皮疹显露,瘰疬,胁下痞块,舌质红,苔黄糙,脉洪数。

治法:清气凉营,解毒利咽。

主方:清瘟败毒饮加减。

常用药:生石膏、知母、甘草、黄连、黄芩、栀子、水牛角、生地黄、赤芍、牡丹皮、连翘、玄参、桔梗。

加减:胁下痞块者,可予清肝化痰丸加减;发热目黄,皮肤黄染者,可予茵陈蒿汤加减;咳嗽气急,鼻煽,口唇紫绀者,可予麻杏石甘汤加减;出现颈项强直,神识不清,肢体抽动,或瘫痪,口眼㖞斜,吞咽困难,失语,斜视,痴呆,迟钝等症状,可予犀地

and nape, unconsciousness, convulsion in the limbs, or paralysis, deviated eyes and mouth, difficulty in swallowing, aphasia, squinting, dullness, slow reaction, etc, add *Rhinoceros Horn and Rehmannia Collateral-Clarifying Decoction* (Xi Di Qing Luo Yin) with modification.

清络饮加减。

(3) Deficiency of Vital Energy and lingering of evils

(3) 正虚邪恋

Manifestations: Prolonged duration, gradual fading of fever, or low-grade fever, scrofula, obvious diminishing lumps in the rib-side, shortness of breath, lack of strength, thirst with less drinks, scanty and brown urine, dry and constipated stool, pale or red tongue, scanty or patchy peeled tongue coating, thready and weak pulse.

证候:病程日久,发热渐退,或见低热,瘰疬、胁下痞块明显缩小,气短乏力,口渴少饮,小便短赤,大便干结,舌质淡或红,苔少或花剥,脉细弱。

Therapeutic method: To boost qi, engender body fluid, clear away and resolve residual heat.

治法:益气生津,清解余热。

Main formula: *Sweet Wormwood and Turtle Shell Decoction* (Qing Hao Bie Jia Tang) with modification.

主方:青蒿鳖甲汤加味。

Commonly used herbs: *Artemisiae Annuae Herba* (Qing Hao), *Trionycis Carapax Et Rhizoma* (Bie Jia), *Rehmanniae Radix Cruda* (Sheng Di Huang), *Anemarrhenae Rhizoma* (Zhi Mu), *Moutan Cortex Radicis* (Mu Dan Pi), *Persicae Semen* (Tao Ren), *Paeoniae Radix Rubra* (Chi Shao).

常用药:青蒿、鳖甲、生地黄、知母、牡丹皮、桃仁、赤芍。

Modification: For dry and constipated stool, add *Richosanthis Fructus* (Gua Lou). For poor appetite, add *Setariae Fructus Germinatus* (Gu Ya), *and Hordei Fructus Germinatus* (Mai Ya). For swollen and intractable scrofula, add *Scrophulariae Radix* (Xuan Shen), *Ostreae Concha* (Mu Li), *Bulbus Fritillariae Thumbergii* (Zhe Bei Mu), *Prunella Spica* (Xia Ku Cao), and *Taraxaci Herba* (Pu Gong

加减:大便干结者,加瓜蒌;食欲不振者加谷芽、麦芽;瘰疬肿大经久不消者,加玄参、牡蛎、浙贝母、夏枯草、蒲公英;胁下痞块较大者,加丹参、郁金、三棱、莪术;小便黄赤,淋漓不尽者加白茅根、大蓟、小蓟、蒲黄。

Ying). For relatively large lumps in the rib-side, add *Salviae Miltiorrhizae Radix Et Rhizoma* (Dan Shen), *Curcumae Radix*(Yu Jin), *Sparganii Rhizoma* (San Leng), and *Curcuma Rhizoma* (E Zhu). For brown and yellow urine, and dribbling urintion, add *Imperatae Rhizoma* (Bai Mao Gen), *Cirsii japonica herba* (Da Ji), *Cirsii Herba*(Xiao Ji), and *Typhae Pollen* (Pu Huang).

4　Other therapies

4.1　Chinese Patent medicine

(1) *Purple Snow Elixir* (Zi Xue Dan) is appropriate for infectious mononucleosis in pattern of heat penetrating into the heart and liver.

(2) *Pulse-Engendering Decoction* (Sheng Mai Yin) is appropriate for infectious mononucleosis in pattern of deficiency in both qi and yin.

4.2　External therapy

(1) *Agreeable Golden Yellow Powder* (Ru Yi Jin Huang San): Mix it with tea or vinegar to make paste, apply to the swollen lymph nodes, twice a day, with the effects to clear away heat, resolve toxin, disperse accumulation and diminish swelling.

(2) *Tin-like Powder* (Xi Lei San), spray in appropriate amount at the throat, three times a day. This can be effective in resolving toxin and disinhibiting throat.

4　其他治疗

4.1　中成药

（1）紫雪丹:适用于传染性单核细胞增多症热陷心肝证。

（2）生脉饮:适用于传染性单核细胞增多症恢复期气阴两虚证。

4.2　外治疗法

（1）如意金黄散:用茶或醋调敷在肿大的淋巴结上,每日换敷 2 次,有清热解毒,散结消肿之效。

（2）锡类散:适量喷吹于咽部,每日 3 次,有解毒利咽之效。

Section 6　Hand-foot-mouth Disease

第 6 节　手足口病

Hand-foot-mouth disease is an acute eruptive contagious disease, caused by Coxsackievirus A16

手足口病是由肠道病毒引起的急性出疹性传染病,以

(CoxA 16) and enterovirus 71 (EV 71), and clinically characterized by maculopapules and herpes in the hand, foot and mouth. Often it occurs in the preschool children, and the highest incidence is in children under 3 years old. The patients and carriers are regarded as the resource of infection. It is mainly transmitted through the digestive tract, respiratory tract and intimate contact, etc. It occurs in the summer and autumn, and its prognosis is favourable. A few of critical cases may be complicated with carditis, cerebritis, and cerebrospinal meningitis (CSM), etc. The severe ones may threaten life. The fatal causes are related to brain stem encephalitis and neurogenic pulmonary edema.

柯萨奇A组16型(CoxA 16)、肠道病毒 71 型(EV 71)多见,临床以手、足、口腔等部位的斑丘疹、疱疹为特征。常见于学龄前儿童,3 岁以下发病率最高。患者和隐性感染者均为传染源,主要通过消化道、呼吸道和密切接触等途径传播。多见于夏秋季节,一般预后较好,少数重症患儿可并发心肌炎、脑炎、脑脊髓膜炎等,甚或危及生命,致死原因主要为脑干脑炎及神经源性肺水肿。

In traditional Chinese medicine, it belongs to the category of "seasonal pestilence" and "febrile diseasea".

本病属中医学"时疫""温病"等范畴。

1 Etiology and pathogenesis

It is caused by infection of exogenous seasonal evil of hand-foot-mouth disease. The involved organs are mainly the lung and spleen. Due to delicacy in the lung of the infants, the interstices are loose. Because of frequent insufficiency in the spleen, the spleen is damaged. If nursing care is inappropriate, the seasonal evil of hand-foot-mouth disease would enter through the mouth and nose, affecting the lung and spleen. If the lung qi fails in its diffusing ability and Wei-defensive qi is obstructed, exterior pattern of Wei-defensive ability of the lung would be present. The lung governs the skin and hair. The spleen governs the flesh. If the lung and spleen are damaged, water and dampness would be accumulated internally to combat with seasonal evil toxin,

1 病因病机

由外感手足口病时邪所致,其病变脏腑主要在肺脾。小儿肺脏娇嫩,腠理疏松;脾常不足,易受损伤。若调护失宜,手足口病时邪由口鼻而入,伤及肺脾。肺气失宣,卫阳被遏,则见肺卫表证;肺主皮毛,脾主肌肉,肺脾受损,水湿内停,与时行邪毒相搏,熏灼口腔,蕴蒸肌肤,则口咽部、手、足、臀部发生疱疹。一般邪轻病浅,预后良好。若素体虚弱,或感邪较重,邪盛正衰,湿热蒸盛,内燔气营,病情较重,甚则邪毒

burning the oral cavity and steaming the skin, and which lead to herpes in the mouth, throat, hand, foot, and buttocks. Generally, if the evil is mild, the disease would be shallow and the prognosis is favorable. If the body constitution is weak originally, or infected severely with the evil, and the evel is exuberant and Vital Energy declines, dampness and heat would be accumulated, to blaze Qi-energy system and Ying-nutrient system internally, leading to critical condition or even the transmuted pattern of coma, delirious speech and convulsion due to inward penetration of evil toxin. In severe cases, life may be threatened, due to yang injury by yin injury and collapse of the heart yang. The pathological location mainly lies in the lung and spleen and may involve the heart and liver.

内陷而见神昏谵语、抽搐等变证。严重者可因阴损及阳,心阳虚脱而危及生命。病位主要在肺脾,可波及心肝。

2 Key to diagnosis

(1) There is a contact history of hand-foot-mouth disease 1～2 weeks before the onset. The latent period is mostly 2～10 days, in an average of 3～5 days.

(2) Clinical manifestations

1) Ordinary cases: Acute onset, fever, herpes scattered in the oral mucosa, maculopapules and herpes on the hand, foot and buttocks, surrounded by inflammatory flush. There is little fluid inside herpes, probably accompanied by cough, runny nose and poor appetite, etc. In some cases, it is just manifested as skin rash or herpes angina. Mostlty, it will heal in a week, and the prognosis is favorable. In some cases, the skin rash is not typical. For instance, a single location is perhaps just manifested as maculopapules.

2 诊断要点

(1) 病前 1～2 周有手足口病接触史。潜伏期多为 2～10 日,平均 3～5 日。

(2) 临床表现

1) 普通病例:急性起病,发热,口腔黏膜出现散在疱疹,手、足和臀部出现斑丘疹、疱疹,疱疹周围可有炎性红晕,疱内液体较少。可伴有咳嗽、流涕、食欲不振等症状。部分病例仅表现为皮疹或疱疹性咽峡炎。多在 1 周内痊愈,预后良好。部分病例皮疹表现不典型,如单一部位或仅表现为斑丘疹。

2) Critical cases: In a few cases (especially under 3 years old), the pathological situation develops rapidly, and in 1～5 days after the onset, there can be meningitis, encephalitis (of which, brain stem encephalitis is most dangerous), cerebrospinal meningitis (CSM), pulmonary edema, and circulatory disturbance, etc. In fewer cases, the severely critical situation may cause death. The survivors may have sequelae.

2）重症病例：少数病例（尤其是小于3岁者）病情进展迅速，在发病1～5日出现脑膜炎、脑炎（以脑干脑炎最为凶险）、脑脊髓炎、肺水肿、循环障碍等，极少数病例病情危重，可致死亡，存活病例可留有后遗症。

(3) Routine blood test shows normal count of white blood cell count, and relative increase in the ratio between lymphocyte and monocyte.

3）血常规检查示白细胞计数正常，淋巴细胞和单核细胞比值相对增高。

3 Pattern differentiation and treatment

3 辨证论治

To identify its severity: Mild pattern is characterized by short duration, herpes merely in the palms, soles and mouth, sparsely scattered, red in color, no obvious flush at the bottom of herpes, clear fluid in herpes, mild general symptoms, or accompanied by pattern of failure of the lung in Wei-defensive and diffusing ability and pattern of failure of the spleen in transportation and transformation, with the symptoms of fever, runny nose, cough, nausea, vomiting, and diarrhea. Severe pattern is characterized by long duration, herpes on the four limbs, buttocks and other parts besides the palms, soles and mouth, densely distributed in clusters, in dark purple color, obvious red flush at the bottom, turbid fluids inside, and severe general symptoms, or accompanied by pattern of toxin scorching Qi-enegy system and Ying-nutrient system, with the symptoms of high fever, vexation and agitation, sore throat, refusal of food intake, brown urine, constipated stool, etc. The severe cases may present

辨轻重：轻证病程短，疱疹仅现于手足掌心及口腔部，稀疏散在，疹色红润，根盘红晕不著，疱液清亮。全身症状轻微，或伴低热、流涕、咳嗽、恶心、呕吐、泄泻等肺卫失宣、脾失健运证；重证病程长，疱疹除见手足掌心及口腔部外，四肢、臀部等其他部位也常累及，且分布稠密，或成簇出现，疹色紫暗，根盘红晕显著，疱液混浊，全身症状较重，常伴高热、烦躁、口咽疼痛、拒食、尿赤便结等毒炽气营证。严重者可因邪陷心肝，或邪毒犯心而出现心、肝经证候。

the symptoms and signs in the heart meridian and liver meridian, caused by penetration of evils into the heart and liver or invasion of evils into the heart.

The basic therapeutic principle is to clear away heat, dispel dampness, and resolve toxin. The mild patterns should be treated by diffusing the lung qi and resolving the exterior, clearing away heat and dissolving dampness. The severe patterns should be treated by clarifying qi, cooling down Ying-nutrient system, resolving toxin and dispeling dampness. The penetration of evil toxin into the heart and liver, and invasion of evil toxin into the heart should be treated in combination of the method to clarify the heart, open the orifices, extinguish wind, and relieve convulsion, and the method to boost qi, nourish yin, activate blood and disperse blood stasis.

以清热祛湿解毒为基本治则。轻证治以宣肺解表，清热化湿；重证治以清气凉营，解毒祛湿。出现邪毒内陷或邪毒犯心者，又当配伍清心开窍、息风镇惊；益气养阴、活血祛瘀等法。

(1) Invasion of evils into the lung and spleen

Manifestations: Slight fever or no fever, runny nose, cough, sore throat, poor appetite, nausea, vomiting and diarrhea, blisters in the mouth, present about one to two days later or at the same time, small ulcers after rupture of blisters, pain and salivation, no appetite, and rice-size or gram-size maculopapules in the palms and soles, present with development of the disease, and quickly turning into herpes, scattered sparsely, red in color, and no obvious flush at the bottom, clear fluids, red tongue, thin, yellow and slimy tongue coating, rapid and floating pulse.

Therapeutic method: To diffuse the lung qi, resolve the exterior, clear away heat and melt dampness.

(1) 邪犯肺脾

证候：发热轻微，或无发热，流涕咳嗽，咽红疼痛，或纳差恶心，呕吐泄泻，1～2 日后或同时出现口腔内疱疹，破溃后形成小的溃疡，疼痛流涎，不欲进食。随病情进展，手足掌心部出现米粒至绿豆大小斑丘疹，并迅速转为疱疹，分布稀疏，疹色红润，根盘红晕不著，疱液清亮，舌质红，苔薄黄腻，脉浮数。

治法：宣肺解表，清热化湿。

Main formula: *Sweet Dew Toxin-Dispersing Elixir* (Gan Lu Xiao Du Dan) with modification.

Commonly used herbs: *Lonicerae Flos Japonicae* (Jin Yin Hua), *Forsythia Furctus* (Lian Qiao), *Scutellariae Radix*(Huang Qin), *Menthae Haploalycis Herba* (Bo He), *Amomi Furctus Rotundus* (Dou Kou), *Pogostmonis Herba*(Huo Xiang), *Acori Rhizoma Tatarinowii* (Shi Chang Pu), *Talcum* (Hua Shi), *Artemisiae Scopariae Herba*(Yin Chen), *Isatidis Radix* (Ban Lan Gen), *Belamecandae Rhizoma* (She Gan), *Bulbus Fritillariae Thumbergii* (Zhe Bei Mu).

Modification: For nausea and vomiting, add *Perillae Caulis* (Zi Su Geng), *Bambusae Caulis in Taenias* (Zhu Ru). For diarrhea, add *Alismatis Rhizoma* (Ze Xie), and *Coicis Semen* (Yi Yi Ren). For high fever, add *Puerariae Radix* (Ge Gen), *Bupleuri Radix* (Chai Hu). For severe itching, add *Cicadae Periostracum* (Chan Tui), *Dictamni Cortex* (Bai Xian Pi). For aversion to cold, add *Ledebouriellae Radix* (Fang Feng), and *Schizonepetae Herba* (Jing Jie). For fever, thirst, nausea, vomiting, diarrhea, red tongue with yellow tongue coating, use *Pueraria, Scutellaria, and Coptis Decoction* (Ge Gen Huang Qin Huang Lian Tang) together.

(2) Accumulation and steaming of dampness and heat

Manifestations: Continuous high fever, vexation and agitation, thirst, herpes distributed densely or in clusters in the mouth, on hands and feet, limbs and buttocks, dark purple in color, obvious flush at the bottom and turbid fluid inside, foul breath, salivation, scorching pain, refusal of food, brown and yellow urine, constipated stool, crimson tongue,

主方:甘露消毒丹加减。

常用药:金银花、连翘、黄芩、薄荷、豆蔻、藿香、石菖蒲、滑石、茵陈、板蓝根、射干、浙贝母。

加减:恶心呕吐者,加紫苏梗、竹茹;泄泻加泽泻、薏苡仁;高热者,加葛根、柴胡;肌肤痒甚者,加蝉蜕、白鲜皮;恶寒者,加防风、荆芥;若发热、口渴、恶心呕吐、泄泻、舌红苔黄,合葛根黄芩黄连汤。

(2) 湿热蕴蒸

证候:持续高热,烦躁口渴,口腔、手足、四肢、臀部疱疹,分布稠密,或成簇出现,疹色紫暗,根盘红晕显著,疱液混浊,口臭流涎,灼热疼痛,甚或拒食,小便黄赤,大便秘结,舌质红绛,苔黄厚腻

slimy, thick and yellow or dry and yellow tongue coating, rapid and slippery pulse.

或黄燥，脉滑数。

Therapeutic method: To clear away heat, cool down Ying-nutrient system, resolve toxin and dispel dampness.

治法：清热凉营，解毒祛湿。

Main formula: *Scourge-Clearing and Toxin-Vanquishing Decoction* (Qing Wen Bai Du Yin) with modification.

主方：清瘟败毒饮加减。

Commonly used herbs: *Coptidis Rhizoma* (Huang Lian), *Scutellariae Radix* (Huang Qin), *Gardeniae Fructus* (Zhi Zi), *Forsythia Furctus* (Lian Qiao), *Gypsum Fibrosum* (Sheng Shi Gao), *Anemarrhenae Rhizoma* (Zhi Mu), *Rehmanniae Radix Cruda* (Sheng Di Huang), *Paeoniae Radix Rubra* (Chi Shao), *Moutan Cortex Radicis* (Mu Dan Pi), *Isatidis Folium Folium* (Da Qing Ye), *Arnebiae Radix* (Zi Cao), *Plantaginis Herba* (Che Qian Cao).

常用药：黄连、黄芩、栀子、连翘、生石膏、知母、生地黄、赤芍、牡丹皮、大青叶、紫草、车前草。

Modification: For much dampness, remove *Anemarrhenae Rhizoma* (Zhi Mu), and *Rehmanniae Radix Cruda* (Sheng Di Huang), add *Pogostmonis Herba* (Huo Xiang), *Talcum* (Hua Shi), and *Lophatheri Herba* (Dan Zhu Ye). For constipated stool, add *Rhei Radix Et Rhizoma* (Da Huang), and *Natrii Sulfas Exsiccatus* (Xuan Ming Fen). For fullness and distention in the abdomen, add *Aurantii Fructus Immaturus* (Zhi Shi), and *Magnoliae Officinalis Cortex* (Hou Pu). For thirst with preference for drinks, add *Ophiopogonis Radix* (Mai Dong), and *Phragmitis Rhizoma* (Lu Gen). For vexation and agitation, add *Sojae Semen Praeparatum* (Dan Dou Chi), and *Nelumbinis Plumula* (Lian Zi Xin). For severe itching, add *Dictamni Cortex* (Bai Xian Pi), and *Kochiae Fructus* (Di Fu

加减：偏于湿重者，去知母、生地黄，加藿香、滑石、淡竹叶；大便秘结者，加大黄、玄明粉；腹胀满者，加枳实、厚朴；口渴喜饮者，加麦冬、芦根；烦躁不安者，加淡豆豉、莲子心；瘙痒重者，加白鲜皮、地肤子。若邪毒炽盛，内陷厥阴，而见壮热、神昏、抽搐者，宜送服安宫牛黄丸或紫雪丹。若邪毒犯心，而见心悸、胸闷、气短者，又当参照病毒性心肌炎节施治。

Zi). For penetration of preponderant evil toxin into Jueyin, manifested by high fever, coma, and convulsion, it is appropriate to take *Peaceful Palace Bovine Bezoar Pill* (An Gong Niu Huang Wan) or *Purple Snow Elixir* (Zi Xue Dan). For invasion of evil toxin into the heart, manifested by palpitation, oppression in the chest, and shortness of breath, refer to Section of Viral Myocarditis for treatment.

4 Other therapies

4.1 Chinese Patent medicine

(1) *Heat-Clearing and Toxin-Resolving Oral Liquid* (Qing Re Jie Du Kou Fu Ye) is appropriate for hand-foot-mouth disease in pattern of invasion of evil into the lung and spleen.

(2) *Dual Coptis Oral Liquid* (Shuang Huang Lian Kou Fu Ye) is appropriate for hand-foot-mouth disease in pattern of invasion of evil into the lung and spleen.

(3) *Infantile Quick Heat-Clearing Oral Liquid* (Xiao Er Re Su Qing Kou Fu Ye) is appropriate for hand-foot-mouth disease in pattern of invasion of evil into the lung and spleen.

(4) *Gardenia Flower Oral Liquid* (Huang Zhi Hua Kou Fu Ye) is appropriate for hand-foot-mouth disease due to preponderance of heat toxin.

(5) *Stomach-Clearing Coptis Pill* (Qing Wei Huang Lian Wan) is appropriate for hand-foot-mouth disease in pattern of steaming and preponderance of dampness and heat.

4.2 External therapy

(1) *Mirabilitum Praeparatum* (Xi Guan Shuang), *Borneol and Borax Powder* (Bing Peng San), *Pearl and Bezoar Powder* (Zhu Huang San),

4 其他疗法

4.1 中成药

（1）清热解毒口服液：适用于手足口病邪犯肺脾证。

（2）双黄连口服液：适用于手足口病邪犯肺脾证。

（3）小儿热速清口服液：适用于手足口病邪犯肺脾证。

（4）黄栀花口服液：适用于手足口病偏于热毒炽盛者。

（5）清胃黄连丸：适用于手足口病湿热蒸盛证。

4.2 外治疗法

（1）西瓜霜、冰硼散、珠黄散、喉风散、锡类散，任选1种，涂搽口腔患处，每日3

Throat Wind Powder (Hou Feng San), and *Tin-like Powder* (Xi Lei San), select one of these, and apply to the affected area, three times a day.

次。

(2) *Golden Yellow Powder* (Jin Huang San), *Indigo Powder* (Qing Dai San), *Purple Gold Spindle* (Zi Jing Ding), select one of the three, mix it with sesame oil, apply to the affected areas on hand and foot, three times a day.

（2）金黄散、青黛散、紫金锭，任选 1 种，麻油调，敷于手足疱疹患处，每日 3 次。

(3) Decoct *Lonicerae Flos Japonicae* (Jin Yin Hua) 15g, *Isatidis Radix* (Ban Lan Gen) 15g, *Taraxaci Herba* (Pu Gong Ying)15g, *Plantaginis Herba* (Che Qian Cao) 15g, *Spirodelae Herba* (Fu Ping) 15g, *Phellodendri Cortex Chinensis(Huang Bo)* 10g, wash the affected parts on the hand and foot with herbal decoction, used for severe condition.

（3）金银花 15 克，板蓝根 15 克，蒲公英 15 克，车前草 15 克，浮萍 15 克，黄柏 10 克。水煎外洗手足疱疹处。适用于手足疱疹重者。

(4) Grind *Calcinatum Gypsum Fibrosum* (Duan Shi Gao) 30g, *Phellodendri Cortex Chinensis* (Huang Bo) 15g, *Concha Meretricis seu Cyclinae* (Ge Ke) 15g, *Angelicae Radix Dahuricae* (Bai Zhi) 10g, *Minium* (Huang Dan) 3g, into fine powder together. Mix it with oil and apply onto the affected parts on the hand and foot, used for a large number of herpes, severe pain and itching.

（4）煅石膏 30 克，黄柏 15 克，蛤壳 15 克，白芷 10 克，黄丹 3 克。共为细粉，油调外敷手足疱疹处。适用于疱疹多而痛痒甚者。

Chapter 11 Parasitic Diseases

第 11 章 寄生虫病

Section 1 Roundworm Disease

Roundworm disease, the most common intestinal parasitic disease in childhood, is caused by adult roundworm living in the intestines of the human body.

1 Etiology and pathogenesis

The disease is caused by swallowing infectious roundworm eggs, which grow into adult roundworms and live in the intestines. While lodging in the intestines, worms would disturb frequently, leading to restlessness in the intestines and inhibiting qi dynamic. Therefore, abdominal pain would be present while worms move, and abdominal pain would disappear while worms do not move. If roundworms disturb the intestines, the stomach qi would flow upward reversely, causing vomiting, nausea and drooling. While living in the intestines, roundworms would steal the essences of grain and water. When the spleen fails in transportation and transformation, the functions of the stomach would be hindered, resulting in indigestion, and abnormal appetite, emaciation due to failed nourishment of the skin and flesh by diet, sallow facial complexion and emaciated body and fatigued spirit in severe

第 1 节 蛔虫病

蛔虫病，是儿童时期最常见的肠道寄生虫病，由蛔虫成虫寄生于人体肠道而引起。

1 病因病机

因吞入感染性蛔虫卵，发育为成虫寄生肠道。虫踞肠内，频频扰动，致肠腑不宁，气机不利，故虫动则腹痛，虫静而痛止。蛔扰胃腑，胃气上逆，见呕恶流涎。蛔虫居于肠内，劫取水谷精微，脾失健运，胃滞不化，故食欲异常，饮食不荣肌肤而见消瘦，重者面黄肌瘦，精神疲乏，甚至肚腹胀大，四肢瘦弱，形成蛔疳。虫聚肠内，脾胃失和，内生湿热，熏蒸于上，可见烦躁、龂齿等症。病位主要在脾胃、肠腑，亦可影响到胆腑。

condition, and even distending sensation in the abdomen, thin and weak limbs, forming so-called roundworm sign. While worms gather in the intestines, the spleen and stomach would be disharmonious, dampness and heat would develop internally and steam upward, causing vexation, agitation, and grinding of the teeth. The pathological location mainly lies in the spleen, stomach, intestines, and may also involve the gallbladder.

2　Key to diagnosis

(1) Abdominal pain around the umbilicus occurs repeatedly, alleviated by rubbing and pressing, accompanied by poor appetite, allotriophagia, susceptible to nausea, vomiting, diarrhea or constipation, and vexation, listless spirit and grinding of teeth during sleep in some cases, and malnutrition, anemia, and even retarded growth in severe cases.

(2) Roundworm eggs are found in feces. There is a history of vomiting or defecating worm.

3　Pattern identification and treatment

It is principally based upon pattern identification in accordance with the theory of six hollow organs. The disease is mianly related to the small intestines, stomach, gallbladder, and large intestines. The ordinary pattern is most common. The lodgement of roundworms in the intestines belongs mostly to excess pattern, mainly manifested by recurrent abdominal pain around the umbilicus. The transmuted patterns, respectively termed roundworm syncope pattern, and roundworm conglomeration pattern, are induced because roundworms enter the diaphragm and go to the gallbladder, presenting abdominal pain in the subcostal area or

2　诊断要点

（1）腹痛，位于脐周，反复发作，喜揉按；食欲不振，异食癖；易发生恶心、呕吐、腹泻或便秘；部分患儿烦躁，精神萎靡，龂齿；病情严重者可造成营养不良、贫血，甚至生长发育迟缓。

（2）粪便中查到蛔虫卵，吐虫史或排虫史。

3　辨证论治

以六腑辨证为纲，病在小肠、胃腑、胆腑、大肠。常证最为多见，虫踞肠腑，多为实证，以发作性脐周腹痛为主要症状。变证有蛔厥证和虫瘕证；蛔厥证，为蛔虫入膈，窜入胆腑，腹痛在剑突下或右上腹，呈阵发性剧烈绞痛，痛时肢冷汗出，多有呕吐，且常见呕吐胆汁和蛔虫；虫瘕者，虫团聚结肠腑，腹部剧痛不止，阵发性加重，腹部可扪及活动性条索感或团状

right upper abdomen, in severe paroxysmal colic pain, accompanied by cold limbs and cold sweating, or frequently by vomiting, and vomiting with bile and roundworm. In roundworm conglomeration pattern, roundworms gather and tangle in the intestines, leading to incessant severe pain that is aggravated paroxysmally, and palpable mobile stripe-like or lump-like mass in the abdomen, and accompanied by severe vomiting and frequent constipation.

包块，伴有剧烈呕吐，大便多不通。

The treatment is designed to deal with the causastive reason and clinical symptoms respectively. The method to deal with the causastive reason is supposed to kill and expel roundworms, in combination with the therapy to regulate the spleen and stomach. Those with strong body constitution should be treated by eliminating the worms in priority, and then regulating the spleen and stomach. Those with weak body constitution should be treated by expelling the worms and supporting the Vital Energy simultaneously. Those with body deficiency should be treated by regulating the spleen and stomach before eliminating the worms. In the transmuted patterns of roundworm syncope pattern, and roundworm conglomeration pattern, because the pathological condition is comparatively severe, and abdominal pain is serious, the treatment should be given by the medicinal products in sour, acrid and bitter flavor to calm down the worms and stop pain for dealing with the symptoms, in order to seek opportunity to expel worms for dealing with the causative reason. Both the causative reason and clinical symptoms could be treated simultaneously by calming down the worms, expelling the worms, and promoting purgation, so as to dredge and benefit six

治疗分治本和治标。治本之法为杀虫驱蛔，需结合调理脾胃。体壮者，当先驱虫，后调脾胃；体弱者，驱虫扶正并举；体虚甚者，应先调理脾胃，继而驱虫。发生蛔厥、虫瘕等变证时，病情较重，腹痛剧烈，可先予酸、辛、苦等药味，以安蛔止痛治标，其后再择机驱虫治本；也可以标本兼施，安蛔、驱虫、通下并用，使六腑通利，腹痛较快缓解。

hollow organs and to alleviate abdominal pain more quickly.

(1) Pattern of roundworm in the intestines

Manifestations: Intermittent pain in the umbilicus and abdomen, irregular defecation or constipation, diarrhea, or roundworm in stool, no appetite for food or preference for strange food, restless sleep, sallow complexion and emaciation, distending and enlarged belly, palpable stripe-like stuff in the abdomen in severe condition, red tongue tip, white or slimy tongue coating, slippery and string-taut pulse.

Therapeutic method: To kill and expel roundworm, regulate the spleen and stomach.

Main formula: *Quisqualis Powder* (Shi Jun Zi San) with modification.

Commonly used herbs: *Quisqualis Fructus* (Shi Jun Zi), *Ulmi Semen* (Wu Yi Ren), *Arecae Semen* (Bing Lang), *Arecae Semen* (Da Fu Zi).

Modification: For obvious abdominal pain, add *Corydalis Rhizoma* (Yan Hu Suo), and *Toosendan Fructus* (Chuan Lian Zi) to circulate qi and relieve pain. For distending sensation in the abdomen and constipation, add *Rhei Radix Et Rhizoma* (Da Huang) and *Rehmanniae Radix Praeparata* (Shu Di Huang) to kill worms and promote purgation. For nausea and vomiting, add *Bambusae Caulis in Taenias* (Zhu Ru), and *Zingiberis Rhizoma Recens* (Sheng Jiang) to rectify reversely-flowing qi and check nausea.

(2) Roundworm Syncope Pattern

Manifestations: Sudden colic pain in the abdomen with body coiled and bent, restlessness, cold limbs, sweating, nausea, vomiting of bile or round-

(1) 肠虫证

证候:脐腹疼痛,时作时止;大便不调,或便秘,或泄泻,或便下蛔虫;不思饮食,或嗜异食;夜寐不安;面黄消瘦,肚腹胀大,严重者腹部可扪及条索状物。舌尖红,苔白或腻,脉弦滑。

治法:驱蛔杀虫,调理脾胃。

主方:使君子散加减。

常用药:使君子、芜荑仁、槟榔、大腹子。

加减:腹痛明显者,加延胡索、川楝子行气止痛;腹胀便秘者,加大黄、槟榔杀虫泻下;呕吐者,加竹茹、生姜降逆止呕。

(2) 蛔厥证

证候:突然腹部绞痛,弯腰曲背,辗转不宁,肢冷汗出,恶心,呕吐胆汁或蛔虫;

worm, continuous abdominal pain in paroxysmal aggravation in severe cases, probably accompanied by aversion to cold, fever, even jaundice.

重者腹痛持续而阵发性加剧，可伴畏寒发热，甚至出现黄疸。

Therapeutic method: To calm down roundworm, stop pain, and expel roundworm.

治法：安蛔定痛驱虫。

Main formula: *Mume Pill* (Wu Mei Wan) with modification

主方：乌梅丸加减。

Commonly used herbs: *Mume Fructus* (Wu Mei), *Asari Radix Et Rhizoma* (Xi Xin), *Zingiberis Rhizoma* (Gan Jiang), *Coptidis Rhizoma* (Huang Lian), *Angelicae Sinensis Radix* (Dang Gui), *Aconiti Lateralis Radix Praeparata* (Fu Zi), *Pericarpium Zanthoxyli* (Shu Jiao), *Cinnamomi Ramulus* (Gui Zhi), *Ginseng Radix* (Ren Shen), *Phellodendri Cortex Chinensis* (Huang Bo).

常用药：乌梅、细辛、干姜、黄连、当归、附子、蜀椒、桂枝、人参、黄柏。

Modification: For fever and jaundice, take out warm and dry herbs like *Zingiberis Rhizoma* (Gan Jiang), *Aconiti Lateralis Radix Praeparata* (Fu Zi), and *Cinnamomi Ramulus* (Gui Zhi), add *Artemisiae Scopariae Herba* (Yin Chen), *Gardeniae Fructus* (Zhi Zi), *Scutellariae Radix* (Huang Qin), and *Rhei Radix Et Rhizoma* (Da Huang) to clear away dampness and heat, calm down roundworm and remove jaundice. If diagnosed as dead roundworm in the biliary tract, it is advisable to prescribe *Major Qi-Coordinating Decoction* (Da Cheng Qi Tang) plus *Artemisiae Scopariae Herba* (Yin Chen) to relax the bowels, benefit the gallbladder and expel roundworm.

加减：发热黄疸者，去干姜、附子、桂枝等温燥之品，加茵陈、栀子、黄芩、大黄清利湿热，安蛔退黄。如确诊为胆道死蛔，直接予大承气汤加茵陈通腑利胆排蛔。

Chapter 12 Disease of the Newborn

第 12 章 新生儿疾病

Section 1 Jaundice of the Newborn

第 1 节 新生儿黄疸

Jaundice of the newborn refers to stained yellow color in the cutaneous mucosa or other organs, caused by accumulation of bilirubin in the body. If bilirubin in the blood of the newborn is over 5～7 mg/dl, jaundice by the naked eye would be present. Jaundice of the newborns can be physiological and pathologic. In this section, only the pathologic jaundice is mainly discussed. When the unconjugated bilirubin is too high in the blood, bilirubin encephalopathy (nuclear jaundice) would be induced, propably resulting in sequela of the nervous system in varying degrees. Those in critical conditions may die.

新生儿黄疸是因胆红素在体内积聚而引起的皮肤黏膜或其他器官黄染。若新生儿血中胆红素超过 5～7 毫克/分升即可出现肉眼可见的黄疸。新生儿黄疸可分为生理性和病理性，本节主要讨论病理性黄疸。当血中未结合胆红素过高时，可引起胆红素脑病（核黄疸），可留有不同程度的神经系统后遗症，重者甚至死亡。

In traditional Chinese medicine, it is held to be related to fetal constitution, so it is called "fetal jaundice".

中医学认为本病与胎禀因素有关，故称为"胎黄"或"胎疸"。

1 Etiology and pathogenesis

1 病因病机

The main pathogenic factors are dampness and heat, and cold and dampness. There is constitutional preponderance of dampness or internal accumulation of dampness and heat in the pregnant woman left to the fetus. There are infants infected with

湿热与寒湿是其主要致病因素。孕母素体湿盛或内蕴湿热之毒，遗于胎儿，或因胎产之时，出生之后，婴儿感受湿热邪毒。或因小儿先天

dampness and heat during the birth or after birth. There are dampness and turbidity produced internally by deficiency of spleen yang due to insufficiency of the prenatal natural endowment. And there are infants invaded by damp evil after birth. Moreover, due to constitutional insufficiency of natural endowment in the infants, the collaterals are obstructed, or there is stagnation of qi and blood due to retention of dampness and heat in the liver meridian for long time, which leading to jaundice.

禀赋不足，脾阳虚弱，湿浊内生；或生后为湿邪所侵。另外，部分小儿禀赋不足，脉络阻滞，或湿热蕴结肝经日久，气血郁阻而发黄。

2 Key to diagnosis

2 诊断要点

(1) Jaundice appears early (within 24 hours after birth), develops fast, with obvious yellow color. It may reappear after abatement, or jaundice appears late but lingers persistently. There could be enlargement in the liver and spleen, fatigued spirit, no desire to suck breast-milk, gray and white stool.

（1）黄疸出现早（出生24小时内），发展快，黄色明显，可消退后再次出现，或黄疸出现迟，持续不退。肝脾可见肿大，精神倦怠，不欲吮乳，大便或呈灰白色。

(2) Serum bilirubin and jaundice index is obviously in increase.

（2）血清胆红素、黄疸指数显著增高。

(3) Urine bilirubin is positive; urobilinogen test is positive or negative.

（3）尿胆红素阳性，尿胆原试验阳性或阴性。

(4) Blood type is determined in both mother and child, in order to exclude dynamic jaundice caused by incompatibility of ABO or RH blood type.

（4）母子血型测定，以排除ABO或Rh血型不合引起的溶血性黄疸。

(5) Liver functions may be normal.

（5）肝功能可正常。

(6) The examination of antigen and antibody system related to hepatitis should be done for hepatitis syndrom.

（6）肝炎综合征应作肝炎相关抗原抗体系统检查。

3 Pattern identification and treatment

3 辨证论治

In pattern identification of this disease, it is necessary to differentiate between physiological jaundice and pathological jaundice first, and then to

本病辨证首先要区分生理性黄疸与病理性黄疸，然后再对病理性黄疸辨其阴黄

differentiate between yin jaundice and yang jaundice in pathological jaundice. For its transmuted pattern, it is necessary to note the difference between fetal yellow stirring wind and collapse of fetal jaundice.

阳黄，针对其变证要注意胎黄动风与胎黄虚脱的区别。

The pathological jaundice should be treated by removing dampness and abating jaundice, which is the basic therapeutic principle. According to differences of yang jaundice and yin jaundice, the treatment should be given respectively to abate jaundice by clearing away heat and removing dampness, by warming up the Middle Energizer and dissolving dampness, and to disperse blood stasis and eliminate accumulation for pattern of qi stagnation and blood stasis.

病理性黄疸的治疗以利湿退黄为基本原则。根据阳黄与阴黄的不同，分别治以清热利湿退黄和温中化湿退黄，气滞血瘀证以化瘀消积为主。治疗过程中尚须顾护初生儿脾胃，避免苦寒伤正。

(1) Accumulation and steaming of damp and heat

（1）湿热郁蒸

Manifestations: Yellow color in the face, eyes and skin, bright like orange, loud crying with no desire to suck milk, thirst with dry lips, fever, constipated stool, dark yellow urine, red tongue, slimy and yellow tongue coating.

证候：面目皮肤发黄，色泽鲜明如橘，哭声响亮，不欲吮乳，口渴唇干，或有发热，大便秘结，小便深黄，舌质红，苔黄腻。

Therapeutic method: To clear away heat and remove dampness.

治法：清热利湿。

Main formula: *Virgate Wormwood Decoction* (Yin Chen Hao Tang) with modifications.

主方：茵陈蒿汤加减。

Commonly used herbs: *Artemisiae Scopariae Herba* (Yin Chen Hao), *Gardeniae Fructus* (Zhi Zi), *Rhei Radix Et Rhizoma* (Da Huang).

常用药：茵陈蒿、栀子、大黄。

Modification: For severe fever, add *Polygoni Cuspidati Rhizoma Et Radix* (Hu Zhang), and *Gentianae Radix Et Rhizoma* (Long Dan Cao) to clear away heat and drain fire. For severe dampness, add *Polyporus* (Zhu Ling) and *Talcum* (Hua Shi) to

加减：热重者，加虎杖、龙胆草清热泻火；湿重者，加猪苓、滑石渗湿利水；呕吐者，加半夏、竹茹和中止呕；腹胀者，加厚朴、枳实行气消

eliminate dampness and water. For vomiting, add *Pinelliae Rhizoma* (Ban Xia) and *Bambusae Caulis in Taenias* (Zhu Ru) to harmonize the Middle Energizer and check vomiting. For abdominal distention, add *Magnoliae Officinalis Cortex* (Hou Pu) and *Aurantii Fructus Immaturus* (Zhi Shi) to circulate qi and disperse distention.

胀。

(2) Obstruction of cold and dampness

(2) 寒湿阻滞

Manifestations: Yellowing face, eyes and skin, dull in color, prolonged yellowing without abating, listlessness of spirit, limbs lack of warmth, torpid intake, thin sloppy stool grey in color, short voidings of urine, pale tongue, slimy white tonguecoating.

证候:面目皮肤发黄,色泽晦暗,持久不退,精神萎靡,四肢欠温,纳呆,大便溏薄色灰白,小便短少,舌质淡,苔白腻。

Therapeutic method: To warm up the Middle Energizer and melt dampness.

治法:温中化湿。

Main formula: *Virgate Wormwood Qi-Rectifying Decoction* (Yin Chen Li Zhong Tang) with modifications.

主方:茵陈理中汤加减。

Commonly used herbs: *Artemisiae Scopariae Herba* (Yin Chen), *Atractylodis Macrocephalae Rhizoma* (Bai Zhu), *Ginseng Radix* (Ren Shen), *Zingiberis Rhizoma* (Gan Jiang).

常用药:茵陈、白术、人参、干姜。

Modification: For severe cold, add *Aconiti Lateralis Radix Praeparata Secta* (Fu Pian) to warm up yang. For enlargement of the liver and spleen, and obstruction of the collaterals, add *Sparganii Rhizoma* (San Leng) and *Curcuma Rhizoma* (E Zhu) to activate blood and disperse blood stasis. For poor appetite, add *Massa Fermentata Medicinalis* (Shen Qu) and *Amomi Fructus* (Sha Ren) to circulate qi and arouse the spleen.

加减:寒盛者,加附片温阳;肝脾肿大,络脉瘀阻者,加三棱、莪术活血化瘀;食少纳呆者,加神曲、砂仁行气醒脾。

(3) Qi Stagnation and Blood Stasis

(3) 气滞血瘀

Manifestations: Yellow color in the face, eyes

证候:面目皮肤发黄,颜

and skin, in dark luster and persistant existence, hard lumps under right rib-side, abdominal distention, exposed green-blue veins, blood stasis patches, epistaxis, dark red lips, blood stasis speckles on the tongue, yellow tongue coating.

色逐渐加深，晦暗无华，右胁下痞块质硬，肚腹膨胀，青筋显露，或见瘀斑、衄血，唇色暗红，舌见瘀点，苔黄。

Therapeutic method: To disperse blood stasis and diminish accumulation.

治法：化瘀消积。

Main formula: *Blood Mansion Stasis-Expelling Decoction* (Xue Fu Zhu Yu Tang) with modification.

主方：血府逐瘀汤加减。

Commonly used herbs: *Angelicae Sinensis Radix* (Dang Gui), *Rehmanniae Radix Cruda* (Sheng Di Huang), *Persicae Semen* (Tao Ren), *Carthami Flos* (Hong Hua), *Aurantii Fructus* (Zhi Qiao), *Paeoniae Radix Rubra* (Chi Shao), *Bupleuri Radix* (Chai Hu), *Glycyrrhizae Radix Et Rhizoma Cruda* (Gan Cao), *Platycodonis Radix* (Jie Geng), *Chuanxiong Rhizoma* (Chuan Xiong), *Achyranthis Bidentatae Radix* (Niu Xi).

常用药：当归、生地黄、桃仁、红花、枳壳、赤芍、柴胡、甘草、桔梗、川芎、牛膝。

Modification: For dry and constipated stool, add *Rhei Radix Et Rhizoma* (Da Huang) to relax the bowels. For blood stasis speckles on the skin and bloody stool, add *Moutan Cortex Radicis* (Mu Dan Pi) and *Agrimoniae Herba* (Xian He Cao) to activate blood and check bleeding. For abdominal distention, add *Aucklandiae Radix* (Mu Xiang) and *Cortex Citri medica* (Xiang Yuan Pi) to rectify qi. For hard lump in the rib-side, add *Manis Squama* (Chuan Shan Jia) and *Whitmania pigra Whitman* (Shui Zhi) to activate blood and disperse blood stasis.

加减：大便干结者，加大黄通腑；皮肤瘀斑、便血者，加牡丹皮、仙鹤草活血止血；腹胀者，加木香、香橼皮理气；胁下痞块质硬者，加穿山甲、水蛭活血化瘀。

Chapter 13 Other Diseases

第 13 章 其他病证

Section 1 Sweating Pattern

Sweating pattern refers to a disease of excessive or even profuse sweating in the local or whole body of the child, under normal environment and in quiet state.

Due to lack of full development in the physique and qi and loose and thin interstices, plus vigorous life activities and diffusion of the clear yang, the children are more likely to sweat than adults, especially on the head. If there is excessive sweating in hot weather, thick clothes and quilts, quick milk-feeding or strenuous activities, without other abnormal signs, it is not pathological. Sweating patterns in children are divided into spontaneous sweating and night sweating. Sweating starting in sleeping and ending after waking up is night sweating. Sweating starting with no reason in waking up or sleeping is spontaneous sweating. Spontaneous sweating and night sweating are often seen simultaneously in children.

1 Etiology and pathogenesis

Sweat is one of the five kinds of body fluids in the human body, transformed from steaming and evaporation of body fluids by yang qi. Sweat is fluid

第 1 节 汗证

汗证是指小儿在正常环境和安静状态下，全身或局部无故出汗过多，甚则大汗淋漓的一种病证。

小儿由于形气未充、腠理疏薄，加之生机旺盛、清阳发越，故较成人易出汗，且头汗最多。若在天气炎热，衣被过厚，或喂奶过急，活动剧烈的情况下汗多，但无其他异常，则不属病态。小儿汗证有自汗、盗汗之分。睡中出汗，醒时汗止者，称为盗汗；不分寤寐，无故出汗者，称为自汗；小儿汗证往往自汗、盗汗并见。

1 病因病机

汗是人体五液之一，由阳气蒸化津液而来。汗为心之液，卫气为阳，营血为阴，

of the heart. Wei-defensive qi is yang. Ying-nutrient qi is yin. When yin and yang are balanced, and Ying-nutrient qi and Wei-defensive qi are in harmony, body fluids could be contained internally. If imbalance exists between qi and blood, between yin and yang, and between solid organs and hollow organs, and if disharmony exists between Ying-nutrient qi and Wei-defensive qi, and dysfunction exists in Wei-defensive yang, the interstices would fail to perform its opening and closing ability, leading to discharge of sweating. Sweating pattern in children is mostly related to weak body constitution.

阴阳平衡，营卫调和，则津液内敛。若阴阳脏腑气血失调，营卫不和，卫阳不固，腠理开阖失司，则汗液外泄。小儿汗证的发生，多责之于体虚。

Sweating pattern in children is caused by imbalance between yin and yang, and divided into deficiency pattern and excess pattern. Clinically, deficiency pattern is commonly seen, manifested by insecurity of the exterior due to deficiency, by poor astringency due to yin deficiency, and by deficiency in both qi and yin. The excess pattern is often related to accumulated heat in the heart and spleen.

小儿汗证为阴阳失衡所致，有虚实之分，临床以虚证多见。虚证中常见表虚不固、阴虚不守、气阴两虚；实证为心脾积热。

2 Key to diagnosis

(1) It is mainly manifested by general or local excessive sweating under the normal environment and quiet state.

(2) Sweating starting in sleeping and ending after waking up is night sweating. Sweating both at nighttime and daytime is spontaneous sweating.

(3) By exclusion of improper nursing, sweating induced by such objective factor of climatic change and other pathogenic factors.

2 诊断要点

(1) 小儿在正常环境和安静状态下，以全身或局部多汗为主要表现。

(2) 寐则汗出，醒时汗止者为盗汗；不分寐寤而汗出者为自汗。

(3) 排除护理不当，气候变化等客观因素及其他疾病因素所引起的出汗。

3 Pattern identification and treatment

Spontaneous sweating and night sweating in children often exist simultaneouly. The key is to

3 辨证论治

小儿自汗、盗汗常同时并存，重点应辨其虚实。若

differentiate between their deficiency and excess. General sweating, susceptibility to cold at normal times, poor appetite, lassitude, or sweating after prolonged disease, is mostly attributed to deficiency pattern. Sweating mainly on the head, or excessive sweating on the four limbs, strong physique, dry stool, scanty and yellow urine or scanty and brown urine, is attributed to excess pattern.

全身出汗,平时易反复感冒,纳呆乏力,或见于久病之后,多属虚证;若以头汗为主,或四肢汗多,形体壮实,便干,尿黄少或短赤等则为实证。

The basic therapeutic principle is to regulate yin and yang. Besides administration of oral medicine, the umbilical treatment of the external therapies can be used for assistance.

以调和阴阳为基本治则。除内服药外,可配合脐疗等外治法。

(1) Insecurity of the exterior due to deficiency

(1) 表虚不固

Manifestations: Mainly spontaneous sweating, plus night sweating, sweating all over the body, aggravated by exertion, lusterless facial complexion, poor appetite, fatigued spirit and lack of strength, recurrent cold at the normal times, pale tongue, thin and white tongue coating, thready and weak pulse.

证候:以自汗为主,兼有盗汗,汗出遍及全身,动则更甚,面色少华,纳呆,神疲乏力,平时常反复感冒,舌质淡,苔薄白,脉细弱。

Therapeutic method: To boost qi, secure the exterior and constrain sweating.

治法:益气固表敛汗。

Main formula: *Jade Wind-Barrier Powder* (Yu Ping Feng San) and *Oyster Shell Powder* (Mu Li San) with modification.

主方:玉屏风散合牡蛎散加减。

Commonly used herbs: *Astragali Radix* (Huang Qi), *Ledebouriellae Radix* (Fang Feng), *Atractylodis Macrocephalae Rhizoma* (Bai Zhu), *Ostreae Concha Calcinata* (Duan Mu Li), *Ephedrae Herba* (Ma Huang Gen), *Tritici Levis Fructus* (Fu Xiao Mai).

常用药:黄芪、防风、白术、煅牡蛎、麻黄根、浮小麦。

Modification: For fatigued spirit and poor appetite, add *Codonopsis Radix* (Dang Shen), *Hordei Fructus Germinatus Ustus* (Jiao Mai Ya), *Crataegi Fructus Ustus* (Jiao Shan Zha), and *Massa Fermentata*

加减:神疲纳差者加党参、焦三仙。亦可用黄芪桂枝五物汤。

Medicinalis Ustus (Jiao Shen Qu). *Astragalus Cinnamon Twig Five Agents Decoction* (Huang Qi Gui Zhi Wu Wu Tang) can also be used.

(2) Deficiency of Both Qi and Yin

Manifestations: Night sweating often after febrile disease or prolonged disease, often accompanied by spontaneous sweating, emaciation, fatigued spirit, lack of strength, vexation, poor sleep, low fever, flushed cheeks, thirst with preference for drinks, feverish sensation in the chest, palms and soles, light red tongue, scanty or patchy peeled tongue coating, rapid, weak and thready pulse.

Therapeutic method: To boost qi and nourish yin.

Main formula: *Pulse-Engendering Powder* (Sheng Mai San) with modification.

Commonly used herbs: *Pseudostellariae Radix* (Tai Zi Shen), *Ophiopogonis Radix* (Mai Dong), *Schisandrae Fructus Chinensis* (Wu Wei Zi), *Tritici Levis Fructus* (Fu Xiao Mai), *Ostreae Concha Calcinata* (Duan Mu Li), *Rehmanniae Radix Cruda* (Sheng Di Huang).

Modification: For lusterless facial complexion, add *Astragali Radix* (Huang Qi); for low fever and flushed cheeks, add *Anemarrhenae Rhizoma* (Zhi Mu), and *Lycii Cortex* (Di Gu Pi); for incessant excessive sweating, add Ephedrae Radix Et Rhizoma (Ma Huang Gen) and *Os Draconis Calcinata* (Duan Long Gu); for vexation and poor sleep, add *Polygalae Radix* (Yuan Zhi), *Ziziphi Spinosi Semen* (Suan Zao Ren), *Polygoni Multiflori Caulis* (Shou Wu Teng).

(3) Accumulated Heat in Heart and Spleen

Manifestations: Spontaneous sweating or night

(2) 气阴两虚

证候:多见于热病或久病后,以盗汗为主,也常伴自汗,汗出遍及全身,形体消瘦,神疲乏力,心烦少寐,或低热颧红,口渴喜饮,手足心热,舌质淡红,苔少或剥苔,脉细弱而数。

治法:益气养阴。

主方:生脉散加减。

常用药:太子参、麦冬、五味子、浮小麦、煅牡蛎、生地黄。

加减:面色少华者,加黄芪;低热颧红者,加知母、地骨皮;汗多不止者,加麻黄根、煅龙骨;心烦少寐者,加远志、酸枣仁、首乌藤。

(3) 心脾积热

证候:自汗或盗汗,出汗

sweating, mainly on the head and limbs, hot skin after sweating, yellow and sour-smelling sweat stain, foul breath or sores on the mouth and tongue, flushed face and lips, dry mouth, thirst, vexation and agitation, poor sleep, yellow urine, dry stool, red tongue, yellow tongue coating, rapid and slippery pulse.

Therapeutic method: To clarify the heart and drain fire from the spleen.

Main formula: *Red-Abducting Powder* (Dao Chi San) and *Yellow-Draining Powder* (Xie Huang San) with modification.

Commonly used herbs: *Pogostmonis Herba* (Huo Xiang), *Gardeniae Fructus* (Zhi Zi), *Gypsum Fibrosum* (Sheng Shi Gao), *Glycyrrhizae Radix Et Rhizoma* (Gan Cao), *Ledebouriellae Radix* (Fang Feng), *Tetrapanacis Medulla* (Tong Cao), *Rehmanniae Radix Cruda* (Sheng Di Huang), *Ephedrae Herba* (Ma Huang Gen), *Lophatheri Herba* (Dan Zhu Ye).

Modification: For scanty urine and slimy and yellow tongue coating, add *Talcum* (Hua Shi), and *Plantaginis Herba* (Che Qian Cao); for yellow and heavy sour-smelling sweat stain, add *Artemisiae Scopariae Herba* (Yin Chen), and *Eupatorii Herba* (Pei Lan); for vexation, agitation and poor sleep, add *Polygoni Multiflori Caulis* (Shou Wu Teng), *Ziziphi Spinosi Semen* (Suan Zao Ren).

4 Other therapies

4.1 Chinese Patent Medicine

(1) *Jade Wind-Barrier Granules* (Yu Ping Feng) is used for sweating in pattern of insecurity of the exterior due to deficiency.

以头部或四肢为主,汗出肤热,汗渍色黄酸臭,口气臭秽或见口舌生疮,面赤唇红,口干渴,烦躁少寐,尿黄便干,舌质红,苔黄,脉滑数。

治法:清心泻脾。

主方:导赤散合泻黄散加减。

常用药:藿香、栀子、生石膏、甘草、防风、通草、生地黄、麻黄根、淡竹叶。

加减:尿少、舌苔黄腻者,加滑石、车前草;汗渍色黄酸臭重者,加茵陈、佩兰;烦躁少寐者,加首乌藤、酸枣仁。

4 其他疗法

4.1 中成药

(1) 玉屏风颗粒:适用于汗证表虚不固。

(2) *Checking Deficiency Sweating Granules* (Xu Han Ting) is used for sweating in pattern of insecurity of the exterior due to deficiency.

(2) 虚汗停颗粒:适用于汗证表虚不固。

(3) *Pulse-Engendering Decoction Oral Liquid* (Sheng Mai Yin Kou Fu Ye) is used for sweating in pattern of deficiency in both qi and yin in.

(3) 生脉饮口服液:适用于汗证气阴两虚。

4.2 External therapy

4.2 外治疗法

(1) Take appropriate amount of *Samuc Gallnut Powder* (Wu Bei Zi Fen). Mix it with water or vinegar to make paste. Apply onto the umbilicus every night before sleep, covered with sticking plaster. This is used for night sweating.

(1) 五倍子粉适量,混水或醋调成糊状,每晚临睡前敷脐中,用橡皮膏固定。适用于盗汗。

(2) Apply externally an appropriate amount of *Os Draconis Pulverata* (Long Gu Fen), *Ostreae Concha Pulverata* (Mu Li Fen), used for spontaneous and night sweating.

(2) 龙骨、牡蛎粉适量,每晚临睡前外扑。适用于自汗、盗汗。

Section 2　Infantile Convulsion

第 2 节　惊风

Infantile convulsion is a common acute and severe infantile disease, clinically manifested by convulsion and coma. Infantile convulsion is also a type of symptoms and could appear in many diseases. Its signs and symptoms can be generalized as "four signs and eight symptoms". The "four signs" are phlegm, heat, fright and wind. The "eight symptoms" are twitching, holding, pulling, trembling, turning over, guiding, scurrying, and seeing". In seizure of infantile convulsion, the four signs of phlegm, heat, wind and fright would occur at the same time. The occurrence of the eight symptoms indicates the ongoing of convulsion. In seizure of infantile convulsion, it does not mean that all the eight symptoms would appear all together.

惊风是小儿常见的一种急重病证,临床以抽搐、昏迷为主要症状。惊风又是一种证候,可发生于多种疾病之中。惊风的证候可概括为"四证八候","四证"即痰、热、惊、风;"八候"指搐、搦、掣、颤、反、引、窜、视。惊风发作时,往往痰、热、风、惊四证并见;八候的出现表示惊风已在发作,但惊风发作时,不一定八候全都出现。

There are two kinds of infantile convulsion: acute convulsion and chronic convulsion. Acute and sudden onset, rapid and serious eight symptoms, excess, yang and heat in nature of disease are regarded as acute infantile convulsion. Slow onset, deficiency in the Middle Energizer after prolonged disease, slow and mild eight symptoms, and deficiency, yin and cold in the nature of disease are attributed to chronic infantile convulsion. The critical signs and symptoms of pure yin without yang are present in chronic infantile convulsion, it is called chronic spleen convulsion.

惊风分为急惊风和慢惊风两大类。凡起病急暴，八候表现急速强劲，病性属实属阳属热者，为急惊风；起病缓，病久中虚，八候表现迟缓无力，病性属虚属阴属寒者，为慢惊风。慢惊风中若出现纯阴无阳的危重证候，称为慢脾风。

In Western medicine, it is also called infantile convulsion. It is not obviously seasonal, more frequently occurs in children from one to five years old, and in many diseases like high fever, toxic bacterial diseases, B encephalitis, meningitis, and primary epilepsy, etc.

西医学称为小儿惊厥，无明显季节性，1～5 岁儿童多见，可发生于高热、中毒性细菌性疾病、乙型脑炎、脑膜炎、原发性癫痫等多种疾病中。

Acute Infantile convulsion

急惊风

The onset of acute infantile convulsion is sudden, quick and serious, manifestd by high fever, spasm, and coma, together with four signs of phlegm, heat, fright and wind.

急惊风来势急骤，以高热、抽风、昏迷为主要表现，痰、热、惊、风四证俱备。

1 Etiology and pathogenesis

1 病因病机

Acute infantile convulsion is mainly related to infection of exogenous wind and heat, infection of epidemic toxin and sudden exposure to fright and fear.

急惊风的病因主要为外感风热、感受疫毒及暴受惊恐。

Because of thin and weak skin of children and insufficiency in the exterior and Wei-defensive ability, if exogenous wind and heat are infected, the extreme heat engenders wind, or the exuberant heat produces phlegm, or exuberant phlegm stirs up

小儿肌肤薄弱，卫外不固，外感风热，热极生风，或热盛生痰，痰盛动风，发为急惊风。感受温热疫毒，不能及时清解，内陷厥阴；或感受

wind, acute infantile convulsion would be resulted. Infantile convulsion can be induced by the following factors: infection of pestilent warm and heat toxin unable to fade away on time, leading to penetration into Jueyin, or infection of pestilent summer-heat toxin, scorching Qi-energy system and Ying-nutrient system, misting the clear orifice, and stirring up the liver wind, or ingestion of contaminated and poisonous food, accumulation of pestilent dampness and heat toxin in the intestines and hollow organs, penetrating into the heart and liver, and harassing the mind. Because Yuan-original qi is insufficient and the spirit qi is timid in children, if they are exposed to sudden fright and fear, their qi dynamic would be reversely chaotic, causing infantile convulsion. The diseased location is mainly in the heart and liver. The key pathogenesis is penetration of evil into Jueyin, misting the orifices of the heart and stirring up the liver wind.

暑热疫毒,邪炽气营,蒙蔽清窍,引动肝风;或饮食秽毒,湿热疫毒蕴结肠腑,内陷心肝,扰乱神明,均可发为惊风。小儿元气未充,神气怯弱,若暴受惊恐,致气机逆乱,发为惊风。病位主要在心肝;病机关键为邪陷厥阴,蒙蔽心窍,引动肝风。

2 Key to diagnosis

(1) The disease mostly occurs in children under 3 years old, and gradually decreases in those over 5 years old.

(2) Often there is a history of infection of pestilent wind and heat toxin or exposure to sudden fright and fear.

(3) Clinical manifestations are high fever, spasm, and coma.

(4) There are obvious primary diseases like cold, pneumonia, panting and cough, epidemic bacillary dysentery, epidemic mumps, epidemic encephalitis B, etc. In infection of the central nervous system, pathologic reflex in the examination of the

2 诊断要点

(1) 以 3 岁以下婴幼儿为多,5 岁以上逐渐减少。

(2) 常有感受风热、疫毒之邪或暴受惊恐病史。

(3) 临床以高热、抽风、昏迷为主要表现。

(4) 有明显的原发疾病,如感冒、肺炎喘嗽、疫毒痢、流行性腮腺炎、流行性乙型脑炎等。中枢神经系统感染者,神经系统查体病理反射

nervous system is positive.

(5) If necessary, the following tests can be taken to assist diagnosis: routine stool test, blood culture, cerebrospinal fluid (CSF), electroencephalogram (EEG), and brain CT.

阳性。

（5）必要时可行大便常规、大便培养、血培养、脑脊液、脑电图、脑 CT 等检查协助诊断。

3 Pattern identification and treatment

It is necessary to differentiate the severity and nature of the evils. Few seizures of infantile convulsion, short duration (within 5 min), and no mental, sensory and motor disorder after seizure, belong to mild pattern. Frequent seizures more than twice, or relatively long duration, and unconsciousness, motor and sensory disorder after seizure, belong to severe pattern. Infantile convulsion caused by infection of exogenous wind and heat is usually manifested by high fever, spasm due to fright, often accompanied by exterior pattern of wind and heat. Infantile convulsion caused by infection of pestilent warmth and heat toxin is often characterized by a contact history of epidemic diseases, such as measles and mumps. Infantile convulsion caused by infection of pestilent summer-heat toxin is manifested by evils scorching Qi-energy system and Ying-nutrient system, such as epidemic encephalitis B. The pestilent dampness and heat toxin tends to obstruct the intestines and hollow organs, and directly attack Jueyin, causing coma, spasm, and abnormal stool, common in bacillary dysentery. Infantile convulsion caused by fright and fear is often characterized by a history of being frightened and feared and manifested by restlessness due to fright and fear, and crying after fright, etc.

3 辨证论治

主要辨疾病的轻重及病邪的性质。惊风发作次数较少，持续时间较短，一般在 5 分钟以内，发作后无神志、感觉、运动障碍者，属轻症。若发作次数较多，一般在 2 次以上，或抽搐时间较长，发作后神志不清，甚至有感觉、运动障碍者，属重症。外感风热导致者，表现为高热惊厥，多伴风热表证；温热疫毒所致者多有麻疹、流行性腮腺炎等疫病接触史及特征表现；暑热疫毒引起者易见邪炽气营表现，常见于流行性乙型脑炎；湿热疫毒易阻滞肠腑，直中厥阴，出现神昏抽搐、大便异常，多见于中毒性痢疾；因于惊恐者，常有惊吓病史，及惊惕不安、惊叫急啼等表现。

The basic therapeutic principle is to remove

急惊风的治疗以豁痰、

phlegm, clear away heat, extinguish wind, and relieve convulsion for acute infantile convulsion. In the treatment, it is important to extinguish wind and relieve convulsion, and not to neglect the management of primary diseases as well, and to be sure about priority of the causative reason and clinical symptoms.

清热、息风、镇惊为基本治则。治疗中既要重视息风镇惊,又不可忽视原发疾病的处理,分清标本缓急。

(1) Infection of exogenous wind and heat

(1) 外感风热

Manifestations: Sudden onset, fever, nasal obstruction, runny nose, sore throat, cough, headache, vexation and agitation, coma, convulsion, red tongue, yellow and thin tongue coating, rapid and floating pulse, green-blue or purple fingerprints.

证候:起病急骤,发热,鼻塞,流涕,咽赤,咳嗽,头痛,烦躁,神昏,抽搐,舌质红,苔薄黄,脉浮数,指纹青紫。

Therapeutic method: To expel wind, clear away heat, extinguish wind and relieve convulsion.

治法:疏风清热,息风镇惊。

Main formula: *Lonicera and Forsythia Powder* (Yin Qiao San) with modification.

主方:银翘散加减。

Commonly used herbs: *Lonicerae Flos Japonicae* (Jin Yin Hua), *Forsythia Fructus* (Lian Qiao), *Menthae Haploalycis Herba* (Bo He), *Schizonepetae Spica* (Jing Jie Sui), *Ledebouriellae Radix* (Fang Feng), *Arctii Fructus* (Niu Bang Zi), *Uncariae ramulus Cum uncis* (Gou Teng), *Bombyx Batryticatus* (Jiang Can), *Cicadae Periostracum* (Chan Tui).

常用药:金银花、连翘、薄荷、荆芥穗、防风、牛蒡子、钩藤、僵蚕、蝉蜕。

Modification: For lingering high fever, add *Gypsum Fibrosum* (Sheng Shi Gao), and *Antelopis Tataricae Cornu* (Ling Yang Jiao) (Grind into powder, take infused with water). For rale in the throat, add *Bambusae Concretio Silicea* (Tian Zhu Huang) and *Arisaema Cum Bile* (Dan Nan Xing); for sore throat and constipated stool, add *Scutellariae Radix* (Huang Qin), and *Rhei Radix Et Rhizoma* (Da Huang); for severe coma and convulsion, add

加减:高热不退者,加生石膏、羚羊角(研末冲服);喉间痰鸣者,加天竺黄、胆南星;咽喉肿痛,大便秘结者,加黄芩、大黄;神昏抽搐较重者,加水牛角、全蝎、蜈蚣。

Bubali Cornu (Shui Niu Jiao), *Scorpio* (Quan Xie), *Scolopendra* (Wu Gong).

(2) Pestilent warm and heat toxin

Manifestations: In epidemic measles and mumps, there is lingering high fever, coma, convulsion, headache, vomiting, vexation, agitation, thirst, red tongue, yellow coating, rapid pulse.

Therapeutic method: To balance the liver and extinguish wind, clarify the heart and open orifices.

Main formula: *Antelope Horn and Uncaria Decoction* (Ling Jiao Gou Teng Tang) with modification.

Commonly used herbs: *Antelopis Tataricae Cornu* (Ling Yang Jiao), *Uncariae ramulus Cum uncis* (Gou Teng), *Acori Rhizoma Tatarinowii* (Shi Chang Pu), *Bulbus Fritillariae Cirrhosae* (Chuan Bei Mu), *Mori Folium* (Sang Ye), *Chrysanthemi Flos* (Ju Hua), *Paeoniae Radix Albae* (Bai Shao), *Bombyx Batryticatus* (Jiang Can), *Gardeniae Fructus*(Zhi Zi).

Modification: For severe fever, add *Purple Snow Elixir* (Zi Xue Dan); for coma and manic agitation, add *Peaceful Palace Bovine Bezoar Pills* (An Gong Niu Huang Wan); for copious phlegm, add *Bambusae Concretio Silicea*(Tian Zhu Huang), *Arisaema Cum Bile* (Dan Nan Xing); for constipated stool, add *Rhei Radix Et Rhizoma* (Da Huang); for frequent convulsion, add *Scorpio* (Quan Xie), *Scolopendra* (Wu Gong).

(3) Pestilent Summer-heat and heat toxin

Manifestations: Sudden onset, persistent high fever, recurrent convulsion, headache, stiff neck, vomiting, somnolence, rash and macules on the skin, thirst, constipation, red tongue, yellow coat-

（2）温热疫毒

证候:麻疹、流行性腮腺炎等疫病过程中,出现高热不退,神昏,四肢抽搐,头痛呕吐,烦躁口渴,舌质红,苔黄,脉数。

治法:平肝息风,清心开窍。

主方:羚角钩藤汤加减。

常用药:羚羊角、钩藤、石菖蒲、川贝母、桑叶、菊花、白芍、僵蚕、栀子。

加减:热重者,加紫雪丹;昏迷狂躁者,加安宫牛黄丸;痰盛者,加天竺黄、胆南星;大便秘结者,加大黄;抽搐频繁者,加全蝎、蜈蚣。

（3）暑热疫毒

证候:起病急骤,持续高热,神昏谵语,反复抽搐,头痛项强,呕吐,或嗜睡,或皮肤出疹发斑,口渴便秘,舌质

ing, rapid and string-taut pulse. Those in severe condition may have critical signs of difficult breathing.

红,苔黄,脉弦数。严重者可发生呼吸困难等危象。

Therapeutic method: To clear away heat, dispel summer-heat, open the orifices and extinguish wind.

治法:清热祛暑,开窍息风。

Main formula: *Scourge-Clearing and Toxin-Vanquishing Decoction* (Qing Wen Bai Du Yin).

主方:清瘟败毒饮加减。

Commonly used herbs: *Gypsum Fibrosum* (Sheng Shi Gao), *Rehmanniae Radix Cruda* (Sheng Di Huang), *Coptidis Rhizoma* (Huang Lian), *Bubali Cornu* (Shui Niu Jiao), *Gardeniae Fructus* (Zhi Zi), *Scutellariae Radix* (Huang Qin), *Anemarrhenae Rhizoma* (Zhi Mu), *Paeoniae Radix Rubra* (Chi Shao), *Scrophulariae Radix* (Xuan Shen), *Forsythia Fructus* (Lian Qiao), *Moutan Cortex Radicis* (Mu Dan Pi), *Antelopis Tataricae Cornu* (Ling Yang Jiao)(Grind into powder and take after infused with water), *Uncariae Ramulus Cum Uncis* (Gou Teng), *Bombyx Batryticatus* (Jiang Can).

常用药:生石膏、生地黄、黄连、水牛角、栀子、黄芩、知母、赤芍、玄参、连翘、牡丹皮、羚羊角(研末冲服)、钩藤、僵蚕。

Modification: For severe coma, *Bovine Bezoar and Heart-Clearing Pill* (Niu Huang Qing Xin Wan), *Peaceful Palace Bovine Bezoar Pill* (An Gong Niu Huang Wan), or *Purple Snow Elixir* (Zi Xue Dan) can be used. For constipated stool, add *Rhei Radix Et Rhizoma* (Da Huang), and *Natrii Sulfas Exsiccatus* (Xuan Ming Fen); for vomiting, add *Pinelliae Rhizoma* (Ban Xia); for blood stasis macules on the skin, add *Isatidis Folium* (Da Qing Ye), *Salviae Miltiorrhizae Radix Et Rhizoma* (Dan Shen), *Arnebiae Radix* (Zi Cao).

加减:昏迷较甚者,可选用牛黄清心丸、安宫牛黄丸或紫雪丹;大便秘结者,加大黄、玄明粉;呕吐者,加半夏;皮肤瘀斑者,加大青叶、丹参、紫草。

(4) Pestilent dampness and heat toxin

(4) 湿热疫毒

Manifestations: Persistent high fever, frequent convulsion, coma, delirious ravings, vexation and

证候:持续高热,频繁抽搐,神志昏迷,谵妄烦躁,腹

agitation, abdominal pain, vomiting, sticky stool, or stool with pus and blood, red tongue, slimy and yellow tongue coating, rapid and slippery pulse.

痛呕吐，大便黏腻或夹脓血，舌质红，苔黄腻，脉滑数。

Therapeutic method: To clear away heat, dissolve dampness, resolve toxin and extinguish wind.

治法：清热化湿，解毒息风。

Main formula: *Coptis Toxin-Resolving Decoction* (Huang Lian Jie Du Tang) and *Pulsatilla Decoction* (Bai Tou Wen Tang) with modification.

主方：黄连解毒汤合白头翁汤加减。

Commonly used herbs: *Coptidis Rhizoma* (Huang Lian), *Phellodendri Cortex Chinensis* (Huang Bo), *Gardeniae Fructus* (Zhi Zi), *Scutellariae Radix* (Huang Qin), *Pulsatillae Radix* (Bai Tou Wen), *Cortex Fraxini* (Qin Pi), *Uncariae Ramulus Cum Uncis* (Gou Teng), *Scorpio* (Quan Xie), *Paeoniae Radix Rubra* (Chi Shao).

常用药：黄连、黄柏、栀子、黄芩、白头翁、秦皮、钩藤、全蝎、赤芍。

Modification: For severe stool with pus and blood, use enema therapy with *Rhei Radix Et Rhizoma* (Da Huang) decoction; for coma and recurrent convulsion, choose *Purple Snow Elixir* (Zi Xue Dan) or *Supreme Jewel Elixir* (Zhi Bao Dan). For internal blockage and external collapse, use *Ginseng, Aconite, Dragon Bone, Oyster Shell Counterflow Decoction* (Shen Fu Long Mu Jiu Ni Tang) for oral administration instead.

加减：大便脓血较重者，可用大黄水煎灌肠；昏迷不醒，反复抽搐者，选用紫雪丹、至宝丹。若出现内闭外脱者，改用参附龙牡救逆汤灌服。

(5) Exposure to Sudden Fright and Fear

(5) 暴受惊恐

Manifestations: Original timidness and easily frightened, restlessness, tremble in the body, convulsion and coma after exposure to sudden fright and fear, green stool, irregular pulse and stagnant purple fingerprints.

证候：平素胆小易惊，暴受惊恐后出现惊惕不安，身体颤栗，甚则抽搐、神志不清。大便色青，脉律不整，指纹紫滞。

Therapeutic method: To relieve fright, tranquilize the mind, balance the liver and extinguish wind.

治法：镇惊安神，平肝息风。

Main formula: *Amber Dragon-Embracing Pill*

主方：琥珀抱龙丸合朱

(Hu Po Bao Long Wan) and *Cinnabar Spirit-Quieting Pill* (Zhu Sha An Shen Wan) with modification.

砂安神丸加减。

Commonly used herbs: *Succinum* (Hu Po) (take after infused with water), *Arisaema Cum Bile* (Dan Nan Xing), *Cinnabaris* (Zhu Sha) (take after infused with water), *Realgar* (Xiong Huang), *Bambusae Concretio Silicea* (Tian Zhu Huang), *Coptidis Rhizoma* (Huang Lian), *Angelicae Sinensis Radix* (Dang Gui), *Scorpio* (Quan Xie), *Uncariae Ramulus Cum Uncis* (Gou Teng), *Acori Rhizoma Tatarinowii* (Shi Chang Pu).

常用药:琥珀(冲服)、胆南星、朱砂(冲服)、雄黄、天竺黄、黄连、当归、全蝎、钩藤、石菖蒲。

Modification: For trembling limb in sleeping and restlessness due to fright, add *Magnetitum* (Ci Shi); for vomiting, add *Bambusae Caulis in Taenias* (Zhu Ru), and *Pinelliae Rhizoma* (Ban Xia); for fatigued spirit, lack of strength, and pale nails, add *Astragali Radix* (Huang Qi), *Angelicae Sinensis Radix* (Dang Gui), and *Ziziphi Spinosi Semen* (Suan Zao Ren).

加减:寐中肢体颤动,惊惕不安者,加磁石;呕吐者,加竹茹、半夏;神疲乏力、唇甲色淡者,加黄芪、当归、酸枣仁。

4 Other therapies

4 其他疗法

4.1 Chinese Patent medicine

4.1 中成药

(1) *Peaceful Palace Bovine Bezoar Pills* (An Gong Niu Huang Wan) is used for acute infantile convulsion.

(1) 安宫牛黄丸:适用于急惊风热证。

(2) *Bovine Bezoar Fright-Settling Pill* (Niu Huang Zhen Jing Wan) is used for acute infantile convulsion by exposure to sudden fright and fear.

(2) 牛黄镇惊丸:适用于急惊风暴受惊恐者。

(3) *Antelope Horn Powder* (Ling Yang Jiao Fen) is used for acute infantile convulsion.

(3) 羚羊角粉:适用于急惊风热证。

(4) *Child Return-of-Spring Elixir* (Xiao Er Hui Chun Dan) is used for acute infantile convulsion in pattern of infection of exogenous of wind and heat.

(4) 小儿回春丹:适用于急惊风外感风热者。

4.2 Acumoxatherapy

(1) Body acupuncture: For acute infantile convulsion by infection of exogenous of wind and heat, select Renzhong (GV 26), Hegu (LI 4), Taichong (LR 3), Twelve Jing-Well Points (Shaoshang (LU 11), Shangyang (LI 1), Zhongchong (PC 9), Guanchong (TE 1), Shaochong (HT 9) Shaoze(SI 1), Shixuan (EX 20), and Dazhui (GV 14). For infection of pestilent dampness and heat toxin, select Renzhong (GV 26), Zhongwan (CV 12), Fenglong (ST 40), Hegu (LI 4), Neiguan (PC 6), Shenmen (HT 7),Taichong (LR 3), Quchi (LI 11), etc. For exposure to sudden fright and fear, select Yintang (EX-HN3), Neiguan (PC 6), Shenmen (HT 7), Yanglingquan (GB 34), Sishencong (EX-HN 1), and Baihui (GV 20), etc.

(2) Three-edged needle: Prick and bleed Shixuan (Extra 30), Twelve Jing-Well Points.

(3) Acupressure: For coma and clenched jaw, press Renzhong (GV 26) by fingernail.

4.2 针灸疗法

（1）体针：急惊风中外感风热者，取穴人中、合谷、太冲、手十二井（少商、商阳、中冲、关冲、少冲、少泽）、或十宣、大椎。感受湿热疫毒者，取穴人中、中脘、丰隆、合谷、内关、神门、太冲、曲池等。暴受惊恐所致者，取穴印堂、内关、神门、阳陵泉、四神聪、百会等。

（2）三棱针：取十宣或十二井点刺出血。

（3）指针：神志昏迷，牙关紧闭者，用指甲掐人中。

Chronic Infantile Convulsion

Chronic infantile convulsion occurs with slow onset, manifested by weak convulsion, intermittent seizure and protracted condition, and often accompanied by the symptoms like coma and paralysis, etc.

慢惊风

慢惊风来势缓慢，抽搐无力，时作时止，反复难愈，常伴昏迷、瘫痪等症。

1 Etiology and pathogenesis

It is mostly caused by serious illnesses and prolonged illnesses, such as fulminant vomiting, fulminant diarrhea, prolonged vomiting or prolonged diarrhea.

Fulminant vomit, fulminant diarrhea, prolonged vomiting, prolonged diarrhea, or adminis-

1 病因病机

慢惊风多由大病、久病，如暴吐、暴泻，久吐、久泻等形成。

暴吐暴泻，久吐久泻，或他病过用峻利之品，妄用汗、

tration of harsh and fierce medicine for other diseases and abuse of the sweating and purgative method may cause damage to the spleen and stomach and induce stirring-up wind due to deficiency in the earth and hyperactivity in the wood, leading to chronic infantile convulsion. If the prolonged damage of spleen yang involves the kidney, yang deficiency in the spleen and kidney would be induced and the internal yin and cold would be preponderant, failing to warm up the tendons and leading to frequent convulsion due to dysfunction of the spleen. The prolonged infection of exogenous febrile disease or long-term retention of heat evil and depletion of yin humor after acute infantile convulsion, or influences from other problems would cause insufficiency of essence and blood in the liver and kidney, failing to nourish the meridians and tendons, stirring up internal wind, and there is chronic infantile convulsion. The diseased location lies mainly in the spleen, kidney and liver. The nature of illness is mainly in deficiency.

下之法致脾胃受损，土虚木亢风动，致慢惊风。脾阳损伤，日久及肾，脾肾阳虚，阴寒内盛，不能温煦筋脉，而致时时搐动之慢脾风证；外感热病迁延日久，或急惊风后，热邪久羁，阴液亏耗，或他病影响，致肝肾精血不足，筋脉失于濡养，虚风内动而致慢惊风。病位主要在脾、肾、肝，病性以虚为主。

2　Key to diagnosis

(1) There is a medical history of recurrent vomiting, prolonged diarrhea, acute infantile convulsion, rickets, etc.

(2) It is characterized by slow onset, relatively long duration, and pale facial complexion, somnolence, low spirit, intermittent feeble convulsion, or trembling hands, thready and feeble pulse.

(3) The primary disease should be diagnosed with the clinical manifestations of the sick child, in combination of blood biochemical test, electroencephalogram (EEG), cerebrospinal fluid test, and

2　诊断要点

（1）具有反复呕吐、长期泄泻、急惊风、佝偻病等病史。

（2）起病缓慢，病程较长。症见面色苍白，嗜睡无神，抽搐无力，时作时止，或两手颤动，脉细无力。

（3）根据患儿的临床表现，结合血液生化、脑电图、脑脊液、头颅 CT 等检查，以明确诊断原发病。

head CT.

3 Pattern identification and treatment

Chronic infantile convulsion mostly is in deficiency pattern. The key is to differentiate between the solid organs and hollow organs, and between yin and yang.

Fatigue in the body and spirit, withered and yellow facial complexion, intermittent feeble convulsion, somnolence, half-opened eyes in sleeping, no desire for food, loose stool indicate the involvement of the liver and spleen. Listless spirit and lethargic sleep, pale and lusterless complexion, extreme cold sensation in the four limbs, trembling hand and foot, clear urine, loose stool, pale tongue, faint and deep pulse indicate the involvement of spleen and kidney. Trembling hand and foot, pale and lusterless complexion, extreme cold sensation in the four limbs, clear urine, loose stool, pale tongue, white and thin tongue coating, faint and deep pulse, all these after fulminant and prolonged diarrhea are mostly attributed to yang deficiency. The muscular spasm and stiffness of the limbs, after acute infantile convulsion, accompanied by exhausted spirit, low fever, vexation deu to deficiency, feverish sensation in the chest, palms and soles, dry and constipated stool, crimson tongue with scanty fluid, scanty tongue coating or no tongue coating, rapid and thready pulse, belong to yin deficiency.

The treatment is mainly given to correct deficiency and treat the causative reason, including the common-used clinical methods to warm up the Middle Energizer and fortify the spleen, to warm up

3 辨证论治

慢惊风多属虚证，重在辨脏腑，分阴阳。

形神疲惫，面色萎黄，抽搐无力，时作时止，嗜睡露睛，不欲饮食，大便稀溏，为病在肝脾；神萎昏睡，面白无华，四肢厥冷，手足震颤，溲清便溏，舌淡，脉沉微，为病在脾肾。若暴泻久泻之后，见手足震颤，面白无华，四肢厥冷，溲清便溏，舌质淡，苔薄白，脉沉微者，多属阳虚；若急惊风后，肢体拘挛或强直，伴精神疲惫，低热虚烦，手足心热，大便干结，舌绛少津，苔少或无苔，脉细数者，多属阴虚。

治疗以补虚治本为主，临床常用治法有温中健脾、温阳逐寒、育阴潜阳、柔肝息风等，若有虚中夹实者，宜攻

yang and expel cold, to foster yin and subdue yang, to soothe the liver and extinguish wind. For deficiency mixed with excess, it is appropriate to apply the attacking and supplementing methods simultaneously for dealing with both the causative reason and clinical symptoms.

补兼施，标本兼顾。

(1) Spleen deficiency and liver effulgence

(1) 脾虚肝旺

Manifestations: Listless spirit, somnolence with half-closed eyes, withered facial complexion, no desire for drink and food, loose stool in green-blue color, occasional borborygmus, lack of warmth in limbs, intermittent feeble convulsion, pale tongue, white tongue coating, thready and deep pulse.

证候：精神萎靡，嗜睡露睛，面色萎黄，不欲饮食，大便稀溏，色带青绿，时有肠鸣，四肢不温，抽搐无力，时作时止，舌质淡，苔白，脉沉细。

Therapeutic method: To warm up the Middle Energizer, fortify the spleen, soothe the liver and rectify the spleen.

治法：温中健脾，缓肝理脾。

Main formula: *Liver-relaxing and Spleen-Rectifying Decoction* (Huan Gan Li Pi Tang) with modification.

主方：缓肝理脾汤加减。

Commonly used herbs: *Ginseng Radix* (Ren Shen), *Atractylodis Macrocephalae Rhizoma* (Bai Zhu), *Poria* (Fu Ling), *Citri Reticulatae Pericarpium* (Chen Pi), *Dioscoreae Rhizoma* (Shan Yao), *Lablab Semen Album* (Bai Bian Dou), *Glycyrrhizae Radix Et Rhizoma* (Gan Cao), *Paeoniae Radix Albae* (Bai Shao), *Uncariae ramulus Cum uncis* (Gou Teng), *Zingiberis Rhizoma* (Gan Jiang), *Cinnamomi Cortex* (Rou Gui).

常用药：人参、白术、茯苓、陈皮、山药、白扁豆、甘草、白芍、钩藤、干姜、肉桂。

Modification: For poor appetite, add *Amomi Fructus Rotundus* (Dou Kou), *Amomi Fructus* (Sha Ren). For lack of warmth in limbs and loose stool, use *Aconite Center-Rectifying Decoction* (Fu Zi Li Zhong Tang) instead.

加减：纳呆食少者，加豆蔻、砂仁；四肢不温者，大便稀溏改用附子理中汤。

(2) Yang Deficiency in the Spleen and Kidney

Manifestations: Withered spirit, lethargic sleep, pale and lusterless complexion, sweating on the forehead, lack of warmth, extreme cold sensation in the limbs, clear urine, sloppy stool, trembling hand and foot, pale tongue, thin and white tongue coating, deep and feeble pulse.

Therapeutic method: To warm up and supplement the spleen and kidney, return yang and stop counterflow.

Main formula: *True Securing Decoction* (Gu Zhen Tang) with modification.

Commonly used herbs: *Ginseng Radix* (Ren Shen), *Atractylodis Macrocephalae Rhizoma* (Bai Zhu), *Dioscoreae Rhizoma* (Shan Yao), *Poria* (Fu Ling), Astragali Radix (Huang Qi), *Glycyrrhizae Radix Et Rhizoma*(Gan Cao), *Aconiti Lateralis Radix Praeparata* (Fu Zi), *Cinnamomi Cortex* (Rou Gui), Baked *Zingiberis Rhizoma Recens* (Pao Jiang), *Caryophylli Flos*(Ding Xiang).

Modification: For excessive sweating, add *Os Draconis* (Long Gu), *Ostreae Concha* (Mu Li), and *Schisandrae Fructus Chinensis* (Wu Wei Zi); for vomiting and nausea, add *Euodiae Fructus* (Wu Zhu Yu), *Piperis Fructus* (Hu Jiao) and *Pinelliae Rhizoma* (Ban Xia).

(3) Stirring-Up Wind due to Yin Deficiency

Manifestations: Muscular spasm and rigidity of the limbs, convulsion in varying degrees, low spirit, withered facial complexion, or occasional flushed cheeks, vexation due to deficiency, low fever, feverish sensation in the chest, palms and soles, easy sweating, dry and constipted stool, crimson tongue with scanty fluid, scanty tongue coating or no

（2）脾肾阳虚

证候:神萎昏睡，面白无华，额汗不温，四肢厥冷，溲清便溏，手足震颤，舌质淡，苔薄白，脉沉微。

治法:温补脾肾，回阳救逆。

主方:固真汤加减。

常用药:人参、白术、山药、茯苓、黄芪、甘草、附子、肉桂、炮姜、丁香。

加减:汗多者，加龙骨、牡蛎、五味子；恶心呕吐者，加吴茱萸、胡椒、半夏。

（3）阴虚风动

证候:肢体拘挛或强直，抽搐时轻时重，精神疲惫，面色萎黄，或时有潮红，虚烦低热，手足心热，易出汗，大便干结，舌质绛少津，苔少或无苔，脉细数。

tongue coating, rapid and thready pulse.

Therapeutic method: To foster yin, subdue yang, enrich water to moisten the wood.

治法:育阴潜阳,滋水涵木。

Main formula: *Wind-Stabilizing Pill* (Da Ding Feng Zhu) with modification.

主方:大定风珠加减。

Commonly used herbs: *Colla Corii Asini* (E Jiao), *Rehmanniae Radix Cruda* (Sheng Di Huang), *Ophiopogonis Radix* (Mai Dong), *Paeoniae Radix Albae* (Bai Shao), *Carapax et Testudinis Carapax Et Plastrum* (Gui Jia), *Trionycis Carapax Et Rhizoma* (Bie Jia), *Cannabis Fructus* (Huo Ma Ren), *Ostreae Concha* (Mu Li), *Schisandrae Fructus Chinensis* (Wu Wei Zi), *Glycyrrhizae Radix Et Rhizoma* (Gan Cao).

常用药:阿胶、生地黄、麦冬、白芍、龟甲、鳖甲、火麻仁、牡蛎、五味子、甘草。

Modification: For persistent convulsion, add *Gastrodiae Rhizoma* (Tian Ma), and *Zaocys* (Wu Shao She); for muscular spasm and motor impairment, add *Astragali Radix* (Huang Qi), *Codonopsis Radix* (Dang Shen), *Spatholobi Caulis* (Ji Xue Teng), and *Mori Ramulus* (Sang Zhi).

加减:抽搐不止者,加天麻、乌梢蛇;筋脉拘急,屈伸不利者,加黄芪、党参、鸡血藤、桑枝。

4　Other therapies

4　其他疗法

4.1　Acumoxatherapy

4.1　针灸治疗

(1) Body Acupuncture: Baihui (GV 20), Yintang (EX-HN 3), Qihai (CV 4), Zusanli (ST 36). For spleen deficiency and liver hyperactivity, add Pishu (BL 20), Taichong (LR 3); for yang deficiency in the spleen and kidney, add Pishu (BL 20), Shenshu (BL 23), and Guanyuan (CV 4); for stirring wind due to yin deficiency, add Taixi (KI 3), Taichong (LR 3), and Fengchi (GB 20). Puncture all these acupoints with the needling technique for supplementation.

(1) 体针:取百会、印堂、气海、足三里。脾虚肝旺者,加脾俞、太冲;脾肾阳虚者,加脾俞、肾俞、关元;阴虚风动者,加太溪、太冲、风池。诸穴均用补法。

(2) Ear Acupuncture: Puncture Pt. Sympathet-

(2) 耳针:取交感、神门、

ic, Pt. Ear-Shenmen, Pt. Subcortex, Pt. Heart, Pt. Liver and Pt. Spleen, with the filiform needles by moderate stimulation, or embed the points with *Semen Vaccariae* (Wang Bu Liu Xing Zi).

皮质下、心、肝、脾，毫针中刺激，或王不留行子贴压。

(3) Moxibustion: Select Dazhui (GV 14), Pishu (BL 20), Mingmen (GV 4), Guanyuan (CV 4), Qihai (CV 4), Baihui (GV 20), Zusanli (ST 36), for chronic infantile convulsion in pattern of spleen deficiency and liver hyperactivity, and pattern of yang deficiency in the spleen and kidney.

(3) 灸治：取穴大椎、脾俞、命门、关元、气海、百会、足三里。适用于慢惊风脾虚肝亢证、脾肾阳虚证。

4.2 Tuina Therapy

4.2 推拿疗法

Knead Pt. Wujing, push Pt. Pitu, rub Pt. Pitu, rub Pt. Wuzhijie, knead Pt. Neibagua, and push yin and yang divergently, push Pt. Sanguan, and rub Yongquan (KI 1) and Zusanli (ST 36).

运五经，推脾土，揉脾土，揉五指节，运内八卦，分阴阳，推上三关，揉涌泉，揉足三里。

Section 3 Enuresis

第3节 遗尿

Enuresis refers a disease characterized by inability to control urination voluntarily, frequent enuresis during sleep without awareness till wake-up, in children over five years old. It mostly occurs in children under 10 years old.

遗尿是指5岁以上的小儿不能自主控制排尿，经常睡中小便自遗，醒后方觉的一种病证。多见于10岁以下的儿童。

1 Etiology and pathogenesis

1 病因病机

The production of urine is closely related to the regulatory abilities of water metabolism in the lung, the spleen, and the kidney. After its production, urine is discharged from the bladder, depending upon qi transformation of the Triple Energizer and bladder. Enuresis is often related to dysfunction in qi transformation of the bladder and kidney, especially to insufficiency of kidney qi and deficiency and cold of the bladder.

尿液的生成与肺脾肾三脏对水液代谢的调节密切相关。尿液生成后由膀胱排出，有赖于三焦与膀胱的气化，遗尿多与膀胱和肾的气化功能失调有关，尤其以肾气不足，膀胱虚寒为多见。

The prenatal insufficiency of natural endowment or original weak constitution, insufficiency of the kidney qi, deficiency and cold of the lower body, and failure of the kidney qi in containing ability, or deficiency of the lung qi which fail in governing the managing and regulating ability, or deficiency of the spleen qi which fail to control water, or accumulation of dampness and heat in the liver meridian which leads to failure of the liver in maintaining smooth flow of qi, or downward infusion of dampness and heat which transmits heat to the bladder, all could induce dysfunction of the bladder and hence enuresis.

先天禀赋不足或素体虚弱，肾气不足，下元虚寒，肾气失于固摄；肺气虚弱，治节失司，脾气虚弱，不能制水；湿热之邪蕴郁肝经，致肝失疏泄，或湿热下注，移热于膀胱；均可致膀胱失约而遗尿。

2　Key to diagnosis

(1) The disease occurs in children over 5 years old.

(2) Sleep soundly, difficult to wake up, and wet the bed every night or once several dayrs, and wet the bed several times every night.

(3) Routine urine test and urine culture are normal.

(4) Under X-ray scan, spina bifida occulta can be seen in some sick children.

2　诊断要点

(1) 发病年龄在 5 岁以上。

(2) 睡眠较深，不易唤醒，每夜或隔几日发生尿床，甚则 1 夜尿床数次。

(3) 尿常规及尿培养均无异常。

(4) X 线摄片检查，部分患儿可发现有隐性脊柱裂。

3　Pattern identification and treatment

The key is to differentiate between the solid organs and hollow organs, between deficiency and excess, and between heat and cold nature, based upon the duration, frequency, volume and smell of urine, and accompanying symptoms. Long-term enuresis, in clear and profuse urine, large volume and frequent, accompanied by cold body and cold limbs, pale face and fatigued spirit, lack of strength, and spontaneous sweating, is in deficiency and cold.

3　辨证论治

重在辨别脏腑虚实寒热：根据病程、尿次、尿量、气味及伴随症状辨别。遗尿日久，小便清长，量多次频，兼见形寒肢冷、面白神疲、乏力自汗者多为虚寒；遗尿初起，尿黄短涩，量少灼热，形体壮实，睡眠不宁者多为实热。

New enuresis, scanty and yellow urine, in scanty volume, burning sensation, strong physique, and restless sleep, could be mostly excess and heat.

The basic therapeutic principle is to warm up and supplement the lower origin and secure the bladder. For deficiency pattern, it is mainly to support the Vital Energy and build up the lower origin, to warm up the kidney and promote the containing ability, to supplement the lung and fortify the spleen. For accumulation of dampness and heat in the liver meridian, it is appropriate to clear away heat and remove dampness, in combination of the methods of clarifying the heart and enriching the kidney, arousing the mind and opening the orifices accordingly.

以温补下元，固涩膀胱为基本治则。虚证以扶正培本为主，温肾固摄、补肺健脾。肝经湿热，宜清热利湿；此外，清心滋肾，醒神开窍之法亦可酌情配合使用。

(1) Insufficiency of Kidney Qi

Manifestation: Frequent enuresis during sleep, without awareness of enuresis until waking up, and even several enuresis per night, clear and profuse urine, fatigued spirit, lassitude, pale facial complexion, cold body and cold limbs, weakness in the lower limbs, weakness and soreness in the lumbus and legs, sleep in curled-up posture, pale tongue, deep slow and feeble pulse.

Therapeutic method: To warm up and supplement kidney yang, secure urine and check enuresis.

Main formula: *Cuscuta Powder* (Tu Si Zi San) with modification.

Commonly used herbs: *Cuscutae Semen* (Tu Si Zi), *Radix Morindae Officinalis* (Ba Ji Tian), *Cistanchis Herba* (Rou Cong Rong), *Aconiti Lateralis Radix Praeparata* (Fu Zi), *Corni Fructus* (Shan Zhu Yu), *Schisandrae Fructus Chinensis* (Wu Wei Zi), *Euryales Semen* (Qian Shi), *Ostreae Concha* (Mu Li),

(1) 肾气不足

证候：睡中经常遗尿，醒后方觉，甚者一夜数次，小便清长，神疲乏力，面色苍白，形寒肢冷，下肢乏力，腰腿疲软，蜷卧而睡，舌质淡，脉沉迟无力。

治法：温补肾阳，固涩止遗。

主方：菟丝子散加减。

常用药：菟丝子、巴戟天、肉苁蓉、附子、山茱萸、五味子、芡实、牡蛎、桑螵蛸。

Mantidis Oötheca (Sang Piao Xiao).

Modification: For frequent enuresis, add *Halloysitum Rubrum* (Chi Shi Zhi); for deep sleep and difficulty to wake up, add *Arisaema Cum Bile* (Dan Nan Xing), *Acori Rhizoma Tatarinowii* (Shi Chang Pu), *Polygalae Radix* (Yuan Zhi), and *Ephedrae Herba* (Ma Huang); for poor appetite, and loose stool, add *Codonopsis Radix* (Dang Shen), *Atractylodis Macrocephalae Rhizoma* (Bai Zhu), *Poria* (Fu Ling), and *Crataegi Fructus* (Shan Zha). For mild condition, *Stream-Reducing Pill* (Suo Quan Wan) can be used to warm up the kidney and fortify the spleen.

加减:尿床次数频繁者加赤石脂;困寐不醒者加胆南星、石菖蒲、远志、麻黄;纳差便溏者,加党参、白术、茯苓、山楂。对于病证较轻者,可单用缩泉丸以温肾健脾。

(2) Qi deficiency in the lung and spleen

(2) 肺脾气虚

Manifestations: Enuresis during sleep, frequent urination in the daytime, lusterless facial complexion, weakness in the four limbs, poor appctite, loose stool, spontaneous sweating, susceptible to cold, pale tongue, white and thin tongue coating, slow and weak pulse.

证候:睡中遗尿,白天尿频,面色少华,四肢乏力,食欲不振,大便溏薄,自汗,易感冒,舌质淡,苔薄白,脉缓弱。

Therapeutic method: To supplement the lung and fortify the spleen, secure urine and check enuresis.

治法:补肺健脾,固摄止遗。

Main formula: *Center-Supplementing and Qi-Boosting Decoction* (Bu Zhong Yi Qi Tang) and *Stream-Reducing Pill* (Suo Quan Wan) with modification.

主方:补中益气汤合缩泉丸加减。

Commonly used herbs: *Codonopsis Radix* (Dang Shen), *Astragali Radix* (Huang Qi), *Atractylodis Macrocephalae Rhizoma* (Bai Zhu), *Citri Reticulatae Pericarpium* (Chen Pi), *Angelicae Sinensis Radix* (Dang Gui), *Cimicifugae Rhizoma* (Sheng Ma), *Alpiniae Oxyphyllae Fructus* (Yi Zhi), *Dioscoreae Rhizoma* (Shan Yao), *Linderae Radix* (Wu Yao),

常用药:党参、黄芪、白术、陈皮、当归、升麻、益智、山药、乌药、甘草。

Glycyrrhizae Radix Et Rhizoma(Gan Cao).

Modification: For deep sleep, add *Ephedrae Herba* (Ma Huang), and *Acori Rhizoma Tatarinowii* (Shi Chang Pu); for excessive sweating, add *Os Draconis Calcinata* (Duan Long Gu), *Ostreae Concha Calcinata* (Duan Mu Li); for loose stool, add *Baked Zingiberis Rhizoma Recens* (Pao Jiang); for poor appetite, add *Crataegi Fructus Ustus* (Jiao Shan Zha), *Massa Medicata Fermentata Usta* (Jiao Shen Qu).

加减:寐深者,可加麻黄、石菖蒲;多汗者,加煅龙骨、煅牡蛎;大便稀溏者,加炮姜;纳呆者,加焦山楂、焦神曲。

(3) Accumulation of dampness and heat in the liver meridian

(3) 肝经湿热

Manifestations: Enuresis during sleep, yellow and sticky urine, bad temper, red face and lips, bitter taste in the mouth, red eyes, red tongue, yellow tongue coating, rapid and slippery pulse.

证候:睡中遗尿,色黄味臊,性情急躁,夜梦或夜间龂齿,面赤唇红,口苦,或目睛红赤,舌质红,苔黄,脉滑数。

Therapeutic method: To clear away heat and remove dampness.

治法:清热利湿。

Main formula: *Gentian Liver-Draining Pill* (Long Dan Xie Gan Tang).

主方:龙胆泻肝汤加减。

Commonly used herbs: *Gentianae Radix Et Rhizoma* (Long Dan Cao), *Scutellariae Radix* (Huang Qin), *Gardeniae Fructus*(Zhi Zi), *Bupleuri Radix* (Chai Hu), *Rehmanniae Radix Cruda* (Sheng Di Huang), *Plantaginis Semen* (Che Qian Zi), *Alismatis Rhizoma* (Ze Xie), *Tetrapanacis Medulla* (Tong Cao), *Glycyrrhizae Radix Et Rhizoma*(Gan Cao).

常用药:龙胆草、黄芩、栀子、柴胡、生地黄、车前子、泽泻、通草、甘草。

Modification: For restless sleep at night, obvious teeth grinding in sleep, add *Coptidis Rhizoma* (Huang Lian), and *Poria Cum Ligno Hospite* (Fu Shen); for enduring illness, kidney yin damage, and red tongue, use *Anemarrhena, Phellodendron, and Rehmanni Pill* (Zhi Bo Di Huang Wan).

加减:夜卧不宁,龂齿梦呓较显著者,加黄连、茯神;久病不愈,肾阴耗伤,舌质红者,可用知柏地黄丸。

4 Other therapies

4.1 Chinese Patent medicine

(1) *Gold Lock Essence-Securing Pill* (Jin Suo Gu Jing Wan) is used for pattern of kidney qi insufficiency.

(2) *Center-Supplementing Qi-Boosting Pills* (Bu Zhong Yi Qi Wan) is used for pattern of qi deficiency in the lung and spleen.

(3) *Gentian Liver-Draining Pill* (Long Dan Xie Gan Wan) is used for pattern of accumulation of dampness and heat in the liver meridian.

4.2 Acumoxatherapy

(1) Body Acupuncture: Select Guanyuan (CV 4), Qihai (CV 6), Sanyinjiao (SP 6), Yinlingquan (SP 9) and Yintang (EX-HN 3), and puncture 2～3 acupoints each time, in combination of Zusanli (ST 36). For hand acupuncture, puncture Pt. Enuresis Point (midpoint of the second transverse crease of the little finger), retain the needle for 15 minutes.

(2) Ear Acupuncture: Select Pt. Kidney, Pt. Bladder, Pt. Subcortex, Pt. Ear-Shenmen, Pt. Endocrine, Pt. Lung and Pt. Spleen.

(3) Hand Acupuncture: Puncture Pt. Enuresis Point (midpoint of the second transverse crease of the little finger), retain the needle for 15 minutes, once every other day, seven sessions as one course.

4.3 Tuina Therapy

Rub Pt. Dantian for 200 times, massage the abdomen for 20 minutes, rub Guiwei (GV 1) for 30 times. For elder children, use scrubing method, chafe Shenshu (BL 23), and Shangliao (BL 31), Ciliao (BL 32), Zhongliao (BL 33) and Xiaoliao (BL 34) until it is warm.

4 其他疗法

4.1 中成药

(1) 金锁固精丸:适用于遗尿肾气不足证。

(2) 补中益气丸:适用于遗尿肺脾气虚证。

(3) 龙胆泻肝丸:适用于遗尿肝经湿热证。

4.2 针灸疗法

(1) 体针:取关元、气海、三阴交、阴陵泉、印堂,每次2～3穴,可配足三里。手针取夜尿点(小指二横纹中点),留针15分钟。

(2) 耳针:取肾、膀胱、皮质下、神门、内分泌、肺、脾。

(3) 手针:针刺夜尿点(掌面小指第二指关节横纹中点处),每次留针15分钟。隔日1次,7次为1个疗程。

4.3 推拿疗法

揉丹田200次,摩腹20分钟,揉龟尾30次。较大儿童可用擦法。摩擦肾俞、八髎,以热为度。

4.4 External therapy

(1) Grind *Galla Chinensis* (Wu Bei Zi) 3g, into fine powder. Mix it with warm water and apply onto the umbilicus, and cover it with gauze, once every night, for 3 to 5 days successively.

(2) Grind *Fructus Rubi* (Fu Pen Zi), *Fructus Rosae Laevigatae* (Jin Yin Zi), *Schisandrae Fructus Chinensis* (Wu Wei Zi), *Cuscutae Semen* (Tu Si Zi), *Rhizoma Curculiginis* (Xian Mao), *Psoraleae Fructus* (Bu Gu Zhi), *Corni Fructus* (Shan Zhu Yu), *Mantidis Oötheca* (Sang Piao Xiao), each 60g. *Caryophylli Flos* (Ding Xiang), *Cinnamomi Cortex* (Rou Gui), 30g. into powder and seal it in a bottle for use. Take 1g every time and apply it onto the umbilicus, then drip 1 to 2 drops of white liquor into the navel, fix it with *Navel-Warming Paste* (Nuan Qi Gao) externally, change the dressing once every three days.

(3) Bake *Psoraleae Fructus* (Bu Gu Zhi) for 10 to 20 minutes, grind it into powder. Prescribe 1.5g every time for children from 3 to 9 years old, and 2.4g every time for children from 10 to 12 years old, and take after infused with warm boiled water every night.

4.4 外治疗法

（1）可用五倍子 3 克，研末，温开水调敷于脐部，外用纱布覆盖，每晚 1 次，连用 3～5 次。

（2）覆盆子、金樱子、五味子、菟丝子、仙茅、补骨脂、山茱萸、桑螵蛸各 60 克，丁香、肉桂各 30 克，研末装瓶备用。每次 1 克填入脐中，滴1～2 滴白酒后，外用暖脐膏固定，3 日换药 1 次。

（3）补骨脂炒 10～20 分钟后，研细。3～9 岁每次服 1.5 克，10～12 岁每次服 2.4 克，每晚用温开水冲服。

Section 4 Infantile Eczema

Infantile eczema, also known as fetal tinea, is clinically characterized by red macules over the skin, millet-like papules, papulo-vesicle, blisters, dotted erosion after rupture, oozing exudation, crusts and accompanied severe itching. The disease includes infantile eczema in Western medicine and some of infantile atopic dermatitis in babyhood. It

第 4 节　奶癣

奶癣又称胎癣，临床症状以皮肤红斑、粟粒状丘疹、丘疱疹或水疱，疱破后出现点状糜烂、渗液、结痂并伴剧烈瘙痒为特征。本病包括西医婴儿湿疹及一部分婴儿期的异位性皮炎等疾病。其发

is related to allergic constitution, and can appear generally or regionally. It is not obviously seasonal, and occurs repeatedly, mostly in the babies form one to three months old. It usually heals before 2 years old.

病以过敏体质为多，可泛发或局限，无明显季节性，易反复发作，多始发于1～3个月的婴儿，一般在2岁以内可愈。

In traditional Chinese medicine, it is termed as "fetus closing sore", and is differentiated as "dry closing sore" and "wet closing sore".

中医学也称本病为"胎敛疮"，且有"干敛""湿敛"之区别。

1 Etiology and Pathogenesis

1 病因病机

It is mostly caused by internal retention of dampness and heat, exuberant dampness due to the spleen deficiency, and invasion of wind, dampness and heat evils, which result in a struggle between the internal evils and external evils and present onto the skin. If it lingers for long time to induce wind and dryness due to blood deficiency, and further malnutrition in the muscles and skin, it would occur repeatedly to be an intractable condition. Because the evils are hidden deeply and the problem lingers for long time, the retained dampness would turn into fire to consume and damage body fluid and blood, presenting the symptoms of wind and dryness due to blood deficiency, and malnutrition in the muscles and skin.

奶癣多由湿热内蕴，或脾虚湿盛，复受风、湿、热邪侵袭，内外邪气相搏，发于肌肤所致。若迁延日久，致血虚风燥，肌肤失养，可反复发作，缠绵难愈。由于邪深病久，湿郁化火，耗伤津血，可出现血虚风燥，肌肤失养之证候。

2 Key to diagnosis

2 诊断要点

(1) The skin rash is mostly distributed symmetrically, and occurs mostly over head and face, such as cheeks, forehead, and vertex. The skin rash over the face initially are clustered or scattered in red macules or papules. The skin rash on the head or eyebrows is often with oily scales and yellow crust. The mild condition is manifested by mere light red patches, accompanied by a small amount of pap-

(1) 皮疹分布大多对称，多先发于头面部，如面颊、额部、头顶等处。面部者初为簇集的或散在的红斑或丘疹；头部或眉部者，多有油腻性的鳞屑和黄色结痂。病轻者，仅有淡红的斑片，伴有少量的丘疹、小水疱和小片糜

ules, tiny blisters and small patches of erosion and exudation. The severe condition is manifested mainly by bright red patches, a large number of blisters, erosion and exudation.

烂渗液；病重者，红斑鲜艳，水疱多，以糜烂渗液为主。

(2) The skin lesions are seborrheic, wet and dry. The seborrheic skin lesions often occur 1 to 2 months after birth, in small red macules, attached with yellow scales, on the forehead, cheeks and around the eyebrows, and often accompanied by mild erosion in the neck, under the armpits, and in the inguinal region, and would heal after stop of milk feeding. The wet skin lesions often occur in children at the age of 3 to 6 months old, in red macules, papules, blisters, erosion and exudation, and would tend to have secondary infection easily. The dry skin lesions often occur in children over 1 year old of emaciated physique, manifested by wet and red, dry, scaling skin lesions, or papules and patchy infiltration, repeated occurrence and difficult healing.

(2) 皮损有脂溢性、湿性、干性之分。脂溢性者多发生于出生后1～2月，皮损在前额、面颊、眉周围有小片红斑，上附黄色鳞屑，颈部、腋下，腹股沟常有轻度糜烂，停乳后可痊愈。湿性者常见于3～6月的婴儿，皮损有红斑、丘疹、水疱、糜烂、渗液，容易继发感染。干性者多发生在1岁以上较为消瘦的小儿，皮损潮红、干燥、脱屑，或有丘疹和片状浸润，常反复发作，不易治愈。

(3) In varying severity and intermittent seizure, the skin lesions often disappear suddenly with fever and diarrhea, and may appear again after fever fades away and diarrhea stops, often accompanied by obvious and severe itching, leading to restless sleep and agitation in the sick children.

(3) 皮损时轻时重，时愈时发，常在发热、腹泻时症状突然消失，待热退、腹泻停止后皮损又现。多伴有明显剧烈瘙痒，致使患儿睡卧不安，神情烦躁。

(4) It usually breaks out 1 to 3 months after birth, fades away gradually after one to two years, would heal up naturally in most cases, but would linger and be hard to heal up in a few cases.

(4) 多在婴儿出生后1～3个月发病，一般1～2周岁之后逐渐减轻，大多可自愈，少数可迁延不愈。

(5) There is a family history of asthma, and allergic rhinitis in some sick children.

(5) 部分患儿及家族有哮喘、过敏性鼻炎等病史。

3 Pattern identification and treatment

3 辨证论治

The skin rashes manifested mainly by dryness

皮疹以干燥、脱屑为主

and scaling are often related to wind and dryness due to blood deficiency and often seen in the infants with emaciation and malnutrition. The skin rashes manifested mainly by blisters, erosion and exudation are mostly seen in the fat infants with preponderance of both dampness and heat. The skin rashes mainly manifested by blisters, erosion and exudation are in those with exuberant dampness due to the spleen deficiency. The preponderance of both dampness and heat is mostly manifested by eczema, accompanied by infection, fever, red macules, erosion, scanty and brown urine, dry and constipated stool.

的多因血虚风燥，多见于形体消瘦、营养不良的小儿。若皮疹以水疱、糜烂、渗液为主，多见于湿热俱盛的肥胖婴儿。脾虚湿盛者皮疹以水疱、糜烂、渗液为主；湿热俱盛者多见湿疹伴继发感染、发热、红斑、糜烂、小便短赤、大便干结。

The basic therapeutic principle is to dispel wind and eliminate dampness, assisted by the methods to clear away heat, nourish blood, fortify the spleen according to different characteristics of the signs and symptoms.

以祛风除湿为基本治则，并根据证候特点佐以清热、养血、健脾等法。

(1) Preponderance of both dampness and heat

(1) 湿热俱盛

Manifestations: Skin rash in red macules, papules, blisters, erosion, or crusting and severe itching, mostly on the head, face, body trunk and flexion sides of the limbs, accompanied by vexation, restlessness, poor appetite, scanty and brown urine, dry and constipated stool, red tongue, slimy and yellow tongue coating, slippery pulse, green-blue fingerprints.

证候：皮疹见红斑、丘疹、水疱、糜烂，或有结痂，瘙痒难忍，多发于头面部及躯干、四肢的屈侧面，伴有烦躁不安，纳呆，小便短赤，大便干结，舌质红，苔黄腻，脉滑，指纹青紫。

Therapeutic method: To clear away heat, remove dampness, dispel wind and relieve itching.

治法：清热利湿，祛风止痒。

Main formula: *Wind-Dispersing and Red-Abducting Decoction* (Xiao Feng Dao Chi San) with modification.

主方：消风导赤汤加减。

Commonly used herbs: *Rehmanniae Radix Cruda* (Sheng Di Huang), *Coptidis Rhizoma* (Huang

常用药：生地黄、黄连、金银花、茯苓、白鲜皮、薄荷、

Lian), *Lonicerae Flos Japonicae* (Jin Yin Hua), *Poria* (Fu Ling), *Dictamni Cortex* (Bai Xian Pi), *Menthae Haploalycis Herba* (Bo He), *Tetrapanacis Medulla* (Tong Cao), *Junci Medulla* (Deng Xin Cao), *Arctii Fructus* (Niu Bang Zi), *Glycyrrhizae Radix Et Rhizoma* (Gan Cao).

通草、灯心草、牛蒡子、甘草。

Modification: For skin rash over the upper body or spreading over the whole body, add *Mori Folium* (Sang Ye), *Chrysanthemi Flos* (Ju Hua), and *Xanthii Fructus* (Cang Er Zi). For skin rash over the trunk or pathway along the liver meridian, add *Gentianae Radix Et Rhizoma* (Long Dan), *Gardeniae Fructus* (Zhi Zi), and *Scutellariae Radix* (Huang Qin). For skin rash over the lower limbs, add *Plantaginis Semen* (Che Qian Zi). For severe itching, add *Radix Cynanchi Paniculati* (Xu Chang Qing), and *Kochiae Fructus* (Di Fu Zi). For scorching redness and heat, add *Paeoniae Radix Rubra* (Chi Shao), and *Moutan Cortex Radicis* (Mu Dan Pi).

加减:发于上部或弥漫全身者,加桑叶、菊花、苍耳子;发于躯干或肝经所行部位者,加龙胆、栀子、黄芩;发于下肢者,加车前子;瘙痒甚者,加徐长卿、地肤子;皮损焮红灼热者,加赤芍、牡丹皮。

(2) Exuberance of dampness due to spleen deficiency

(2) 脾虚湿盛

Manifestations: Dark red skin rash, covered by blisters and exudations, dryness and crust in some parts, accompanied by poor appetite, thin and loose stool, abdominal distention, vomiting of milk, pale tongue, slow and soggy pulse, pale red fingerprints.

证候:皮疹颜色暗红不鲜,表面有水疱、渗液,部分干燥结痂,伴有纳差,大便稀溏,腹胀,吐乳,舌质淡,苔白腻,脉濡缓,指纹淡红。

Therapeutic method: To fortify the spleen and eliminate dampness.

治法:健脾除湿。

Main formula: *Dampness-Eliminating and Stomach-Calming Poria Five Decoction* (Chu Shi Wei Ling Tang) with modification.

主方:除湿胃苓汤加减。

Commonly used herbs: *Atractylodis Rhizoma* (Cang Zhu), *Magnoliae Officinalis Cortex* (Hou

常用药:苍术、厚朴、陈皮、猪苓、泽泻、茯苓、白术、

Pu), *Citri Reticulatae Pericarpium* (Chen Pi), *Polyporus* (Zhu Ling), *Alismatis Rhizoma* (Ze Xie), *Poria* (Fu Ling), *Atractylodis Macrocephalae Rhizoma* (Bai Zhu), *Talcum* (Hua Shi), *Ledebouriellae Radix* (Fang Feng), *Cinnamomi Cortex* (Rou Gui), *Glycyrrhizae Radix Et Rhizoma* (Gan Cao).

滑石、防风、肉桂、甘草。

Modification: For no appetite or vomiting of milk, add *Pogostmonis Herba* (Huo Xiang), and *Eupatorii Herba* (Pei Lan). For thin and loose stool, add *Baked Zingiberis Rhizoma Recens* (Pao Jiang), and *Puerariae Radix* (Ge Gen); for itching, add *Kochiae Fructus* (Di Fu Zi), and *Dictamni Cortex* (Bai Xian Pi).

加减:胃纳不香或吐乳者,加藿香、佩兰;大便稀溏者,加炮姜、葛根;瘙痒者,加地肤子、白鲜皮。

(3) Wind and dryness due to blood deficiency

(3) 血虚风燥

Manifestations: Recurrent skin lesions, thick and rough skin, dry rash, scaling, pigmentation, moss-like change, limited distribution, severe itching, a little exudation by scratching, accompanied dry mouth, restless sleep, dry and constipated stool, pale tongue, thin white tongue coating, or scanty tongue coating, rapid and thready pulse, light-colored fingerprints.

证候:皮损反复发作,皮肤肥厚粗糙,皮疹干燥、脱屑,色素沉着,苔藓样改变,分布局限,瘙痒剧烈,抓破有少量渗液,伴口干,夜寐不安,大便干结,舌质淡,苔薄白或少苔,脉细数,指纹淡。

Therapeutic method: To nourish blood and moisten dryness, dispel wind and relieve itching.

治法:养血润燥,祛风止痒。

Main formula: *Blood-Nourishing and Wind-Stabilizing Decoction* (Yang Xue Ding Feng Tang) with modification.

主方:养血定风汤加减。

Commonly used herbs: *Rehmanniae Radix Cruda* (Sheng Di Huang), *Angelicae Sinensis Radix* (Dang Gui), *Polygoni Multiflori Radix* (He Shou Wu), *Chuanxiong Rhizoma* (Chuan Xiong), *Paeoniae Radix Rubra* (Chi Shao), *Moutan Cortex Radicis* (Mu Dan Pi), *Radix Asparagi* (Tian Dong), *Ophiopogonis Radix* (Mai Dong), *Bombyx Batryticatus* (Jiang

常用药:生地黄、当归、何首乌、川芎、赤芍、牡丹皮、天冬、麦冬、僵蚕。

Can).

Modification: For skin lesion, coarse and severely thick skin, add *Salviae Miltiorrhizae Radix Et Rhizoma* (Dan Shen), *Spatholobi Caulis* (Ji Xue Teng), *Lumbricus* (Di Long); for severe itching, add *Scolopendra* (Wu Gong), *Zaocys* (Wu Shao She); for dry mouth, dry and constipated stool, add *Trichosanthis Radix* (Tian Hua Fen), and *Scrophulariae Radix* (Xuan Shen); for restless sleep, add *Margaritifera Concha* (Zhen Zhu Mu), and *Ostreae Concha* (Mu Li).

加减：皮损粗糙、肥厚严重者，加丹参、鸡血藤、地龙；瘙痒剧烈者，加蜈蚣、乌梢蛇；口干、大便干结者，加天花粉、玄参；夜寐不安者，加珍珠母、牡蛎。

4 Other therapies

4 其他疗法

4.1 Chinese Patent medicine

4.1 中成药

(1) *Better-than-Gold Toxin-Transforming Powder* (Sai Jin Hua Du San) is used for pattern of exuberance of both dampness and heat.

(1) 赛金化毒散：用于治疗湿热俱盛型奶癣。

(2) *Mysterious Two Pill* (Er Miao Wan) is used for pattern of exuberance of both dampness and heat.

(2) 二妙丸：用于治疗湿热俱盛型奶癣。

4.2 External therapy

4.2 药物外治

For obvious red swelling and exudation, decoct 10% of *Phellodendri Cortex Chinensis* (Huang Bo) solution, or *Sophorae Flavescentis Radix* (Ku Shen), *Scutellariae Radix* (Huang Qin), and *Phellodendri Cortex Chinensis* (Huang Bo), each 10%～15%, or *Portulacae Herba* (Ma Chi Xian) in 30g with water, for wet compressing or wash. For little erosion and exudation, apply *Indigo Powder* (Qing Dai San) mixed with sesame oil. For red macules and papules and no exudation, apply *Three Yellows Wash Preparation* (San Huang Xi Ji) or *Calamine Wash Preparation* (Lu Gan Shi Xi Ji) topically. For skin lesion, infiltration, thickening of the skin, and moss-like

红肿渗液明显者，用10%黄柏水或苦参、黄芩、黄柏各10%～15%或马齿苋30克水煎湿敷或溻洗；少量糜烂渗出者，用青黛散麻油调敷；以红斑、丘疹为主者，无渗液时，用三黄洗剂或炉甘石洗剂外搽；皮损浸润肥厚、苔藓样变者，用加味黄芩膏或黑豆馏油膏外搽。

change, apply externally *Supplemented Scutellaria Paste* (Jia Wei Huang Qin Gao) or *Black Soybean Distillate* (Hei Dou Liu You Gao).

Section 5　Constipation

Constipation refers to a disease manifested by hard and dry stool, constipated and difficult defecation, long intervals between defecations, or difficulty defecation regardless of intention. Functional constipation in Western medicine belongs to scope of this disease.

It may occur in all ages and all seasons. Because of difficulty in defecation, poor appetite and restless sleep could be induced, or because of forced defecation, anal fissure, prolapse of the rectum or hemorrhoid could be induced in some sick infants.

1　Etiology and Pathogenesis

The common causes are related to dietary imbalance, emotional disorder, internal accumulation of dryness and heat, deficiency and depletion of qi and blood.

The infants are often insufficient in the spleen and don't have self-control in milk and food. When there is inappropriate feeding and nursing, or damage of the spleen and stomach due to excessive ingestion of hot-spicy, acrid, fried foods, or uncooked, cold, fatty, and sweet food, or stagnation of the liver qi and dysfunction of qi dynamic by emotional and mental disorder, or retention of residual heat after febrile and heat diseases, or transmission of residual lung heat downward into the large intestines, or consumption and damage of body fluid

第 5 节　便秘

便秘指大便干燥坚硬，秘结不通，排便时间间隔延长，或虽有便意但排出困难的一种病证。西医学的功能性便秘属于本病范畴。

便秘可发生于任何年龄，一年四季均可发病。由于排便困难，部分小儿可发生食欲不振，睡眠不安，或可由于便时努力，引起肛裂、脱肛或痔疮。

1　病因病机

常见病因有饮食失调、情志失和、燥热内结、气血亏虚。

小儿脾常不足，乳食不知自节，若喂养不当，或过食辛辣炙煿、生冷肥甘之品，损伤脾胃；或情志不舒，肝气郁结，气机不利；或温热病后，余热留恋，或肺热下移大肠，或过用辛温药物，伤津耗液；或气血虚衰，气虚则脾胃运化传导无力，血虚则津液不足以滋润大肠；诸因均可致腑气郁滞，致运化失常，引起

due to overuse of warm and acrid medicinal stuffs, or dysfunctions of the spleen and stomach in transportation and transformation by qi deficiency and blood debilitation, or insufficiency of body fluids due to blood deficiency in failure to moisten the large intestines, all these could lead to qi stagnation in the hollow organs, causing dysfunctions in transportation and transformation, and hence constipation. The pathologic location is in large intestines, but it is closely related to the functional disharmony of the spleen, stomach, lung, liver and kidney.

便秘。病位在大肠,与脾胃肺肝肾等脏腑功能失调密切相关。

2 Key to diagnosis

(1) A history of painful defecation or forced defecation.

(2) Hard and dry stool, constipation and difficult defecation regardless of intention.

(3) The interval between defecations is prolonged, defecation ≤ twice per week.

(4) There are lots feces masses retained in the rectum, or there is a history of retention of lots feces.

At least, two of the above symptoms are present for over a month.

2 诊断要点

(1) 有排便疼痛或费力史。

(2) 大便干燥坚硬,秘结不通,或虽有便意但排出困难。

(3) 排便时间间隔延长,每周排便少于等于 2 次。

(4) 直肠内存在大量粪便团块,或有大量粪便潴留史。

至少出现上述 2 条以上症状,持续 1 个月以上。

3 Pattern identification and treatment

It is necessary to differentiate between heat and cold and between deficiency and excess. Excess pattern is mainly caused by retention of milk and food, internal accumulation of dryness and heat, and dysfunction of qi dynamic. It is manifested by dry and hard feces, often accompanied by pain and distention in the abdomen, aggravated pressure, bitter taste in the mouth, foul breathing, oral ulceration and restless sleep. Deficiency pattern is mainly

3 辨证论治

主要辨别病证的寒热虚实　实证多为乳食积滞、燥热内结、气机郁滞所致,粪质干燥坚硬,常伴腹胀拒按,口苦口臭,口腔溃疡,睡眠不安等症状。虚证多因气血亏虚,失于濡养,传导无力所致。病程较长,粪质不甚干结,欲便不出或便出不畅,常

caused by lack of nourishment and feeble transportation due to depletion of qi and blood. It is manifested by long duration and very dry and constipated stool, no defecation regardless of strong intention, and difficult defecation, often accompanied by deficient manifestations like fatigue, lassitude, pale and lusterless complexion, etc. Constipation in heat pattern is often manifested by flushed face, hot sensation in the body, dry mouth, yellow urine, abdominal pain and distention, red tongue and yellow coating, etc. Constipation in cold pattern is often manifested by lack of warmth in the four limbs, profuse and clear urine, and pale tongue coating.

伴神疲乏力，面白无华等虚证表现。热证便秘多有面赤身热，口干，尿黄，腹胀腹痛，舌红苔黄等症状。寒证便秘常见四肢不温，小便清长，舌淡苔白等表现。

Excess pattern is mainly treated by expelling evils, with the methods to clear away heat and eliminate obstruction, to soothe the liver and regulate qi, and to reduce stagnation and disperse accumulation. Deficiency pattern is mainly treated by supporting the Vital Energy in priority, frequently with the methods to fortify the spleen, boost qi, enrich yin and nourish blood, moisten the intestines and promote bowel movement, warm up yang and reinforce the kidney, etc.

治疗实证以驱邪为主，常用清热通导、疏肝理气、消积导滞之法；虚证以扶正为先，多用健脾益气、滋阴养血、润肠通便、温阳益肾等法。

(1) Retention of milk and food

(1) 乳食积滞

Manifestations: Dry and constipated stool, difficulty in defecation, abdominal distention and pain, no desire for milk and food, nausea and vomiting, feverish sensation in the chest, palms and sores, vexation, restless sleep, scanty and yellow urine, red tongue, thick and yellow tongue coating, deep and forceful pulse, stagnant and purple fingerprints.

证候：大便干结，排便困难，腹胀满疼痛，不思乳食，或恶心呕吐，手足心热，心烦，睡眠不安，小便短黄，舌红苔黄厚，脉沉有力，指纹紫滞。

Therapeutic method: To eliminate stagnation and disperse accumulation, clear away heat and re-

治法：消积导滞，清热通便。

lax the bowel.

Main formula: *Unripe Bitter Orange Stagnation-Eliminating Pill* (Zhi Shi Dao Zhi Wan) with modification.

主方:枳实导滞丸加减。

Commonly used herbs: *Rhei Radix Et Rhizoma* (Da Huang), *Aurantii Fructus Immaturus* (Zhi Shi), *Scutellariae Radix* (Huang Qin), *Coptidis Rhizoma* (Huang Lian), *Massa Fermentata Medicinalis* (Liu Shen Qu), *Atractylodis Macrocephalae Rhizoma* (Bai Zhu), *Poria* (Fu Ling), *Raphani Semen* (Lai Fu Zi).

常用药:大黄、枳实、黄芩、黄连、六神曲、白术、茯苓、莱菔子。

Modification: For abdominal distention and pain, add *Arecae Pericarpium* (Da Fu Pi), and *Cyperi Rhizoma* (Xiang Fu); for stagnation and accumulation transforming into heat, add *Forsythia Fructus* (Lian Qiao), and *Picrorhizae Rhizoma* (Hu Huang Lian); for improper feeding, add *Hordei Fructus Germinatus* (Mai Ya); for vomiting and nausea, add *Pogostmonis Herba* (Huo Xiang), and *Bambusae Caulis in Taenias* (Zhu Ru).

加减:腹胀痛者,加大腹皮、香附;积滞化热者,加连翘、胡黄连;伤乳者,加麦芽;呕恶者,加藿香、竹茹。

(2) Internal accumulation of dryness and heat

(2) 燥热内结

Manifestations: Dry and hard stool, difficulty in defecation or even constipation, flushed face and hot sensation in the body, dry mouth and foul breathing, ulcers in the mouth and tongue, abdominal distention and pain, scanty and brown urine, red tongue, dry and yellow tongue coating, rapid and slippery pulse, purple and stagnant fingerprints.

证候:大便干硬,排出困难,甚至秘结不通,面红身热,口干口臭,或口舌生疮,腹胀腹痛,小便短赤,舌质红,苔黄燥,脉滑数,指纹紫滞。

Therapeutic method: To clear away heat and eliminate stagnation, moisten the intestines and relax the bowels.

治法:清热导滞,润肠通便。

Main formula: *Cannabis Fruit Pill* (Ma Zi Ren Wan) with modification.

主方:麻子仁丸加减。

Commonly used herbs: *Cannabis Semen* (Ma Zi Ren), *Rhei Radix Et Rhizoma* (Da Huang), *Aurantii Fructus Immaturus* (Zhi Shi), *Arecae Semen* (Bing Lang), *Armeniacae Semen Amarum* (Ku Xing Ren), and *Paeoniae Radix Albae* (Bai Shao).

常用药：麻子仁、大黄、枳实、槟榔、苦杏仁、白芍。

Modification: For dry mouth and tongue, add *Rehmanniae Radix Cruda* (Sheng Di Huang), and *Scrophulariae Radix* (Xuan Shen); for ulcers in the mouth and tongue, add *Picrorhizae Rhizoma* (Hu Huang Lian) and *Lophatheri Herba* (Dan Zhu Ye); for abdominal distention and pain, add *Aucklandiae Radix* (Mu Xiang).

加减：口干舌燥者，加生地黄、玄参；口舌生疮者，加胡黄连、淡竹叶；腹胀痛者，加木香。

(3) Dysfunction of Qi Dynamic

（3）气机郁滞

Manifestations: Dry and constipated stool, frequent belching, borborygmus and flatus, mass and oppression in the chest and rib-side, distension and pain in the abdomen, red tongue, white and thin tongue coating, string-taut pulse, stagnant fingerprints.

证候：大便闭涩，嗳气频作，肠鸣矢气，胸胁痞闷，腹中胀痛，舌质红，苔薄白，脉弦，指纹滞。

Therapeutic method: To soothe the liver, regulate qi, eliminate stagnation and relax the bowel.

治法：疏肝理气，导滞通便。

Main formula: *Six Milled Ingredients Decoction* (Liu Mo Tang) with modification.

主方：六磨汤加减。

Commonly used herbs: *Aucklandiae Radix* (Mu Xiang), *Linderae Radix* (Wu Yao), *Aquilariae Lignum Resinatum* (Chen Xiang), *Rhei Radix Et Rhizoma* (Da Huang), *Arecae Semen* (Bing Lang), *Aurantii Fructus Immaturus* (Zhi Shi), *Curcumae Radix* (Yu Jin).

常用药：木香、乌药、沉香、大黄、槟榔、枳实、郁金。

Modification: For long-term accumulated qi turning into fire, bitter taste in the mouth and dry throat, add *Scutellariae Radix* (Huang Qin), and *Gardeniae Fructus* (Zhi Zi); for frequent belching,

加减：气郁日久化火，口苦咽干者，加黄芩、栀子；嗳气频作者，加旋覆花、紫苏子；恶心呕吐者去槟榔，加厚

add *Inulae Flos* (Xuan Fu Hua), and *Perillae Fructus* (Zi Su Zi); for nausea and vomiting, take out *Arecae Semen*(Bing Lang), add *Magnoliae Officinalis Cortex* (Hou Pu) and *Pinelliae Rhizoma* (Ban Xia); for mass and fullness in the chest and rib side, add *Richosanthis Fructus* (Gua Lou) and *Cyperi Rhizoma*(Xiang Fu); for abdominal distention and pain, add *Citri Reticulatae Pericarpium Viride* (Qing Pi) and *Raphani Semen*(Lai Fu Zi).

朴、半夏;胸胁痞满者,加瓜蒌、香附;腹胀腹痛者,加青皮、莱菔子。

(4) Depletion and Deficiency of Qi and Blood

(4) 气血亏虚

Manifestations: Dry and hard feces, difficulty in defecation without dry and hard stool but with defecating intention, sweating, shortness of breath, fatigue after defecation, pale and lusterless complexion, pale lips and nails, dreamfulness, pale tongue, white tongue coating, feeble pulse, light-colored fingerprints.

证候:粪质干结,或并不干硬,虽有便意,但难于排出;汗出气短,便后疲乏,面白无华,唇甲色淡,多梦,舌淡,苔白,脉弱,指纹淡。

Therapeutic method: To boost qi, nourish blood, moisten the intestines and relax the bowels.

治法:补气养血,润肠通便。

Main formula: *Astragalus Decoction* (Huang Qi Tang) and *Intestine-Moistening Pill* (Run Chang Wan) with modification.

主方:黄芪汤合润肠丸加减。

Commonly used herbs: *Astragali Radix* (Huang Qi), *Citri Reticulatae Pericarpium* (Chen Pi), *Cannabis Fructus* (Huo Ma Ren), *Codonopsis Radix* (Dang Shen), *Atractylodis Macrocephalae Rhizoma* (Bai Zhu), *Angelicae Sinensis Radix* (Dang Gui), *Rehmanniae Radix Cruda* (Sheng Di Huang), *Persicae Semen* (Tao Ren), *Aurantii Fructus* (Zhi Qiao), *Mel* (Feng Mi).

常用药:黄芪、陈皮、火麻仁、党参、白术、当归、生地黄、桃仁、枳壳、蜂蜜。

Modification: For severe qi deficiency, add *Ginseng Radix* (Ren Shen); for prolapse of the rectum by qi deficiency, use *Astragali Radix* (Huang Qi) in high dose and add *Cimicifugae Rhizoma*

加减:气虚较甚者,加人参;气虚下陷脱肛者,重用黄芪,加升麻、柴胡,或用补中益气汤;面白唇淡者,加何首

(Sheng Ma), *Bupleuri Radix* (Chai Hu), or use *Center-Supplementing and Qi-Boosting Decoction* (Bu Zhong Yi Qi Tang); for pale face and pale lips, add *Polygoni Multiflori Radix* (He Shou Wu), *Lycii Fructus* (Gou Qi Zi), and *Colla Corii Asini* (E Jiao).

乌、枸杞子、阿胶。

4 Other therapies

4.1 Chinese Patent medicine

(1) *Unripe Bitter Orange Stagnation-Abducting Pill* (Zhi Shi Dao Zhi Wan) is used for pattern of retention of milk and food.

(2) *Cannabis Fruit Pill* (Ma Ren Wan) is used for pattern of internal accumulation of dryness and heat.

(3) *Free Wanderer Pill* (Xiao Yao Wan) is used for pattern of dysfunction of dynamic qi.

(4) *Center-Supplementing Qi-Boosting Pill* (Bu Zhong Yi Qi Wan) is used for pattern of failure in transportation due to qi deficiency.

(5) *Intestine-Moistening Pill* (Run Chang Wan) is used for pattern of deficiency of body fluid due to blood deficiency.

4.2 Acumoxatherapy

(1) Body acupuncture: Select the main acupoints of Dachangshu (BL 25), Tianshu (ST 25), Zhigou (TE 6), and Shangjuxu (ST 37). For internal accumulation of dryness and heat, add Hegu (LI 4) and Quchi (LI 11); for dysfunction of qi dynamic, add Zhongwan (CV 12) and Xingjian (LV 2). For qi and blood deficiency, add Pishu (BL 20) and Weishu (BL 21). Use the sedating needling technique for excess pattern, and use the enforcing needling technique for deficiency pattern.

4 其他疗法

4.1 中成药

（1）枳实导滞丸:用于治疗便秘乳食积滞证。

（2）麻仁丸:用于治疗便秘燥热内结证。

（3）逍遥丸:用于治疗便秘气机郁滞证。

（4）补中益气丸:用于治疗便秘气虚不运证。

（5）润肠丸:用于治疗便秘血虚津亏证。

4.2 针灸疗法

（1）体针:主穴取大肠俞、天枢、支沟、上巨虚。燥热内结者加合谷、曲池;气机郁滞者加中脘、行间;气血虚者加脾俞、胃俞。实证用泻法,虚证用补法。

(2) Press seeds on the ear points: The commonly used ear points are Pt. Lower Section of Rectum, Pt. Large Intestines, and Pt. Constipation Spot.

(2) 耳穴压丸:常用穴为直肠下段、大肠、便秘点。

4.3 Tuina Therapy

4.3 推拿疗法

(1) Knead Pt. Dachang, push Pt. Liufu, knead and reinforce Pt. Pitu, rub Pt. Neibagua, rub the abdomen, press and rub Zusanli (ST 36), push Pt. Qijiegu. These are used for constipation of excess pattern.

(1) 清大肠、退六腑、清补脾土、运内八卦、摩腹、按揉足三里、推下七节骨。用于治疗实证便秘。

(2) Knead Pt. Pitu for supplementation, push Pt. Shenshui, rub Pt. Dachang, push Pt. Sanguan, rub the abdomen, pinch up the spine. These are used for constipation of deficiency pattern.

(2) 补脾土、推肾水、清大肠、推上三关、摩腹、捏脊。用于治疗虚证便秘。

4.4 External therapy

4.4 外治疗法

Grind *Rhei Radix Et Rhizoma* (Da Huang) into fine powder. Put the powder into bottle for later use. Take 3g every time, after infused with warm boiled water to make round biscuit-like paste, apply the paste onto Shenque (CV 8) in the umbilicus and cover with adhesive plaster or gauze, applied for constipation of excess pattern.

大黄细末,装瓶备用,每次取 3 克,用温水调成饼状贴于脐部神阙穴,用胶布或纱布固定。用于治疗实证便秘。

Section 6 Anorexia

第 6 节 厌食

Aversion to food is a common disease related to the spleen and stomach in the infants, clinically characterized by long-term poor appetite, no greed for food, and good spirit in spite of reduced ingestion.

厌食是小儿常见的脾胃病证,临床以较长时期食欲不振,食量减少,但精神尚好为特征。

It can occur in all ages, and is mostly seen in the age from 1 to 6 years old, and in higher incidence in children of the cities. It can occur in all seasons. Besides poor appetite in the infants, no special discomforts would be present, and the prognosis is favorable. In lingering and intractable ca-

各年龄均可发生,以 1～6 岁多见,城市儿童发病率较高。发病无明显季节性。患儿除食欲不振外,一般无特殊不适,预后良好。长期不愈者,可使气血生化乏源,抗

ses, the resources for production of qi and blood would be in shortage, and the body resistance would decline, leading to susceptibility to other problems, and even infantile indigestion due to gradual emaciation.

病能力下降，易患他病，甚至日渐消瘦转为疳证。

1 Etiology and pathogenesis

1 病因病机

It is mostly related to inappropriate feeding and nursing, poor recuperation after illness, inhibited emotion, and insufficiency of prenatal natural endowment, and emotional disorder. The key pathogenesis is failure of the spleen in transportation.

多与喂养不当、病后失调、先天禀赋不足以及情志不畅等因素有关，病机关键为脾运失健。

The infants are unable to control themselves for milk and food. Inappropriate feeding and nursing, infection of other diseases, abuse of medications, insufficient fetal constitution, or emotional inbalance, could damage the spleen and stomach, affecting their functions in acceptance, transportation transformation, and hence anorexia.

小儿乳食不知自制，若哺喂不当，或患他病、误用药物，或胎禀不足，或情志不舒，均可损伤脾胃，影响脾胃的受纳运化功能，导致厌食。

The organs of infants are delicate and their physique and qi are not fully developed. The attacking action by evils, or abuse of bitter and cold herbs, or overuse of warm and dry medicinal stuffs, or lack of proper recuperation after illness, all could lead to abnormal accepting, transporting and transforming abilities of spleen and stomach, and hence anorexia. The pathological location is mainly in the spleen and stomach. The pathogenesis is failure of the spleen in normal functions. The lack of the resource for production of qi and blood in long-term illness could influence the growth and development of the infants, and turn into infantile indigestion.

小儿脏腑娇嫩，形气未充，若攻伐，或过用苦寒，或过用温燥，或病后失于调养，均可使脾胃受纳运化失常，而致厌食。病位主要在脾胃，病机为脾失健运。病久因气血生化乏源而影响小儿生长发育，可转为疳证。

2 Key to diagnosis

2 诊断要点

(1) There is a history of inappropriate feeding

(1) 有喂养不当、病后失

and nursing, poor recuperation after illness, insufficiency in prenatal constitution or emotional disorder.

调、先天不足或情志失调等病史。

(2) The main symptoms are relatively longtime poor appetite, obvious reduced food intake, in comparison with normal children of the same age, probably accompanied by lusterless facial complexion, emaciated physique, good spirit and normal movements.

(2) 以较长时期食欲不振，食量明显少于正常同龄儿为主要症状，可伴面色少华，形体偏瘦，但精神尚好，活动如常。

(3) Excluded are other anorexia symptoms caused by diseases due to infection of exogenous pathogens or internal damage.

(3) 除外其他外感、内伤疾病所致的厌食症状。

3 Pattern identification and treatment

3 辨证论治

It is necessary to differentiate between deficiency and excess. Short duration, poor appetite, no pleasure in food ingestion, almost normal physique, and normal tongue and pulse are attributed to excess pattern. Long duration, lusterless facial complexion, emaciated physique, irregular defecation, besides poor appetite and reduced ingestion of food, are attributed to deficiency pattern. Of the above symptoms, if accompanied by lusterless facial complexion, or withered yellow facial complexion, thin and loose stool, pale tongue, and thin tongue coating, it is related to qi deficiency of the spleen and stomach. If accompanied by constipated stool, red tongue with little liquid, scanty tongue coating or peeled tongue coating, it is related to yin deficiency of the spleen and stomach.

重在辨虚实。病程短，仅表现纳呆食少，食而乏味，形体尚可，舌脉正常者为实证；病程长，除食欲不振，食量减少外，伴面色少华，形体偏瘦，大便不调者为虚证。其中伴面色少华或萎黄，大便溏薄，舌淡苔薄者属脾胃气虚；伴大便秘结，舌红少津，苔少或剥脱者为脾胃阴虚。

The treatment is mainly given to normalize the spleen and promote the stomach as the basic therapeutic principle. Methods to normalize the spleen and harmonize the stomach, fortify the spleen and

以运脾开胃为基本治则，根据中医证型分别以运脾和胃、健脾益气、滋养胃阴等法进行治疗。同时，应注

boost qi, nourish the stomach yin, etc, are used respectively in accordance to different patterns in traditional Chinese medicine. Meanwhile, it is necessary to nurse the sick child with proper diet and correct bad dietary habits.

意患儿的饮食调养，纠正不良饮食习惯。

(1) Failure of the spleen in transportation and and transformation

（1）脾失健运

Manifestations: Poor appetite, reduced food intake, experiencing food as lacking in flavor, normal physique and spirit, pale red tongue, white thin or slimy tongue coating, slow and harmonized pulse.

证候：食欲不振，食量减少，食而乏味，形体正常，精神如常，舌淡红，苔薄白或薄腻，脉和缓。

Therapeutic method: To normalize the spleen and promote the stomach.

治法：运脾开胃。

Main formula: *Priceless Qi-Righting Powder* (Bu Huan Jin Zhen Qi San) with modification.

主方：不换金正气散加减。

Commonly used herbs: *Atractylodis Rhizoma* (Cang Zhu), *Magnoliae Officinalis Cortex* (Hou Pu), *Citri Reticulatae Pericarpium* (Chen Pi), *Pogostmonis Herba* (Huo Xiang), *Massa Fermentata Medicinalis* (Liu Shen Qu), *Galli Endothelium Corneum Gigerii* (Ji Nei Jin), *Glycyrrhizae Radix Et Rhizoma* (Gan Cao).

常用药：苍术、厚朴、陈皮、藿香、六神曲、鸡内金、甘草。

Modification: For fullness and distention in the epigastric region and abdomen after meal, add *Aucklandiae Radix* (Mu Xiang), and *Raphani Semen* (Lai Fu Zi); for belching and nausea, add *Bambusae Caulis in Taenias* (Zhu Ru) and *Pinelliae Rhizoma* (Ban Xia); for loose stool, add *Dioscoreae Rhizoma* (Shan Yao), and *Coicis Semen* (Yi Yi Ren); for dry stool, add *Aurantii Fructus Immaturus* (Zhi Shi), and *Arecae Semen* (Bing Lang).

加减：食后脘腹饱胀明显者，加木香、莱菔子；嗳气泛恶者，加竹茹、半夏；大便偏稀者，加山药、薏苡仁；大便偏干者，加枳实、槟榔。

(2) Qi deficiency in the spleen and stomach

（2）脾胃气虚

Manifestations: No thought of milk and food,

证候：不思乳食，食量减

reduced intake of food, lusterless facial complexion, emaciation, fatigued limbs, lack of strength, thin and loose stool with undigested food, pale tongue, white and thin tongue coating, feeble and slow pulse, light red fingerprints.

少，面色少华，形体偏瘦，肢倦乏力，大便溏薄，夹有不消化食物残渣，舌质淡，苔薄白，脉缓无力或指纹淡红。

Therapeutic method: To fortify the spleen and boost qi.

治法：健脾益气。

Main formula: *Special Achievement Powder* (Yi Gong San) with modification.

主方：异功散加减。

Commonly used herbs: *Codonopsis Radix*(Dang Shen), *Atractylodis Macrocephalae Rhizoma* (Bai Zhu), *Poria* (Fu Ling), *Citri Reticulatae Pericarpium* (Chen Pi), *Galli Endothelium Corneum Gigerii* (Ji Nei Jin), *Crataegi Fructus Ustus* (Jiao Shan Zha), *Setariae Fructus Germinatus* (Gu Ya), *Glycyrrhizae Radix Et Rhizoma*(Gan Cao).

常用药：党参、白术、茯苓、陈皮、鸡内金、焦山楂、炒谷芽、甘草。

Modification: For thin stool, add *Atractylodis Rhizoma* (Cang Zhu), *Coicis Semen* (Yi Yi Ren), and *Dioscoreae Rhizoma* (Shan Yao); for profuse sweating and susceptibility to cold, add *Astragali Radix* (Huang Qi), *Ledebouriellae Radix* (Fang Feng), and *Ostreae Concha* (Mu Li); for depression in emotion, add *Bupleuri Radix* (Chai Hu), and *Fructus Sacrodactylis* (Fo Shou).

加减：大便稀薄者，加苍术、薏苡仁、山药；汗多易感冒者，加黄芪、防风、牡蛎；情志抑郁者，加柴胡、佛手。

(3) Yin deficiency in the spleen and stomach

(3) 脾胃阴虚

Manifestations: No thought of food, reduced intake of food, thirst with preference of lots drinks, emaciation, dry stool, vexation and poor sleep, red tongue with little liquid, scanty or peeled tongue coating, thready and rapid pulse.

证候：不思进食，食量减少，口干饮多，形体偏瘦，大便偏干，或心烦少寐，舌质红少津，苔少或剥脱，脉细数。

Therapeutic method: To nourish yin and harmonize the stomach.

治法：养阴和胃。

Main formula: *Stomach-Nourishing and Humor-Increasing* (Yang Wei Zeng Ye Tang) with

主方：养胃增液汤加减。

modification.

Commonly used herbs: *Adenophorae Radix* (Sha Seng), *Ophiopogonis Radix* (Mai Dong), *Dendrobii Herba* (Shi Hu), *Polygonati Odorati Rhizoma* (Yu Zhu), *Paeoniae Radix Albae* (Bai Shao), *Mume Fructus* (Wu Mei), *Glycyrrhizae Radix Et Rhizoma* (Gan Cao).

常用药:沙参、麦冬、石斛、玉竹、白芍、乌梅、甘草。

Modification: For thirst, add *Phragmitis Rhizoma* (Lu Gen), and *Trichosanthis Radix* (Tian Hua Fen); for vexation and poor sleep, add *Picrorhizae Rhizoma* (Hu Huang Lian), and *Ziziphi Spinosi Semen* (Suan Zao Ren); for heat in the palms and soles, and night sweating, add *Moutan Cortex Radicis* (Mu Dan Pi), and *Lycii Cortex* (Di Gu Pi); for constipated stool, add *Cannabis Fructus* (Huo Ma Ren), and *Pruni Semen* (Yu Li Ren).

加减:口干者,加芦根、天花粉;烦躁少寐者,加胡黄连、酸枣仁;手足心热、盗汗者,加牡丹皮、地骨皮;大便秘结者,加火麻仁、郁李仁。

4 Other therapies

4 其他疗法

4.1 Chinese Patent medicine

4.1 中成药

(1) *Child Tangerine Pill* (Xiao Er Xiang Ju Wan) is used for pattern of failure of the spleen in transportation and transformation.

(1) 小儿香橘丸:用于治疗厌食脾失健运证。

(2) *Child Spleen-Fortifying Pill* (Xiao Er Jian Pi Wan) is used for pattern of qi deficiency in the spleen and stomach.

(2) 小儿健脾丸:用于治疗厌食脾胃气虚证。

(3) *Child Healthy and Quiet Oral Liquid* (Er Kang Ning) is used for all patterns of anorexia.

(3) 儿康宁口服液:用于治疗厌食各证。

(4) *Clove Stomach-Opening Paste* (Ding Xiang Kai Wei Tie) is used for all patterns of anorexia.

(4) 丁香开胃贴:用于治疗厌食各证。

4.2 External therapy

4.2 外治疗法

(1) *Alpiniae Officinarum Rhizoma* (Gao Liang Jiang), *Citri Reticulatae Pericarpium Viride* (Qing Pi), *Citri Reticulatae Pericarpium* (Chen Pi), *Piperis Fructus Longi* (Bi Bo), *Atractylodis Rhizoma*

(1) 高良姜、青皮、陈皮、荜拨、苍术、薄荷、蜀椒各等份,研为细末,做成香袋,佩带于胸前。用于治疗厌食各证。

(Cang Zhu), *Menthae Haploalycis Herba* (Bo He), *Pericarpium Zanthoxyli* (Shu Jiao), in equal amount, grind them into fine powder and make a scent bag, to hang in front of the chest. This is appropriate for all kinds of anorexia.

(2) *Caryophylli Flos*(Ding Xiang), and *Euodiae Fructus* (Wu Zhu Yu), each 30g; *Cinnamomi Cortex* (Rou Gui), *Asari Radix Et Rhizoma* (Xi Xin) and *Aucklandiae Radix* (Mu Xiang), each 10g, and *Atractylodis Macrocephalae Rhizoma* (Bai Zhu) and *Galla Chinensis* (Wu Bei Zi), each 20g. Grind these together into powder, and take 5～10g of the powder to make paste with liquor or ginger, and apply topically onto Shenque (CV 8), and change the paste once every 24 hours, for 7～10 days as one course. This is used for pattern of failure of the spleen in transportation and transformation, and pattern of qi deficiency in the spleen and stomach.

（2）丁香、吴茱萸各30克，肉桂、细辛、木香各10克，白术、五倍子各20克，共研末，取药粉5～10克，用酒或生姜汁调糊状，外敷神阙，24小时换药1次，7～10日为1个疗程。用于脾失健运、脾胃气虚证。

4.3 Tuina Therapy

Methods: Knead Pt. Pijing, rub Pt. Neibagua, push Pt. Sihenwen, rub the abdomen, rub the abdomen divergently, rub Zusanli (ST 36), once every day, for 20～30 min every time, with 7～10 days as one course, in combination or without combination of the spine-pinching method. This will help increase appetite.

4.3 推拿疗法

采用补脾经、运内八卦、推四横纹、摩腹、分腹阴阳、揉足三里等手法，每日1次，每次20～30分钟，7～10日为1个疗程。配合或单独应用捏脊疗法，对增进和改善食欲也有帮助。

Shanghai Pujiang Education Press (Former Shanghai University of Traditional Chinese Medicine Press)
1550 Haigang Haigang Ave, Shanghai, P.R.China 201306

图书在版编目(CIP)数据

中医儿科学：英汉对照/虞坚儿主编. —上海：上海浦江教育出版社有限公司,2018.9
(精编实用中医文库/陈凯先,李其忠,何星海总主编)
ISBN 978-7-81121-566-3

Ⅰ.①中… Ⅱ.①虞… Ⅲ.①中医儿科学—英、汉 Ⅳ.①R272

中国版本图书馆 CIP 数据核字(2018)第206251号

上海浦江教育出版社出版
社址:上海海港大道 1550 号上海海事大学校内　　邮政编码:201306
分社:上海蔡伦路 1200 号上海中医药大学内　　邮政编码:201203
电话:(021)38284910(12)(发行)　38284923(总编室)　38284916(传真)
E-mail: cbs@shmtu. edu. cn　URL: http://www. pujiangpress. cn
上海盛通时代印刷有限公司印装　上海浦江教育出版社发行
幅面尺寸:170 mm×240 mm　印张:23. 75　字数:452 千字
2018 年 9 月第 1 版　2018 年 9 月第 1 次印刷
责任编辑:黄　健　张洁怡　封面设计:赵宏义
定价:98. 00 元